AF333055

SURGICAL MANAGEMENT OF
ABDOMINAL WALL HERNIAS

SURGICAL MANAGEMENT OF
ABDOMINAL WALL HERNIAS

Edited by

MARTIN KURZER, British Hernia Centre, London, UK

ALLAN E KARK, British Hernia Centre, London, UK

and

GEORGE E WANTZ, Division of Surgery, Cornell University Medical College,
The New York Hospital, New York, NY, USA

Martin Dunitz

First published in the United Kingdom in 1999
by Martin Dunitz Ltd, The Livery House, 7–9 Pratt Street, London NW1 0AE

A CIP record for this book is available from the British Library.

ISBN 1–85317–477–7

Distributed in the United States by:
Blackwell Science Inc.
Commerce Place, 350 Main Street
Malden, MA 02148, USA
Tel: 1-800-215-1000

Distributed in Canada by:
Login Brothers Book Company
324 Salteaux Crescent
Winnipeg, Manitoba, R3J 3T2
Canada
Tel: 204-224-4068

Distributed in Brazil by:
Ernesto Reichmann Distribuidora de Livros, Ltda
Rua Coronel Marques 335, Tatuape 03440-000
Sao Paulo,
Brazil

Composition by Scribe Design, Gillingham, Kent, UK
Printed and bound in Singapore

CONTENTS

CONTENTS

LIST OF CONTRIBUTORS

Parviz Amid	Lichtenstein Hernia Institute, Inc, 9201 Sunset Boulevard, Suite 505, Los Angeles, CA 90069, USA
Georg Arlt	Surgical University Clinic of the RWTH Aachen, Pauwelisstrasse 30, D-52074 Aachen, Germany
Claude Avisse	Service de Chirurgie Générale et Digestive, Hôpital Robert Debre, Avenue du Général Koenig, F-51092 Reims Cedex, France
Nick Barwell	Royal Cornwall Hospital, Treliske, Truro, Cornwall, UK
Francesco Battocchio	Divisione di Chirurgia Geriatrica, Cattedra di Chirurgia Generale, University of Padua, Ospedale Giustinianeo, via Giustiniani 2, I-35128 Padua, Italy
Philip A Belsham	British Hernia Centre, 87 Watford Way, London NW4 4RS, UK
Robert Bendavid	Shouldice Hospital, 7750 Bayview Avenue, Thornhill, Ontario, Canada L3T 4A3
Alain Burde	Service de Chirurgie Générale et Digestive, Hôpital Robert Debre, Avenue du Général Koenig, F-51092 Reims Cedex, France
Jean-Pierre Conce	Service de Chirurgie Générale et Digestive, Hôpital Robert Debre, Avenue du Général Koenig, F-51092 Reims Cedex, France
Luigi De Santis	Divisione di Chirurgia Geriatrica, Cattedra di Chirurgia Generale, University of Padua, Ospedale Giustinianeo, via Giustiniani 2, I-35128 Padua, Italy
Nial Eames	Department of Orthopaedic Surgery, Queen's University, Musgrave Park Hospital, Stockman's Lane, Belfast BT9 7JB, UK
Jean-Bernard Flament	Service de Chirurgie Générale et Digestive, Hôpital Robert Debre, Avenue du Général Koenig, F-51092 Reims Cedex, France
O Jeremy A Gilmore	Groin and Hernia Clinic, 180 Harley Street, London W1N 2ET, UK

Liam F Horgan Department of General Surgery, Whipps Cross Hospital, Whipps Cross Road, Leytonstone, London E11, UK

Terry Irwin Ward 15/16 Office, Royal Victoria Hospital, Grosvenor Road, Belfast, BT12 6BA, UK

Allan E Kark British Hernia Centre, 87 Watford Way, London NW4 4RS, UK

Andrew Kingsnorth Department of Surgery, Plymouth Postgraduate Medical School, Derriford Hospital, Plymouth PL6 8DH, UK

Martin Kurzer British Hernia Centre, 87 Watford Way, London NW4 4RS, UK

John Lawson Department of Radiology, Belfast City Hospital, Lisburn Road, Belfast BT9 7AB, UK

Marc-Claude Marti Department of Surgery, University Hospital of Geneva, CH-1211, Geneva 4, Switzerland

Erik Nilsson Department of Surgery, Motala Hospital, S-59185 Motala, Sweden

Jean-Pierre Palot Service de Chirurgie Générale et Digestive, Hôpital Robert Debre, Avenue du Général Koenig, F-51092 Reims Cedex, France

Alan W Robbins The Hernia Center, 222 Schanck Road, Suite 100, Freehold, NJ, 07728-2974, USA

Bruno Roche Department of Surgery, University Hospital of Geneva, CH-1211 Geneva 4, Switzerland

Ira M Rutkow The Hernia Center, 222 Schanck Road, Suite 100, Freehold, NJ, 07728-2974, USA

Volker Schumpelick Surgical University Clinic of the RWTH Aachen, Pauwelsstrasse 30, D-52074 Aachen, Germany

John E Skandalakis Emory University School of Medicine, The Robert W Woodruff Health Sciences Center, 1462 Clifton Road, Atlanta, GA, 30322, USA

Renée Stoppa Clinique Chirurgicale de l'Université Hôpital Nord, Place Victor Pauchet, F-80054 Amiens Cedex 1, France

Oreste Terranova Divisione di Chirurgia Geriatrica, Cattedra di Chirurgia Generale, University of Padua, Ospedale Giustinianeo, Via Giustiniani 2, I-35128 Padua, Italy

George E Wantz Division of Surgery, Cornell Medical Center, The New York Hospital, NY, 10023, USA

David Watkin Department of Surgery, Leicester Royal Infirmary, Leicester LE1 5WW, UK

James M Wellwood Department of General Surgery, Whipps Cross Hospital, Whipps Cross Road, Leytonstone, London E11, UK

FOREWORD

Surgical Management of Abdominal Wall Hernias is a representative guide to the current state of the art in the field of hernia repair, as summarized at the International Conference on Hernia Surgery held in London in 1996, which was organized by the British Hernia Centre.

This gathering provided an international forum for the recent major advances in hernia repair; the impetus was our belief that the hitherto rather homely topic of hernia repair had, in reality, become a focal point of surgical interest. The commonest of surgical operations could finally graduate from its surgical practice ground at the end of a long list of ostensibly more important surgical challenges. It had long been known, but seldom emphasized, that there were unacceptably high recurrence rates from a 100-year-old procedure, resulting in huge economic costs in provision of surgery, aftercare and idle morbidity. The documented success of prosthetic repair had finally demanded a wide hearing. The explosion of interest was further aided by the cries of distress from many other directions, notably the wastefulness in hospital health economics, the ever-increasing waiting times (up to two years, in some cases) and the months-long delay in rehabilitation. The scene was thus set for a wide-ranging review of all aspects of an exceedingly common, if relatively ignored, operation.

Hernia surgery has now come of age: we in the hernia field have not only GREPA (Groupe de Recherche Européen sur la Paroi Abdominale) as an organization, but a new international journal (*Hernia*) edited by Professor Chevrel and a newly formed American Hernia Society.

We at the British Hernia Centre are proud to have played a part in helping the spotlight shine on this fascinating specialty and we hope that this book will further enhance these advances.

Dudley J Rogg
Founder and Chief Executive
The British Hernia Centre
London, UK

ACKNOWLEDGEMENTS

In the organization of the International Conference on Hernia Surgery held in London in 1996 and subsequently of this book, we are particularly indebted to Mr Brendan Devlin for his invaluable counsel. It is thanks to his guidance and assistance that we were fortunate enough to be able to call upon many leaders in the field of hernia surgery, although inevitably many other equally notable surgeons were unable to participate or contribute.

We would like to express our appreciation to all the contributors for the professional way in which they submitted their manuscripts. We would like also to thank all the staff at Martin Dunitz Publishers, especially Robert Peden, for his editorial advice and expertise.

Thanks are due to Marlena Stamboulian and Lara Samuels for expertly typing the manuscripts and to Tristan Wright for his skill in producing many of the intraoperative photographs.

Finally, we would like to thank our families for their unfailing encouragement and support.

Martin Kurzer
Allan E Kark
George E Wantz

INTRODUCTION

There have been many recent changes in the surgical world, nowhere more so than in the area of hernia repair. Ten years ago surgeons who used prosthetic mesh routinely in the repair of primary groin hernias were a small minority, their practice frowned upon by most of their colleagues. Today the pendulum has swung the other way with prosthetic mesh being used with increasing frequency by a rapidly rising number of surgeons. At the present the interested general surgeon has a bewildering wealth of choice regarding the 'best' way to repair a hernia. Whether or not to use prosthetic mesh is only one question that needs to be answered. If mesh is used, what type should it be? Should the approach be open or laparoscopic, and if the latter what technique should be employed? With open repair should one utilize local anaesthetic, and allow the patient home the same day; or keep the patient in for one or two nights? And what about the complex cases – the multiple recurrent groin hernias or the massive incisional hernias?

All the above issues and other crucial points of interest were covered at an International Hernia Conference held in London in 1996. Experts on hernia repair from the USA and Europe were asked to address their particular area of interest and their individual approach to hernia repair, with the emphasis very much on practical aspects of the surgery. Many controversial points were raised and many problems resolved in a frank and open manner. Overall the lectures were of such a high standard and so well received that we have taken the opportunity to share the expert views of the speakers with a wider audience in the form of this book. This volume is therefore a compilation of their views and represents the state of the art in hernia surgery today. Its purpose is to give an overview of current thoughts and practice in abdominal wall hernia repair. Inevitably the style and detail of each of the chapters vary, with each reflecting its author's personal approach.

The early part of this book re-examines some fundamental concepts, of relevance to all surgical procedures but often neglected. David Watkin critically evaluates the indications for operating on groin hernias, while Erik Nilsson and Marc-Claude Marti look at the problems of assessing the outcome of hernia surgery and its economic implications.

We then move on to some more practical considerations, with a comprehensive summary of the relevant surgical anatomy from John Skandalakis and a clear exposition of a true Bassini operation from Oreste Terranova in Italy. Nick Barwell then details his method of local anaesthetic groin hernia repair using the Shouldice technique.

Robert Bendavid of the Shouldice Hospital leads into the following four chapters by introducing us to the various types of prosthetic material available. Chapters 8 through 11, two from each side of the Atlantic, demonstrate the different ways in which mesh may be used in open anterior approach groin hernia repair, including Volker Schumpelick's transinguinal preperitoneal placement for large recurrent hernias. Three of these four chapters (Kark, Amid, Rutkow) come from specialized hernia centres.

In Chapters 12 and 13 Jerry Gilmore and Terry Irwin discuss the difficult problem of groin pain in the absence of a palpable lump, the former with particular reference to sportsmen, the latter looking at the role of herniography.

James Wellwood's vast experience of laparoscopic groin hernia repair is presented in Chapter 14, following which there are three chapters on recurrent groin hernia repair. The chapters by Renée Stoppa and George Wantz are complementary, describing bilateral and unilateral repair respectively.

Jean-Bernard Flament and his unit have achieved remarkable results in the repair of massive multi-recurrent incisional hernias – in many instances operating successfully on cases that other surgeons have deemed inoperable. Chapter 18 goes some way towards explaining how they have done this, emphasizing a team approach and meticulous pre-operative and post-operative care.

Finally Andrew Kingsnorth casts his experienced academic eye over the role of clinical trials in hernia surgery, encouraging us to report our results in a more rigorous and scientific manner, and pointing the way to the future.

Martin Kurzer
Allan E Kark
George E Wantz

1 INDICATIONS AND URGENCY

David Watkin

A hernia may be managed either expectantly, or by using a truss or operatively. Congenital umbilical hernias in children generally close without active treatment, but expectant management of groin hernia in adults carries no prospect of cure. At the beginning of the twentieth century, when the operative mortality rate was high, a truss was commonly recommended as the sole treatment for inguinal hernias, but the most recent paper advocating its use was published in 1947.[1] However, the literature is remarkably vague about positive indications for the operative repair of hernias. Original articles are generally concerned with either surgical technique, aftercare or results, with the assumption that the procedure is necessary. Textbooks of surgery tend to either ignore indications for operation for inguinal hernias[2,3] or state that repair is offered to most patients,[4] or to all except those who are unfit[5,6] or elderly.[7] However, Devlin[8] and Green[9] suggest that small reducible direct inguinal hernias in the elderly may be ignored. Abrahamson[10] considers that small wide-necked direct inguinal hernias in old people may be left alone unless they are enlarging, while Kettlewell[11] and Ellis[12] go further, stating that most direct inguinal hernias do not need an operation. All of these statements seem to be opinions rather than reviews of the evidence. In contrast, prompt elective repair is unanimously favoured for femoral hernias due to the high incidence of strangulation.[13,14]

The indications and urgency of operations for groin hernias have been examined from first principles as there is no consensus in the literature. The indications for any operation are based upon either the relief of present symptoms or the prevention of future serious complications. For groin hernias the main continuing symptom is discomfort, but this is not experienced by all patients. Disfigurement is important for some patients, while a few have problems with the scrotal skin or with envelopment of the penis. Surgeons will usually advise repair in patients with these chronic symptoms, as this is a low risk procedure, unless there are strong medical contraindications. However, some groin hernias give no real symptoms. Patients have either been unaware of the swelling until it is discovered at a routine examination, or they notice a painless lump and present out of concern about its possible significance. For such patients, the need for repair is determined by the future development of symptoms or the risk of strangulation which also indicates the urgency of operation. This risk amounts to the incidence of strangulation multiplied by the mortality rate should it happen. As these figures differ between inguinal and femoral hernias they will be considered separately.

INGUINAL HERNIA

The incidence of strangulation among inguinal hernias

The most appropriate measure of the probability of strangulation is its annual incidence in a population of patients with untreated hernias. In the 1890s, Berger asked 10 000 patients attending a truss clinic whether and when they had experienced an episode of incarceration, and he calculated this risk as 0.37% per year.[15] The weakness of this estimate is that these patients had recovered from the episode, while those who had died of strangulation would not have reached him. Neutra studied a population in Colombia where elective hernia repair was virtually unobtainable, and found a very similar rate of strangulation for inguinal hernias of 0.29% per year.[16]

Unfortunately, most series express operations for strangulation as either a percentage of the total operations for hernia, or as a proportion of the cases of intestinal obstruction. For both these methods of calculation, the denominator is subject to other variables – the ease of access to elective repair and the incidence of other causes of intestinal obstruction, respectively. Gallegos and colleagues attempted to estimate the probability of strangulation by reviewing the casenotes of 561 adults undergoing repair of groin hernias to discover the prior length of the history.[17] From this they computed the cumulative probability of strangulation for inguinal hernias as 2.8% at 3 months, 4.5% at 2 years and 8.6% at 5 years, but the series included only 22 strangulated hernias, so the confidence limits were wide (2.6% to 14.6% at 5 years). Furthermore, their results were entirely dependent upon the patients' recall of the length of history and the accurate recording of this in the notes; the Kaplan–Meier plot shows evidence of preference for durations of 2 and 5 years (Fig. 1).

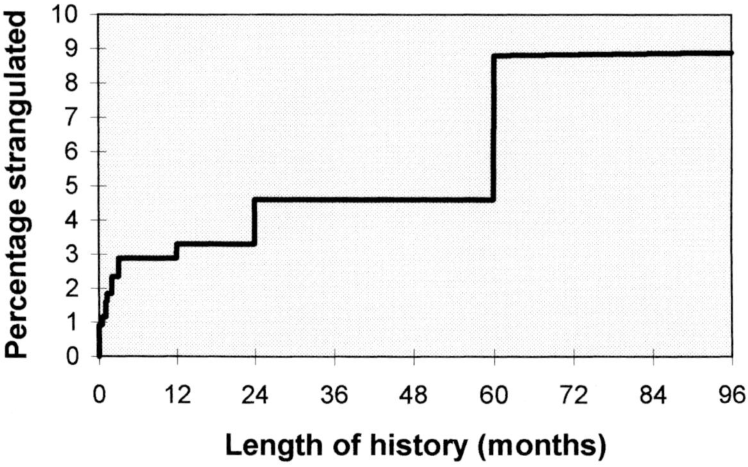

Figure 1. Cumulative proportions of inguinal hernias strangulating related to length of history (after Gallegos *et al.*[17])

The annual probability of strangulation for inguinal hernias thus appears to lie between 0.3% and 2.9%, with some loading of risk in the first 3 months after the hernia is noticed.

Are all inguinal hernias at equal risk of strangulation?

Age, duration of hernia, irreducibility and type of inguinal hernia (direct or indirect) might influence the probability of strangulation, though some practitioners maintain that there are no reliable indicators.[18] Strangulation peaks in the seventh[19,20] or eighth[21] decade, but there is no information about the age distribution of uncomplicated hernias in the same populations, so the relative probability of strangulation, by decades, cannot be calculated. The influence of the length of history was addressed in the previous section, but it should be emphasized that 10% of strangulations occur with no prior history.[19] The risk of strangulation is greater for irreducible hernias.[22]

Direct inguinal hernias strangulate only rarely, but then they are less common. Gallagher and Earley, in a review, estimate the proportion of direct hernias to be 10–30%, with a preference towards the lower figure.[22] Some individual series give higher percentages, ranging from 25% to 51% (Table 1). Overall, approximately 30% of inguinal hernias are reported as direct, but this may be an underestimate because the figures relate to operative findings and some direct hernias may not have been treated.

The percentage of direct hernias among those that strangulate is much lower. Ellis states that, for a direct hernia 'because of its large opening, strangulation is rare'.[12] In a large collected series of 573 adults with strangulated inguinal hernias, Frankau (1931) found that only 14 (2.4%) were direct.[19] Few recent reports analyse strangulated hernias

Source	Date	Indirect	Combined	Direct No.	%
Marsden[23]	1962	1100	—	367	25
Ralphs et al.[24]	1980	78	—	56	42
Glasgow[25]	1984	10 893	1023	5254	30
Devlin[26]	1988	382	21	165	29
Gilbert[27]	1989	556	140	399	37
Serpell et al.[28]	1990	59	—	62	51

Table 1. Type of inguinal hernia at primary elective operation in adults

by type, but McEntee and colleagues reported 33 strangulated indirect hernias with no direct ones.[21] In contrast, Williams and Hale reported that of 48 strangulated inguinal hernias, five were direct.[18] Taking these figures in conjunction with the relative incidence of elective operations in Table 1, it is clear that strangulation is less common among direct hernias by a factor of at least 10.

Is it possible to diagnose direct inguinal hernias correctly?

The clinical distinction between indirect and direct inguinal hernias is a traditional part of surgical teaching.[29] However, Ralphs and colleagues found that when 67 groins of patients aged over 30 years were examined by a pair of 'expert' clinicians and the findings compared with the operative diagnoses, there was only a 67% accuracy at distinguishing between indirect and direct hernias.[24] Apart from this one paper there is only opinion. Kettlewell states that 'it is important to recognise the narrow necked prevesical direct inguinal hernia', while agreeing that wide-necked direct hernias need not be treated in the elderly.[11] Devlin[26] considers that 'the only type of groin hernia that can be identified with any certainty is the broad-based direct sac in the elderly male . . . it is readily apparent when the patient stands and immediately disappears when he lies'. Allen *et al.* reported, with disapproval, that some surgeons, responding to a postal survey, described selecting elderly patients for operation on the basis of the hernia being indirect; they considered that this unreliable information should not influence management.[30] The practice of advising asymptomatic elderly patients with small, apparently direct, inguinal hernias that they do not need an operation is surely widespread, but it has been challenged. Herniography[31] could be used to exclude an indirect hernia and so put this line of management on a sound footing.

What is the mortality rate for strangulated inguinal hernia in adults?

Historically, operations for strangulated hernia carried a mortality of 11–13% and unfortunately this is still the case in some recent series (Table 2). Three factors influence this mortality – age of the patient, duration of strangulation, and the need for a bowel resection; the effects of the latter two being interrelated. Frankau (1931) in a large collected series found a mortality of 5% at ages 21–50 years, 15% aged 51–70 years and 25% for patients over 70 years.[19] Currently, patients with strangulated hernias are older with 40% aged over 75 years,[33] compared to only 15% in Frankau's series, which accounts for the lack of improvement in overall mortality despite technical advances.

The reduction of mortality from strangulated hernia in the elderly remains a challenge,[35] and ideally hernias should be repaired electively before strangulation can occur.

Source	Date	Patients	Died	
			No.	%
Frankau[19]	1931	604	81	13.4
Vick[20]	1932	1378	158	11.5
Requarth and Theis[32]	1948	145	19	13.1
Hjaltason[33]	1981	86	6	7.0
Andrews[34]	1981	66	9	13.6

Table 2. Mortality of strangulated inguinal hernias in adults

Source	Dates of data collection	Population served	Strangulated adult IHs	
			No.	Per 100 000 per annum
Andrews[34]	1975–80	250 000	66	4.65
Hjaltason[33]	1973–80	338 000	88	3.25
Quill *et al.*[36]	1969–80	180 000	154	7.16
Watkin[37]	1984–91	368 000	158	5.60

Table 3. Population incidence of strangulated inguinal hernias (IHs)

Can the incidence of strangulated inguinal hernia in adults, and its associated mortality be reduced by a policy of elective repair?

The incidence of strangulated inguinal hernias in Western Europe is between 3.25 and 7.16 per 100 000 population per year (Table 3) and data from Quill *et al.* did not show any significant change over 12 years,[36] but there was already an adequate elective hernia repair service in 1970 with no wait for operation. Unfortunately there is no data available for the incidence of strangulation over a longer timescale, but it is often stated that strangulated hernias have declined as a percentage of the total cases of intestinal obstruction in developed countries. In 1932 Vick[20] reported that of 6892 cases of acute intestinal obstruction, 49% were due to hernias, but by 1987 McEntee *et al.*[38] found that hernias were responsible in only 20% of cases. In less sophisticated societies, for example in West Africa, strangulated hernia has remained the most common cause of intestinal obstruction.[39]

On balance, it seems likely that the policy of elective repair of inguinal hernias in the UK *has* reduced the incidence of strangulation, but it is not known if this trend can be sustained. In a series of 79 patients with miscellaneous strangulated hernias in Limerick, 58% had been aware of the hernia for at least a month prior to strangulation.[21] Allen *et al.* found that 20 of 25 patients who replied to a questionnaire had known of their hernia for at least a month, while 18 of them had known for over a year.[30]

Thus there is scope for a further reduction in the incidence of strangulation by intensification of the policy of early elective repair. However, this may not be worthwhile in the elderly. Neuhauser calculated that the 'years lost' from the mortality from elective operations for inguinal hernias at age 65 would slightly exceed the years otherwise liable to be lost from the risk of dying from strangulation.[16] The older the patient and the lower the mortality rate from strangulation, the less advantageous does elective repair become.

Recurrent inguinal hernias

It has been suggested that recurrent inguinal hernias are at greater risk of strangulation,[22,33] and that there is then a higher mortality.[34] However, the accuracy of diagnosis of recurrence is crucial to such calculations and this diagnosis is often uncertain. Giles states that 'there is considerable doubt as to the true incidence of recurrence, for the diagnosis rests completely on the physical examination of the patient. It will be recognised that a slight bulge to one observer may be considered a recurrence by another'.[7] Marsden dodges the issue, defining a recurrence as 'a weakness necessitating a further operation or provision of a truss'.[23]

There does not seem to be a sound basis for assuming that all recurrent hernias are at increased risk of strangulation. It is therefore suggested that asymptomatic, easily reducible, direct recurrences may safely be left alone in the same way as primary direct bulges. Surgical pride should not be the reason for re-operation!

SUMMARY OF THE EVIDENCE REGARDING THE RISK OF STRANGULATION IN ADULT INGUINAL HERNIAS

Overall the incidence of strangulation among an untreated population of patients with inguinal hernias is estimated to be between 0.3% and 2.9% per year, with some loading of risk in the first 3 months. Attempting to identify risk factors, there is no convincing effect of age, but irreducibility does increase the incidence of strangulation. Direct hernias account for 30% of the total number of hernias, but are responsible for only about 3% of strangulations. Thus it is acceptable to leave direct inguinal hernias that are asymptomatic and reducible alone provided they can be identified reliably. Many surgeons think they can correctly diagnose 'direct bulges', but the only formal study found only 69% accuracy in distinguishing between direct and indirect hernias. The decision not to advise operation will rest solely on the surgeon's confidence that the hernia is direct; this could be supported by the use of an investigation such as herniography.

The mortality rate for strangulated inguinal hernias is reported to be 7–14%. There has been disagreement as to whether the incidence of strangulation, and hence the population mortality, has been reduced by a policy of elective repair. There is no data to show a decline in mortality from strangulated hernias, but the proportion of all cases of intestinal obstruction which are due to strangulated hernia has fallen from 49% to 20%. On balance, a policy of elective repair probably has reduced the incidence of strangulation, but in the elderly this does not result in an overall gain in life expectancy.

FEMORAL HERNIA

Femoral hernias made up only 11% of 6182 groin hernias in one series,[26] but they account for between 34%[33] and 51%[19] of strangulated hernias. Thus the proportion of femoral hernias presenting with strangulation is much higher – over 50% in some series (Table 4), compared with less than 10% of inguinal hernias.[19] Gallegos *et al.*[17] used data from the casenotes of 37 patients with femoral hernias (including 12 strangulated)

Source	Date	Elective repair of femoral hernia	Strangulated femoral hernia	
			No.	% of total
Waddington[40]	1971	51	77	60
Wheeler[41]	1975	36	44	55
Tasker[13]	1982	39	38	49
Nicholson *et al.*[14]	1990	82	63	44
Total		208	222	52

Table 4. Percentage of femoral hernias presenting with strangulation

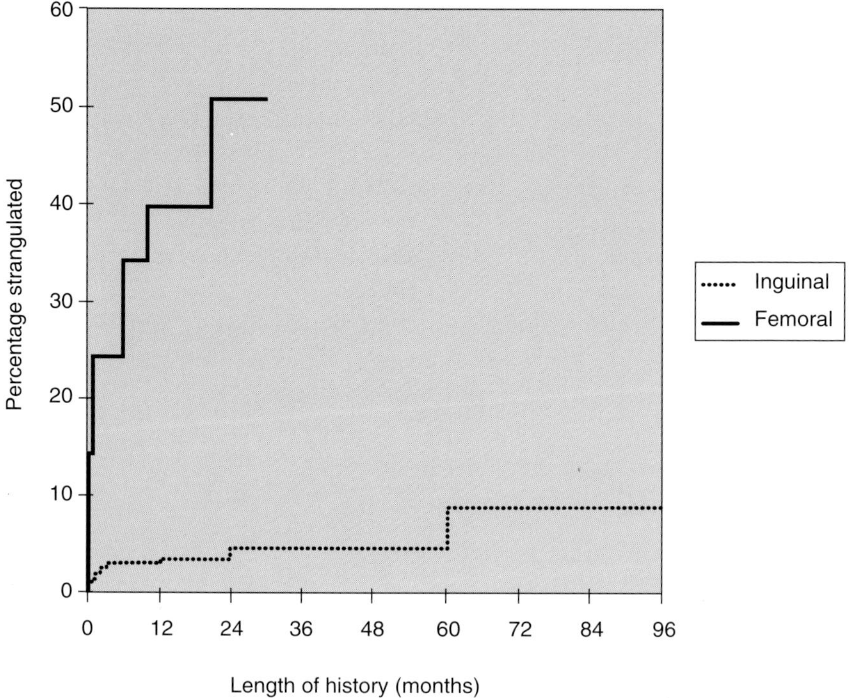

Figure 2. Cumulative proportions of inguinal hernias strangulating related to length of history (after Gallegos *et al.*[17])

to calculate the cumulative probabilities of strangulation at 1 month of 22% and at 21 months of 35% (confidence interval 23–67%). These rates are 10 times those which they found for inguinal hernias (Fig. 2).

The incidence of bowel resection at operation for strangulated femoral hernia is approximately twice that for inguinal hernia[33,34] and this may be expected to increase the mortality rate.[33] Overall, the mortality has been as high as 15% in some series,[13,34] but others have achieved rates of 3% or less.[40,41]

The high incidence of strangulation among femoral hernias, together with the frequency of irreversible gut ischaemia and a significant postoperative mortality, all point to the importance of prompt elective repair. Furthermore, this is a small operation, easily carried out by the low approach, as a day case, under local anaesthesia. It is therefore all the more disappointing that in response to a postal survey, only 38% of general practitioners and 49% of consultant physicians would refer a frail 80-year-old with a femoral hernia to a surgeon.[30]

CONCLUSIONS

1 Indirect inguinal and symptomatic direct inguinal hernias should be repaired surgically, unless the patient's prognosis is short. This eliminates the small long-term risk of strangulation and relieves symptoms.

2 Repair of small, direct, easily reducible inguinal hernias is not mandatory, as they are not at significant risk of strangulation. If asymptomatic, repair should not be advised in the elderly, for whom the risks of operation will outweigh the benefits. This policy could be pursued with more conviction if there was a reliable diagnostic method to determine the type of inguinal hernia; herniography may serve this purpose.

3 Recurrent inguinal hernias should be managed in the same way as primary inguinal hernias.

4 Irreducible inguinal hernias and those presenting with a history of less than 4 weeks should be repaired promptly, as they are at increased risk of strangulation.

5 For other inguinal hernias the risk of strangulation does not justify priority on the waiting list, but employment considerations may require an early operation.

6 All femoral hernias should be repaired urgently to forestall the high risk of strangulation. The difficulty is to identify them and to ensure that they are referred to a surgeon.

REFERENCES

1 Thomas TM. The use and abuse of trusses. *Practitioner* 1947; **159**:388.

2 Nyhus LM, Bombeck CT. Hernias. In Sabiston DC, ed. *Textbook of surgery*, 13th edn. Philadelphia: Saunders 1986.

3 Nyhus LM, Condon RE, eds. *Hernia*, 3rd edn. Philadelphia: Lippincott 1989.

4 Kirk RM, Maynard JD, Henry AN *et al. Surgery*. London: Pitman 1974.

5 Rains AJH, Mann CV, eds. *Bailey and Love's short practice of surgery*, 20th edn. London: Lewis 1988.

6 Ellis H, Calne R. *Lecture notes on general surgery*, 7th edn. Oxford: Blackwell 1987.

7 Giles GR. Hernia. In Cuschieri A, Giles GR, Moosa AR, eds. *Essential surgical practice*, 2nd edn. London: Wright 1988.

8 Devlin HB. In Dudley HAF, ed. *Rob and Smith's atlas of general surgery*. London: Butterworth 1981.

9 Green NA. Hernia. In Macfarlane DA, Thomas LP, eds. *Textbook of surgery*, 5th edn. Edinburgh: Churchill Livingstone 1984.

10 Abrahamson J. Hernias. In Schwartz SI, Ellis H, eds. *Maingot's abdominal operations*, 9th edn. New Jersey: Prentice Hall 1990.

11 Kettlewell MGW. Lumps in the groin and scrotum. *Br J Hosp Med* 1973; **9**:724–30.

12 Ellis H. Inguinal hernia. *Br J Hosp Med* 1970; **4**:9–14.

13 Tasker DG. Femoral hernia: a continuing source of avoidable mortality. *Br J Clin Pract* 1982; **36**:141–4.

14 Nicholson S, Keane TE, Devlin HB. Femoral hernia: an avoidable source of surgical mortality. *Br J Surg* 1990; **77**:307–8.

15 Berger P. La hernie inguino-interstitielle et son traitment par la cure radicale. *Rev Chir Paris* 1902; **21**:1.

16 Quoted in Neuhauser D. Elective inguinal herniorrhaphy versus a truss in the elderly. In Bunker JP, Barnes BA, Mosteller F, eds. *Costs, risks and benefits of surgery*. New York: Oxford University Press 1977.

17 Gallegos NC, Dawson J, Jarvis M, Hobsley M. Risk of strangulation in groin hernias. *Br J Surg* 1991; **78**:1171–3.

18 Williams JS, Hale HW. The advisability of inguinal herniorrhaphy in the elderly. *Surg Gynecol Obstet* 1966; **122**:100.

19 Frankau C. Strangulated hernia: a review of 1487 cases. *Br J Surg* 1931; **19**:176–91.

20 Vick RM. Statistics of acute intestinal obstruction. *BMJ* 1932; **2**:546.

21 McEntee GP, O'Carroll A, Mooney B, Egan TJ, Delaney PV. Timing of strangulation in adult hernias. *Br J Surg* 1989; **76**:725–6.

22 Gallagher J, Earley TK. Adult groin hernias. In Eiseman B, ed. *Prognosis of surgical disease*. Philadelphia: Saunders 1980.

23 Marsden AJ. Inguinal hernia: a three year review of two thousand cases. *Br J Surg* 1962; **49**:384–94.

24 Ralphs DNL, Brain AJL, Grundy DJ, Hobsley M. How accurately can direct and indirect inguinal hernias be distinguished? *BMJ* 1980; **280**:1039–40.

25 Glassow F. Inguinal hernia repair using local anaesthesia. *Ann R Coll Surg Engl* 1984; **66**:382–7.

26 Devlin HB. *Management of abdominal hernias*. London: Butterworth 1988.

27 Gilbert AI. An anatomic and functional classification for the diagnosis and treatment of inguinal hernia. *Am J Surg* 1989; **157**:331–3.

28 Serpell JW, Jarrett PEM, Johnson CD. A prospective study of bilateral inguinal hernia repair. *Ann R Coll Surg Engl* 1990; **72**:299–303.

29 Browse NL. Distinguishing direct and indirect inguinal hernia. *BMJ* 1980; **280**:1207.

30 Allen PIM, Zader M, Goldman M. Elective repair of groin hernias in the elderly. *Br J Surg* 1987; **74**:987.

31 Gullmo A, Broome A, Smedberg S. Herniography. *Surg Clin North Am* 1984; **64**(2):229–44.

32 Requarth W, Theis FV. Incarcerated and strangulated inguinal hernia. *Arch Surg* 1948; **57**:267–75.

33 Hjaltason E. Incarcerated hernia. *Acta Chir Scand* 1981; **147**:263–7.

34 Andrews NJ. Presentation and outcome of strangulated external hernia in a district general hospital. *Br J Surg* 1981; **68**:329–32.

35 Buck N, Devlin HB, Lunn JN. *Report of a confidential enquiry into peri-operative deaths*. Nuffield Provincial Hospitals Trust and the King's Fund for Hospitals: London 1987.

36 Quill DS, Devlin HB, Plant JA *et al*. Surgical operation rates: a twelve year experience in Stockton on Tees. *Ann R Coll Surg Engl* 1983; **65**:248–53.

37 Watkin DFL. Personal communication 1991.

38 McEntee G, Pender D, Mulvin D *et al*. Current spectrum of intestinal obstruction. *Br J Surg* 1987; **74**:976–80.

39 Bador EA. Acute intestinal obstruction in Korle Bu Teaching Hospital, Accra: 1965–69. *Ghana Med J* 1970; **9**:283–7.

40 Waddington RT. Femoral hernias: a recent appraisal. *Br J Surg* 1971; **58**:920–2.

41 Wheeler MH. Femoral hernia: analysis of the results of surgical treatment. *Proc R Soc Med* 1975; **68**:177–8.

2 OUTCOMES

Erik Nilsson

The outcome of any surgical procedure may be evaluated according to the parameters stated in Table 1. In the overall evaluation of a method, *efficacy* refers to the results achieved by experts under optimal circumstances, whereas *effectiveness* refers to its performance in a more general routine situation.[1] Epidemiological analyses of defined populations are usually concerned with effectiveness and this is the approach of the present report. However, for the patient, questions concerning outcome are simple. 'Will I be cured or will the problem recur, what are the risks involved, and can I afford the treatment offered?'

In 1992 the Swedish National Quality Register of Hernia Surgery was established. Like all other quality registers in Sweden it is voluntary and open to all units. It has professional support and permission to use personal identification numbers. Each Swedish citizen has their own unique 10-digit number and this is important for the accuracy and validity of register data. The register functions as follows. Every hernia operation is documented according to a protocol where patient characteristics, type of hernia, method of repair, anaesthesia, postoperative complications, further complaints and reoperation, if applicable, are stated. At the end of each year participating units send all data to the Register Centre located in Motala. Some months later they receive stratified statistics of their own achievements as well as combined data for all aligned units. It should be emphasized that the information returned is detailed and patient specific. Thus each hospital receives the identification codes of patients reoperated upon for recurrence following procedures performed at that hospital since entering the register. In 1992 eight hospitals participated with a combined catchment area of 0.76 million

Symptom relief/recurrence

Complications and sequels

Convalescence and return to normal activity

Cost-effectiveness

Table 1. Factors to be considered when evaluating the outcome of a surgical procedure

inhabitants; by 1995 this had risen to 19 hospitals covering 1.98 million inhabitants, and 29 hospitals had joined by 1997.

By December 1995 there were 8470 operations registered. As Table 2 shows, the operation rate between 1992 and 1995 has declined from 220 to 184 operations per 100 000 people per year. However, the fraction of operations done for recurrent hernias has not declined, remaining a constant and high 16–17%. This figure mainly represents failures of the past. Of the 1406 reoperations registered, 212 (15%) followed procedures performed after the hospitals concerned had joined the hernia register (Table 3). The cumulative incidence of reoperation performed since the start of our register gives a better idea of recent outcome quality. Three years after surgery 4.4% (95%

Year	No. of operations	Operation rate (operations per 100 000 inhabitants per year)	Operations for recurrence (%)	
			Mean	Range
1992	1676	220	16	10–21
1993	1643	216	16	14–19
1994	1831	204	17	15–22
1995	3320	184	17	11–31
Total	8470			
Patients	7764			

Table 2. Number of inguinal hernia repairs carried out between 1992 and 1995 at hospitals participating in the Swedish National Quality Register of Hernia Surgery

Operations	No.	Previous operations performed	
		No.	%
Primary	7064		
Recurrent	1406		
Before 1992		1194	85
1992–95		212	15
Total	8470		

Table 3. Number of primary and recurrent inguinal hernias repaired at the participating hospitals between 1992 and 1995

Definition of recurrence

Method of follow-up

Completeness of follow-up

Time of follow-up

Table 4. Factors of importance in determining recurrence rate following inguinal hernia repair

confidence interval 3.8–5.1%) of all operations have had to be redone because of recurrent hernia, but it should be noted that these are *reoperations* for recurrence, not the total number of recurrences.

Table 4 lists factors that have to be taken into account when determining recurrence rate. In the literature two definitions of recurrence are widely used: the presence of an expansile cough impulse[2] or a weakness of the operation area necessitating a further operation or the provision of a truss.[3] In a recent study it was demonstrated that recurrences exceeded reoperations by 40% at 3 years after surgery.[4] This leads us to the conclusion that the recurrence rate after 3 years would amount to 1.4 times 4.4%, that is roughly 6%. For open hernia techniques without mesh, the recurrence rate 3 years after surgery must be multiplied by a factor of two in order to reach the 10-year rate.[5] The long-term recurrence rate among our patients would thus amount to 12% or higher. This agrees with the fact that 16–17% of all our hernia patients are operated upon for recurrent hernia each year. Yet it has recently been stated that 'For the well-trained surgeon, however, acceptably low recurrence rates (1–3%) can be achieved no matter what method of hernia repair is used'[6] and it is true that recurrence rates as low as this have been demonstrated for the Shouldice method[7] as well as for open mesh techniques.[8,9] Nevertheless, it is obvious that there exists an appreciable difference in outcome quality between our data from the early 1990s and the results that should be expected if we applied modern surgical techniques in the appropriate manner.

One ambition of a quality register must be to reduce this outcome gap between *obtained* and *obtainable* results, to minimize the discrepancy between recent achievements and reasonable expectations. There is also some indication that participation in a register such as the National Quality Register of Hernia Surgery might indeed improve outcome quality. We may analyse this question by taking advantage of the fact that hospitals entered the register at different times. Eight hospitals participated from 1992 and 11 units joined later – one in 1994 and 10 in 1995. It is possible to compare the achievements of the eight initially participating hospitals over the years, and in addition we can compare the 1995 data from these eight hospitals with corresponding figures from the 11 surgical units affiliated later.

Table 5 illustrates the number of operations and reoperations for recurrence of the hernia in the same calendar year at the initially participating eight hospitals. From 1992

Year[a]	No. of operations	Reoperations by 31 December	
		No.	%
1992	1676	13	0.8
1993	1643	17	1.0
1994	1560	15	1.0
1995	1346	3	0.2

[a](1992–1994) vs 1995, P<0.001.

Table 5. Reoperation for early recurrent inguinal hernia (in the same calendar year as primary repair) in 8 initially participating hospitals

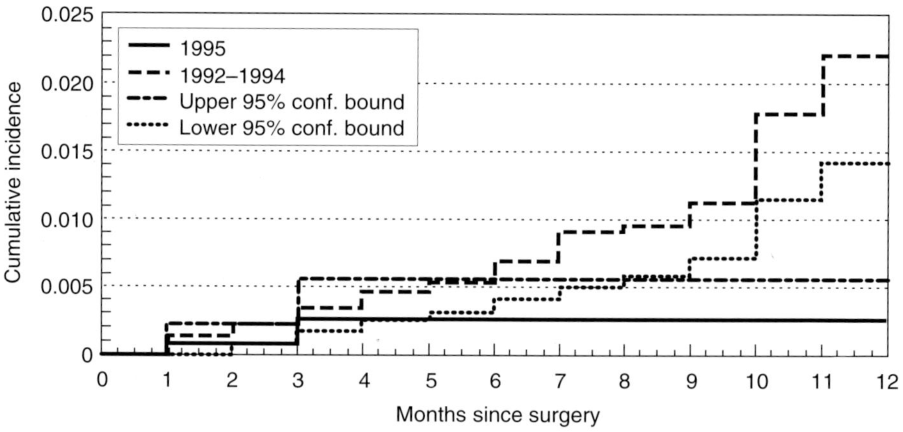

Figure 1. Cumulative risk for reoperation in initial 8 hospitals compared over years

to 1994 between 0.8 and 1.0% of all herniorrhaphies were reoperated at the end of the respective calendar year. But the 1995 figure, when three out of 1346 hernia operations (0.2%) were redone at the end of the year, differs significantly from the others. Figure 1 shows a comparison between the pooled 1992–94 data and the 1995 figures using actuarial analysis. These curves are corrected for deaths of patients and they show an almost 10-fold drop in reoperation rate, which is highly significant. The lower 95% confidence limit for the 1992–95 curve lies above the upper 95% confidence limit for the 1995 data.

Table 6 gives the raw figures and Fig. 2 the corresponding actuarial curves for reoperations performed during 1995 at the two groups of hospitals. There were significantly

Hospital	No of operations	Reoperations by 31 December[a]	
		No.	%
Initial eight	1346	3	0.2
Eleven later	1974	16	0.8

[a]P = 0.002.

Table 6. Reoperation for early recurrent inguinal hernia (in the same calendar year as primary repair): comparison between initial 8 and later 11 hospitals

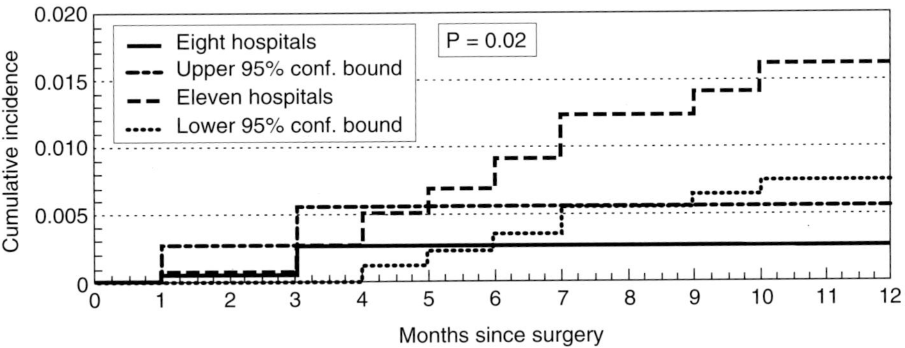

Figure 2. Cumulative risk for reoperation (1995): initial 8 hospitals compared to 11 later aligned hospitals

fewer reoperations at the initial eight hospitals, and a corresponding difference between the actuarial curves, 1.5% and 0.2%, respectively, of the operations being reoperated by 12 months. Analyses of observational data such as these are always open to some criticism. However, they are compatible with the notion that participation in a register and auditing, including benchmarking and improvement in surgical techniques, may reduce reoperation rate in Sweden by at least a factor of five.

With detailed knowledge of 8470 hernia operations and subsequent reoperations due to recurrence, we thought it worthwhile performing risk analyses. As shown in Table 7 the following four variables turned out to be associated with a significantly increased relative risk of recurrence in a Cox proportional hazard model: (1) a postoperative complication, (2) repair of a direct hernia, (3) use of absorbable sutures, and (4) operation for a recurrent hernia. The following variables were tested and were not associated with an increased risk of recurrence: whether the operation was emergency or elective; age of the patient (above median age of group versus below median age); and in-patient stay versus day surgery.

Variable	Operations	Reoperations	RR[a]	95% confidence limit
Postoperative complication	650	34	2.85	1.97–4.12
Direct hernia	3714	139	2.16	1.61–2.88
Absorbable suture	2929	134	2.09	1.48–2.95
Operation for recurrence	1406	69	2.00	1.46–2.72

[a]Adjusted for age of patient, indication for surgery (acute/elective), method of repair, day surgery (yes/no).

Table 7. Factors associated with an increased relative risk (RR) of recurrence of inguinal hernia in 8470 operations in 19 hospitals during 1992–5

Variable	Operation	Reoperation	RR[a]	95% confidence limit
Laparoscopy	1242	23	1.56	0.91–2.69
Mesh, open	978	17	1.43	0.78–2.62
Other 'open' methods	3495	129	1.32	0.92–1.90
Shouldice	1622	40	1.00	1.00

[a]Adjusted for postoperative complications (yes/no), anatomy of hernia, suture material (absorbable/non-absorbable), primary or recurrent hernia, age of patient, indication for surgery, day surgery (yes/no).

Table 8. Operations with an increased relative risk (RR) of recurrence compared with the Shouldice technique

Table 8 compares the methods of repair, and it can be seen that the Shouldice method gave the lowest recurrence rate, but a word of caution is required. These data, in contrast to randomized trials, include the learning curve for laparoscopists and for open mesh surgeons. They do not show what may be achieved but rather what took place. As all 'other open' methods have been in use for a longer period than the Shouldice technique it may be anticipated that the difference between these two groups will increase with time provided no other changes take place. This is also in accordance with a recent meta-analysis.[10]

The hernia patient wants to know what his surgeon can immediately do for him with the present knowledge and the facilities available – not what could be done for him using a new technique at a different location, or when the surgeon has completed his learning curve. For the general hernia patient, effectiveness is more important than efficacy. 'Far better an approximate answer to the right question, which often is vague, than an exact answer to the wrong question, which can always be made precise.'[11] This quotation of a Princeton statistician from over 30 years ago is still appropriate.

One ultimate and rare outcome following hernia surgery is postoperative death within 30 days of operation. Our patients were operated on 8230 occasions. (As some patients were operated bilaterally, this is slightly less than the 8470 herniorrhaphies performed.) Twenty-six patients died, 15 after 509 emergency procedures giving a 3% postoperative mortality rate, and 11 after 7701 elective operations giving a 0.1% mortality rate. These are crude mortality figures and have not been adjusted for whether or not the deaths were related to the hernia operations.

Let us consider the cost-effectiveness of day surgery. All patients undergoing elective hernia repair should be considered for day surgery, although there will always be exceptions. In an economy such as Sweden's where currently 7% of gross national product (GNP) goes to the healthcare sector it is difficult to defend expenditure for overnight stay following elective hernia surgery. In a public healthcare system, money made available by increasing the number of day operations can be used elsewhere.

Year[a]	Operations	Day surgery (%)	Range
1992	1676	33	0–59
1993	1643	46	22–63
1994	1560	53	29–64
1995	1346	56	38–72

[a]1992 vs 1995, P<0.001.

Table 9. Proportion of inguinal hernia repairs carried out as day cases at the 8 initially participating hospitals

Table 9 shows the day surgery rate with means and ranges for the eight hospitals participating initially. During 1992–95 there was a continuous increase in the number of hernias repaired as day cases with a highly significant difference between the 1992 and 1995 figures. This is a general trend in Swedish hernia surgery and it is by no means solely attributable to the existence of the register. However, a comparison between the day surgery rate for 1995 in the eight initially aligned units and the subsequently aligned hospitals demonstrates a highly significant difference of 56% versus 40% (Table 10) leading to a greater cost-effectiveness in the former group.

Hospitals	Operations	Day surgery (%)	Range
Initial 8	1346	56[a]	38–72
11 later	1947	40[a]	6–60
[a]P<0.001.			

Table 10. Proportion of inguinal hernia repairs carried out as day cases at the initial 8 hospitals and the 11 later participating hospitals

CONCLUSION

According to the Swedish National Quality Register of Hernia Surgery, 16–17% of hernia patients are operated on for recurrent hernia. The cumulative incidence of reoperation due to recurrence is 4.4% at 3 years. At participating hospitals that had registered for four years, significantly fewer patients were reoperated upon because of recurrences within 12 months of surgery, and the day surgery rate increased significantly during these years. In 1995 there were marked differences in both reoperation rate and day surgery rate between hospitals that had participated in the register from its start in 1992 and those that had joined later.

The outcome of hernia surgery may be audited from register data of the type presented. While observational data analysis, like this, is helpful in determining areas in need of improvement, it is not a substitute for further surgical research, including randomized trials.[12,13]

Acknowledgement

The register is financially supported by the Swedish National Board of Health and Welfare and the Federation of County Councils in Sweden. I am most grateful to all the hernia surgeons in participating hospitals for allowing me to use their data in this way, for carrying out the surgery and for recording the data.

REFERENCES

1 Institute of Medicine. *Assessing medical technologies.* Washington: National Academy Press 1985; 71.
2 Shuttleworth KED, Davies WD. Treatment of inguinal hernias. *Lancet* 1960; i:126.
3 Marsden AJ. Inguinal hernia. A three-year review of two thousand cases. *Br J Surg* 1962; 49:384.

4   Kald A, Nilsson E, Anderberg B *et al.* Reoperation as surrogate endpoint in hernia surgery: a three year follow-up of 1565 herniorrhaphies. *Eur J Surg* 1998; in press.

5   Devlin HB. Complications of hernia repair. In *Management of abdominal hernias.* London: Butterworths 1988; 187–98.

6   Rutkow IM. The importance of socioeconomic issues in surgical outcome: what is a relevant end point? *Eur J Surg* 1995; **161**:545–8.

7   Bendavid R. The Shouldice repair. In Nyhus LM, Condon RE, eds. *Hernia.* Philadelphia: JB Lippincott 1995; 217–27.

8   Lichtenstein IL, Shulman AG, Amid PK. The tension-free repair of hernias. In Nyhus LM, Condon RE, eds. *Hernia.* Philadelphia: JB Lippincott 1995; 237–47.

9   Rutkow IM, Robbins AW. The mesh plug hernia repair: a follow-up report. *Surgery* 1995; **117**:597–8.

10   Simons MP, Kleijnen J, van Geldere D, Hoitsma HFW, Obertop H. Role of the Shouldice technique in inguinal hernia repair: a systematic review of controlled trials and a meta-analysis. *Br J Surg* 1996; **83**:734–8.

11   Tukey JW. The future of data analysis. *Ann Math Stat* 1962; **33**(1–67):13–14.

12   Black N. Why we need observational studies to evaluate the effectiveness of health care. *BMJ* 1996; **312**:1215–18.

13   Bull AR. Audit and research: complementary but distinct. *Ann R Coll Surg Engl* 1993; **75**:308–11.

3 COST OF HERNIA SURGERY

Marc-Claude Marti and Bruno Roche

While the incidence of groin hernia is not clearly established, the number of hernia operations carried out is known more precisely. We can observe an increase in the number of operations in both the USA and Germany although the same rise has not been observed in the UK.[1,2,3] Hernia repair is the second most frequently performed surgical procedure after appendicectomy: 80 000 hernia repairs are performed yearly in Great Britain, 110 000 in France and 700 000 in the USA.[2,4,5,6] Furthermore, inguinal hernia is the most frequently encountered clinical situation requiring surgery among men. Of these operations, about 90% are performed electively in men, 10% are emergency procedures, and 10% are for a recurrence.

The following different parties are interested in knowing the cost of treatment of hernias:

- patient
- surgeon
- hospital
- insurance provider
- employers
- industry
- politicians.

WHAT IS THE COST OF HERNIA SURGERY?

To answer this question we have to analyse:

- the comparative costs of the different procedures available
- the socioeconomic aspects as they relate to the incidence of groin hernia
- the selection criteria for surgery
- the duration of postoperative disability.

The real cost of a surgical procedure includes various components which differ from one country to another and even from one hospital or institution to another. Some sort of standardization is necessary to overcome these problems.

The components of a surgical procedure which incur costs are as follows:

- pretreatment
- treatment – the operation
- post-treatment medical care
- cost to an employer
- cost to society.

Pretreatment costs

In the pretreatment period, for elective cases, the medical costs consist of the consultation and the preoperative evaluation by the surgeon and by the anaesthetist. These costs are similar for any type of surgery. This also includes the preoperative stay and any investigations.

Treatment costs

The treatment costs include:

Materials
- anaesthesia
- drugs and anaesthetic agents
- reusable materials, e.g. gowns, drapes, endotracheal tubes, etc.
- disposables, e.g. needles, syringes, blades, sutures, staples
- prostheses

Personnel
- anaesthetist
- surgeon and assistant
- nursing staff

Other
- use of operating room (according to duration of the procedure)
- recovery room
- hospital stay
- administration costs.

These different components can be calculated in terms of cash and as a percentage of the total bill. This allows easier comparisons to be made as salaries, billing systems, public charges, and so on, differ between countries and between institutions. How these costs differ according to the selected procedure is discussed later.

Local and regional anaesthesia rather than general anaesthesia are cost beneficial[7] as they result in:

- savings in operating theatre and anaesthetist costs
- reduced incidence of postoperative ileus

- reduced incidence of urinary retention
- shorter recovery room period.

Also, it is well established that outpatient herniorraphy can be accomplished at a lower cost than a traditional in-patient operation without compromising safety.[2] Thus in this case much of the reduction of overall costs does not result from any changes in the actual operative costs but from a shorter recovery room period, reduction of hospital stay and lower administration costs.

Post-treatment costs

Post-treatment costs include the usual postoperative care, wound dressings, administration of pain killers and the treatment of complications that might arise. The incidence and severity of complications vary from procedure to procedure.

During the recovery period different cost-related factors can be identified resulting mainly from time off work. These are as follows:

- cost of medication for postoperative pain
- loss of income to the patient
- loss of productivity to the employer
- cost to the employer of replacing his employee
- cost of disability insurance.

These costs are borne by the employee, the employer, the insurance company and worker's disability compensation insurance, and will vary according to the socioeconomic position of the patient.[4,8]

The time of return to work is influenced by many factors other than postoperative pain and sense of well-being. For instance, patients with worker's compensation take at least four times longer to return to work when compared with age- and sex-matched patients who have private insurance.[4,8]

Recurrence of the original condition induces new costs which are related to the frequency of recurrence, itself linked to the choice of the surgical procedure and the experience of the surgical team.[9] Thus an accurate assessment of the economic impact of inguinal herniorraphy must include evaluation of both short- and long-term medical outcomes.

Short-term outcomes include:

- local wound problems, e.g. infection, haematoma
- urinary retention
- postoperative pain
- other complications, e.g. deep veinous thrombosis, chest infection.

Long-term outcomes include:

- chronic pain
- recurrence of the hernia
- treatment of recurrence.

Repair name	Type	Materials
Bassini	Primary	Suture
Cooper	Primary	Suture
Shouldice	Primary	Suture
Lichtenstein	Mesh patch, plug	Mesh
Laparoscopic	Transabdominal or extraperitoneal	Mesh
		Laparoscopic instruments
Stoppa	Preperitoneal	Mesh

Table 1. Different methods of herniorraphy

Costs related to the choice of surgical procedure

With the recent introduction of laparoscopic procedures, different types of herniorraphy can now be performed (see Table 1). We can compare, for example, the treatment costs of Shouldice procedure and laparoscopic hernia repair (see Table 2).

Excellent results may be achieved now in the treatment of inguinal and femoral hernias with recurrence rates below 1 or 2% particularly in specialized centers, with open techniques, with or without a prosthesis, often on a daycase basis. Nevertheless, 10–17% of inguinal hernia repairs are for recurrences suggesting a much higher recurrence rate outside specialist centers.[2,5,10]

Laparoscopic surgery is more expensive than open herniorraphy because it always requires general anaesthesia. The increase in costs may reach 135% compared with the open technique. This has been confirmed by many authors in the USA,[11,12] in the UK,[13,14] in France[4] and in Germany.[2]

According to several published randomized series,[15] after the surgeon's learning curve for laparoscopic herniorraphy, the complication rate seems equal to or lower than open herniorraphy. What is most impressive is the reduced incidence of groin pain persisting for more than 1 month. Most series to date have looked at relatively few patients of less than 100 per group; a much larger series to include many hundreds of cases is needed. We would urge caution as widely different results for laparoscopic repairs have been published. Ideally data should not be collected by members of the operating team. We do not yet have long enough follow-up periods and in some series as many as 20% of patients have been lost to follow-up.

The frequency of recurrence should be included in cost evaluation as a recurrence doubles the treatment costs and is associated with a longer time off work. Consequently, lowering the recurrence rate by only 1% would have an extremely important economic effect. It is therefore important to identify precisely the procedure which results in the

Item	Shouldice	Laparoscopic
Preoperative stay	=	
Use of operating room	=	=
Anaesthesia*		+
Drugs		+
Reusable materials	=	
Disposables		+
Prosthesis		+
Suture material, staplers		+
Anaesthesiologist*	=	+
Surgeon	=	
Nursing staff	=	
Recovery room		+
Hospital stay		+
Administrative costs		+

=, Costs are equal for both procedures; +, costs are higher for the procedure considered.
*Assuming local anaesthetic for the Shouldice repair.

Table 2. Comparison of treatment cost of Shouldice and laparoscopic hernia repair

lowest recurrence rate. Eypasch *et al.*[2] from Cologne have published an interesting hypothetical calculation:

> With a known number of hernia operations of 500 000 per year in the USA and an estimated low recurrence rate of 2%, 10 000 patients with recurrence would result each year. An operation for recurrent hernia repair costs $3500. If hypothetically laparoscopic hernia repair would be applied to treat all inguinal hernias and again hypothetically there would be no more recurrences at all, then $500 000 000 would have to be spent to prevent 10 000 recurrences. This results in $50 000 for each prevented recurrence. Currently no economy worldwide would be able to tolerate such expenses for a rather simple surgical problem.

It is difficult to measure the costs associated with time off work, which must take into account:

- loss of income to the patient
- loss of productivity to the employer
- cost to the employer of replacing the patient with another worker
- cost of disability insurance
- cost of medication for prolonged postoperative pain.

These costs depend on the type of employment. They can be assessed either to the patient if he is an independent worker or has a private insurance coverage, but they can also be assessed to the employers. In reality the motivation to return to work is also dependent on the health care reimbursement system of the country. For example, in the USA, insurance pays for only a short postoperative recovery time ranging from 3 to 10 days. In Germany and Switzerland, disability of up to 6 weeks is paid for by the employer or by insurance; thus there is no incentive to return to work early either on the part of the worker or because of health insurance.[4,16] This helps to explain why comparisons between countries are so different.

In a randomized study in the UK, Lawrence *et al.*[13] demonstrated that the median time before return to work or to normal activity was 22 days in the group that had laparoscopic repair and 28 days in the group that had open repair. Social class explained 4% of the variance. The type of work undertaken, sedentary or physically active, did not explain a significant amount of variation in time to normal activity. Payne *et al.*[11,12] showed a return to work in 9 days for the laparoscopic group compared with 13 days in the open group, and similar results have been published by other authors.[14,16,17]

In a French study published by Champault *et al.*,[4] employees working for private companies returned to work 10 days earlier after laparoscopic treatment than after open hernia repair; independent liberal active men have a 60% shorter time off work after a Shouldice procedure compared with employees treated by laparoscopy.

As in most western countries, Switzerland now has a high rate of unemployment, and employers prefer to have the salary loss of their workers paid by insurance rather than to pay themselves a salary loss due to a total or partial unemployment. This leads to an artificial prolongation of time off work after hernia repair, as after any surgical procedure.

If larger randomized series confirm that laparoscopic hernia repair results in a shorter time off work than open repair, it will be necessary to prove that the increased costs associated with laparoscopic surgery are balanced by the money saved through an earlier return to work. We can express this concept in a mathematical formula:

$$\text{Nb(cost LHR} - \text{cost OHR)} \leq \text{S(loss of income OHR} - \text{loss of income LHR)} + \text{Nb(RR OHR} - \text{RR LHR) (cost of a recurrence)}$$

where LHR is laparoscopic hernia repair, OHR is open hernia repair, RR is recurrence rate and Nb is the number of patients.

The extra cost resulting from laparoscopic hernia repair as compared to the cost of open hernia repair should be equal to or less than the sum of the reduction of income loss (earlier time to return to work) with laparoscopic surgery plus the reduced cost resulting from a reduced incidence of recurrences.

CONCLUSIONS AND RECOMMENDATIONS

We have reviewed the multiple factors that contribute to the economic costs of hernia management. As groin hernia is a common condition and has such an impact on health-care costs, we should ask how we can reduce these costs?

Several different approaches should be considered:

- avoid unnecessary operations if no benefit is expected—small hernias in elderly patients should be operated on only if they are symptomatic, if they impair the quality of life or if there is a risk of complications;
- avoid unnecessary hospitalization—ambulatory management is economically realistic and safe;[2,18] re-educate surgeons, patients and health insurers in Europe to promote ambulatory surgery; new incentives should be developed;
- use precise standardized procedures of open or laparoscopic hernia repair—this should result in a low recurrence rate of less than 2% or even 1%; surgeons have a responsibility for this quality improvement;
- use laparoscopic treatment if it proves superior to open hernia repair—surgical costs should then be reduced; industry should offer disposable materials, prosthesis and staplers at a more reasonable price; laparoscopic treatment must be cost effective;
- encourage early return to work—new incentives should be developed.

REFERENCES

1 Devlin HB. *Management of abdominal hernias.* London: Butterworths 1988.

2 Eypasch E, Kum CK, Paul A, Trodl H. Socioeconomic aspects of groin hernias: what is the cost of hernia surgery? *Prog Surg* 1995; **21**:8–12.

3 Siewert JR, Bollschweiler E, Hempel K. Wandel der Eingriffshäufigkeit in der Allgemeinchirurgie. *Chirurgie* 1990; **61**:855–63.

4 Champault G, Marachly G, Lauroy J, Boutelier P. Dans quelles conditions le traitement laparoscopique des hernies de l'aine est-il financièrement rentable. *J Chirurgie* 1994; **131**:483–7.

5 Hay J-M, Boudet M-J, Fingerhut A *et al.* Shouldice inguinal hernia repair in the male adult. *Ann Surg* 1995; **222**:719–27.

6 Rutkow IM. Laparoscopic hernia repair: the socioeconomic tyranny of surgical technology. *Arch Surg* 1992; **127**:1271.

7 Behnia R, Hashemi F, Stryker SJ *et al.* A comparison of general versus local anesthesia during inguinal hernioraphy. *Surgery* 1992; **174**:277–80.

8 Salcedo-Wasicek C, Thirlby RC. Postoperative course after inguinal herniorrhaphy. *Arch Surg* 1995; **130**:29–32.

9 Chevrel JP, Perez M, Lumbroso M *et al.* Récidives herniaires. *Presse Méd* 1991; **20**:1543–7.

10 Millikan KW, Kosik ML, Doolas A. A prospective comparison of transabdominal preperitoneal laparoscopic hernia repair versus traditional open hernia repair in a university setting. *Surg Laparosc Endosc* 1994; **4**:247–53.

11 Payne JH, Grininger LM, Izawa MT *et al.* Laparoscopic or open inguinal herniorraphy? *Arch Surg* 1994; **129**:973–81.

12 Payne JH, Ching K, Plotkin E, McCurdy J. Laparoscopic or open herniorrhaphy? A cost analysis of a randomized prospective controlled comparison. *Surg Endosc* 1994; **8**:467.

13 Lawrence K, McWhinnie D, Goodwin A *et al.* Randomised controlled trial of laparoscopic versus open repair inguinal hernia: early results. *BMJ* 1995; **311**:981–5.

14 Stoker DL, Spiegelhalter DJ, Singh R *et al*. Laparoscopic versus open inguinal hernia repair: a randomised prospective trial. *Lancet* 1994; **1**:1243–5.

15 Fitzgibbons RJ, Camps J, Cornet DA *et al*. Laparoscopic inguinal herniorraphy. Results of a multicenter trial. *Ann Surg* 1995; **221**:3–13.

16 Bourke JB, Lear PA, Taylor M. The effect of early return to work after elective repair of inguinal hernia: clinical and financial consequences at one year and three years. *Lancet* 1981; **ii**:623–5.

17 Rider MA, Baker DM, Locker A, Fawcett AN. Return to work after inguinal hernia repair. *Br J Surg* 1993; **80**:745–6.

18 Nilsson E, Anderberg B, Bragmark M *et al*. Hernia surgery in a defined population. Improvements possible in outcome and cost-effectiveness. *Ambulatory Surg* 1993; **1**:150–3.

4 ANATOMICAL ENTITIES OF THE GROIN IN OPEN AND LAPAROSCOPIC REPAIR OF INGUINOFEMORAL HERNIATION

John E Skandalakis

> The imagination voyaging through chaos and reducing it to clarity and order
> is the symbol of all the quests which lend glory to our dust
>
> Lowes, *The Road to Xanadu*

The purpose of this chapter is to describe the important anatomical entities of the groin which are associated with open and laparoscopic herniorrhaphy. The first section will discuss the anatomy from above (from the skin to the anterior surface of the myopectineal orifice of Fruchaud), and the second part will present the anatomy from below (from the peritoneum to the posterior surface of the myopectineal orifice of Fruchaud). It will be seen that the laparoscopic topography and orientation are quite new and different from that of the open method.

ANATOMY OF OPEN HERNIORRHAPHY

The anterior abdominal wall

The corresponding layers of the anterior abdominal wall and inguinal area and scrotum are as follows:

Lower abdominal wall	*Inguinal area and scrotum*
1 Skin	1 Skin
2 Superficial fascia	2 Dartos
3 Innominate fascia	3 External spermatic fascia
4 Internal oblique muscle and aponeurosis	4 Cremasteric fascia and muscle
5 Transversus abdominis muscle and aponeurosis	5 Cremasteric fascia and muscle

cont

Lower abdominal wall	*Inguinal area and scrotum*
6 Transversalis fascia	6 Internal spermatic fascia
7 Preperitoneal fat	7 Preperitoneal fat
8 Peritoneum	8 Tunica vaginalis

External oblique fascia (innominate fascia of Gallaudet)

The external oblique fascia is a thin, tissue-like membrane that covers the external oblique muscle and aponeurosis. In the superficial ring, it forms the intercrural fibers. The innominate fascia follows the spermatic cord and forms the external spermatic fascia as it approaches the scrotum.

External oblique aponeurosis

According to Rizk[1] and Askar,[2,3,4] the aponeurosis of the external oblique is formed by two layers, a superficial layer and a deep layer. These two layers, together with the bilaminar aponeuroses of the internal oblique and transversus abdominis, form the rectus sheath and, by linear decussation, also form the linea alba. If Rizk and Askar are correct, then at the lower abdominal wall, the anterior rectus sheath (since the posterior does not exist) is formed by the fusion of six aponeurotic layers, two from each flat muscle (external oblique, internal oblique, and transversus abdominis). The point where the bilaminar external oblique aponeurosis touches the anterior rectus sheath ('touchdown' point) is always between the linea alba and the lateral border of the rectus sheath (Fig. 1). The external oblique aponeurosis does not extend to the scrotum and is not a covering of the spermatic cord.

The superficial inguinal 'ring' is a triangular opening of the external oblique aponeurosis which is located 1–1.5 cm above and lateral to the pubic tubercle. The opening is formed by a splitting of the external oblique aponeurosis, making the crura of the subcutaneous ring. The inferior (lateral) crus inserts into the tubercle and pecten; the superior (medial) crus inserts anterior to the pubic bone and symphysis. The insertion of the inferior crus is, partly, by way of the lacunar ligament. Fibers from the superior crus cross the midline to insert on the opposite tubercle.

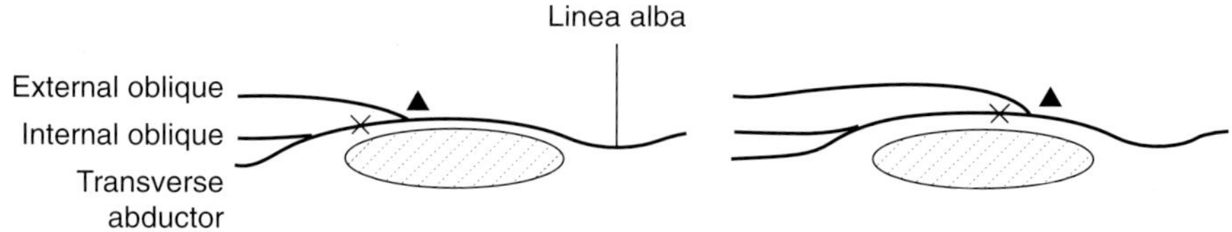

Figure 1. Diagram of the relaxing incision. The X-point of the relaxing incision is at the anterior lamina of the rectus sheath. Triangles mark the 'touchdown' of the external oblique aponeurosis, which is always between the linea alba and semilunar line[5]

In the inguinal area, there are three regional modifications of the external oblique aponeurosis: the inguinal ligament, the lacunar ligament, and the reflected inguinal ligament.

The inguinal ligament (ligament of Poupart). This is the lower edge of the external oblique aponeurosis. It extends from the anterior superior iliac spine to the pubic tubercle. Before the inguinal ligament reaches the pubic tubercle, Gimbernat's ligament and the reflected inguinal ligament are formed. Curiously, Francois Poupart (1661–1709) never published an article or a thesis about the inguinal ligament that bears his name.[6]

The lacunar ligament (ligament of Gimbernat). The lacunar ligament was first described by Antonio de Gimbernat in 1793. According to Madden,[7] the lacunar ligament can be demonstrated only when 'the pyriform fossa is completely exposed' because the ligament practically forms the floor of the fossa.

The ligament of Gimbernat is a triangular extension of the inguinal ligament before its insertion into the pubic tubercle. It is inserted at the pecten pubis, and its lateral end meets the proximal end of the ligament of Cooper. Condon[8] asserted that 'it [the ligament] never forms the medial border of the normal femoral canal.' Other investigators, however, hold the opposite view.

The reflected inguinal ligament. The reflected inguinal ligament is composed of aponeurotic fibers from the inferior crus of the external inguinal ring. The ligament travels upward towards the linea alba.

The internal oblique muscle

The relationship of the internal oblique muscle to other entities in the inguinal region is a subject of disagreement. McVay[8] believed the origin of the muscle was the fascia of the iliopsoas muscle. The medial termination of the internal oblique muscle is the anterior rectus lamina of which it is a part. The internal oblique muscle does not support the lower portion of the posterior inguinal wall because it does not have an insertion into Cooper's ligament.[9] The internal oblique aponeurosis is formed by two fused layers, anterior and posterior. These layers, together with the two other bilaminar aponeuroses form the anterior rectus sheath and the linea alba.

The transversus abdominis muscle and aponeurosis

The origin of the transversus abdominis muscle is the iliopsoas fascia, not from the inguinal ligament, and inserts on Cooper's ligament.[9]

The integrity of the transversus abdominis muscle prevents the formation of hernias and, in this sense, the transversus abdominis muscle forms the most important layer of the abdominal wall. A useful anatomic entity for the repair of inguinal hernias is the transversus abdominis arch. It is formed by the free aponeurotic and muscular lower margin of the muscle. Medially, the arch is aponeurotic; toward the internal ring, it is both muscular and aponeurotic.

In the environment of the internal ring, the internal oblique muscle is muscular and the transversus abdominis muscle is aponeurotic. Medially in the inguinal area, all the aponeurotic layers of the three flat muscles pass anterior to the rectus abdominis muscle to form the anterior lamina of the rectus sheath.

The conjoined tendon

By definition, the conjoined tendon is the fusion of the aponeuronium of the internal oblique aponeurosis with similar fibers from the aponeurosis of the transversus abdominis as they insert on the pubic tubercle and superior ramus of the pubis. Although this description is simple and straightforward, the anatomic configuration described is rare. Hollinshead[10] considered it to exist in 5% of subjects; Condon[11] reported its existence in only 3% of cases; and McVay[9] believed that the 'conjoined tendon' was only an artefact of dissection.

Because of the number of structures juxtaposed in this area and because the term 'conjoined tendon' is extensively used, I propose that the area referred to as the 'conjoined tendon' be replaced by the term 'conjoined area.'

The following are a few other definitions to clarify the local anatomy of the conjoined area (Fig. 2):

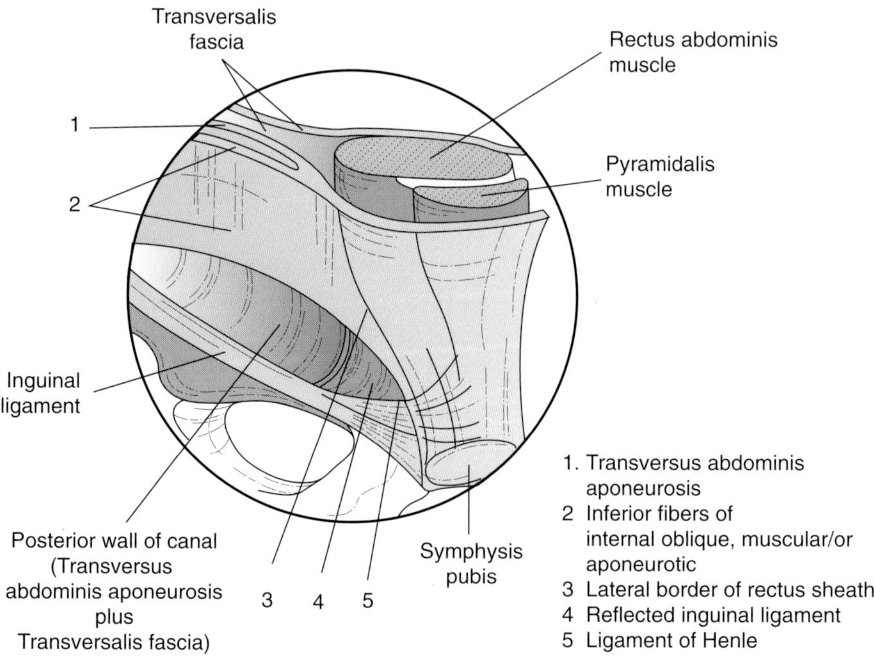

Figure 2. The 'conjoined area'[12]

- As the arch of the transversus abdominis muscle approaches the rectus sheath, it becomes aponeurotic (transversus aponeurosis). Close to the internal ring, the arch is covered by the much more muscular arch of the internal oblique muscle. Always, in the inguinal region, the internal oblique is muscular, and the transversus abdominis aponeurotic.
- The ligament of Henle is the structure that was originally termed 'falx inguinalis.' The ligament is the lateral expansion of the tendon of the rectus abdominis muscle, or an expansion of the rectus sheath, that inserts on the pecten of the pubis. It is present in 30–50% of patients; when present, it is fused with the transversalis fascia.
- The interfoveolar ligament (of Hesselbach) is an apparent thickening of the transversalis fascia at the medial side of the internal inguinal ring. It has the appearance of a spider web and lies in front of the inferior epigastric vessels. The ligament of Hesselbach is not, however, a true ligament.
- The reflected inguinal ligament is composed of aponeurotic fibers from the inferior crus of the external inguinal ring of the French anatomists.

In sum, the conjoined tendon rarely exists.

The rectus abdominis muscle and its sheath

The rectus abdominis muscle is enclosed in a stout sheath formed by the bilaminar aponeuroses of the three flat muscles (internal oblique, external oblique, transversus abdominis) that split and pass around it anteriorly and posteriorly. All three muscles start at the lateral border of the rectus abdominis, form the linea alba, and, in a complicated way, pass to the opposite side of the rectus abdominis muscle.[1,2]

In the lower quarter of the abdominal wall, the aponeuroses pass anteriorly to the rectus abdominis muscle, which is bound posteriorly by the transversalis fascia. The linea semicircularis of Douglas marks the point at which the rectus sheath loses its posterior wall. If the change is gradual, the line is poorly defined; if the change is abrupt, it is well marked.

The transversalis fascia and the internal ring

Although useless by itself for hernia repair, the weak transversalis fascia layer can be used for repair when it is fused with the transversus abdominis aponeurosis.

The transversalis fascia forms a sling around the internal ring. The internal ring is an incomplete ring that consists of a thickening that forms two crura – a long anterior crus and a short posterior crus. The anterior crus is fixed to the transversus abdominis muscle or aponeurosis above, and to the internal ring medially. The posterior crus is fixed to, or inserts on, the iliopubic tract. This arrangement forms an inverted U-shaped sling. When the transversus abdominis muscle is contracted, the sling closes the internal ring under the muscular edge of the internal oblique muscle:

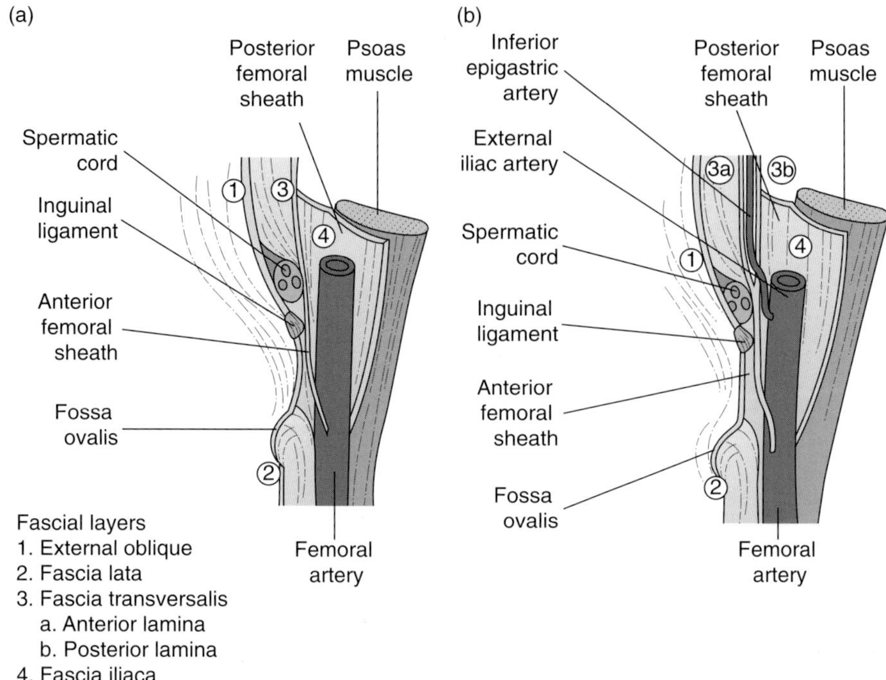

Figure 3. (a) Diagram of the transversalis fascia and femoral sheath (old concept). (b) Diagram of the transversalis fascia and femoral sheath (new concept), emphasizing the bilaminar nature of the transversalis fascia in the inguinal area[13]

Cooper's posterior lamina. Read emphasized the bilaminar formation of the transversalis fascia in the inguinal area, a concept which was described so well by Cooper[14] (Fig. 3).

The iliopubic tract. First described by Alexander Thomson in 1836, the iliopubic tract is an aponeurotic band that extends from the iliopectineal arch to the superior ramus of the pubis. It creates the inferior margin of the deep musculo-aponeurotic layer, which is composed of the transversus abdominis muscle and aponeurosis and the transversalis fascia. The iliopubic tract is frequently referred to by several other names including the ligament of Thomson, deep crural arch, deep femoral arch, anterior femoral sheath, and Bandelette iliopubiene.

The tract attaches laterally to the iliacus and psoas fascia. It continues more laterally to the anterior superior slim spine. Medially, the tract forms the lower border of the internal inguinal ring. It crosses the femoral vessels to form the anterior margin of the femoral sheath. (In reality, perhaps all these anatomic entities originate from the transversalis fascia.) The tract curves around the medial surface of the femoral sheath to attach to the pectineal ligament (Fig. 4).

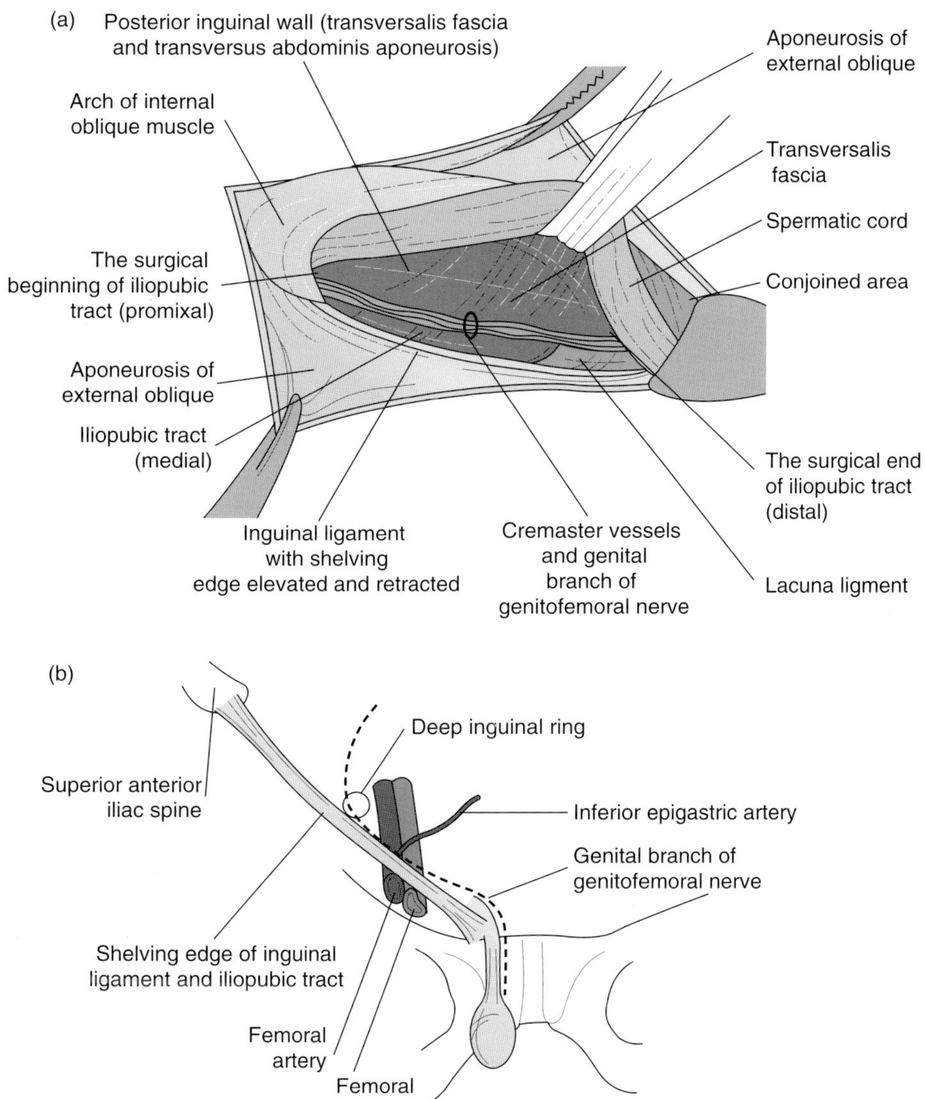

Figure 4. (a) The iliopubic tract and its relations to the genital branch of the genitofemoral nerve. (b) Diagram of the pathway of the genital branch of the genitofemoral nerve from the deep inguinal ring to the medial side of the spermatic cord[15]

Madden[6] reported that the key to understanding the iliopubic tract lies in understanding the pyriform fossa (Fig. 5). This fossa forms part of the posterior wall ('floor') of the inguinal canal. This potential structure is a semi-ovoid space filled with fibrofatty tissue and located at the medial part of the floor. Its borders are the iliopubic tract

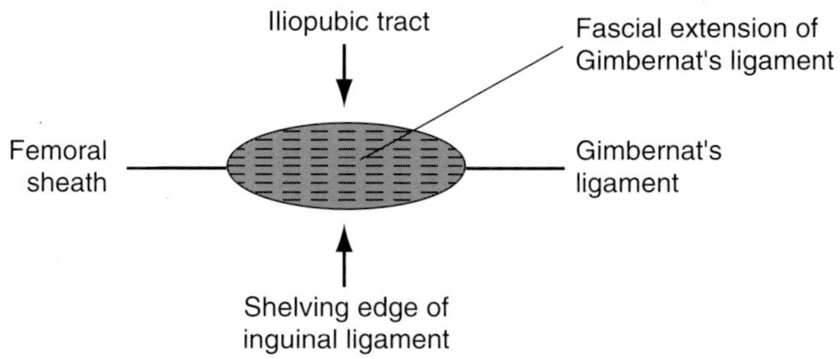

Figure 5. The pyriform fossa of Madden[15]

superiorly, the shelving edge of the inguinal ligament inferiorly, the ligament of Gimbernat medially and femoral sheath laterally.

According to Condon,[16] the iliopubic tract is visible along the inferior margin of the deep inguinal ring, but is covered partially by the inguinal ligament. He pointed out that it is frequently confused with the inguinal ligament, which, although nearby, belongs to the anterior lamina (superficial musculo-aponeurotic layer). Condon[11] found the iliopubic tract present in 98% of dissections. The shelving edge of the inguinal ligament is anterior to the iliopubic arch. The cremaster vessels and the genital branch of the genitofemoral nerve are located very close to the iliopubic tract at the posterior wall of the inguinal canal.

Posterior inguinal wall

The posterior inguinal wall is formed by the fusion of the transversus abdominis aponeurosis and the transversalis fascia. However, a part of the posterior wall (perhaps one-third or a quarter) is not covered by the transversus abdominis aponeurosis. This uncovered portion is located just above the distal part of the ligament of Cooper and the iliopubic tract laterally to the ligament of Gimbernat, and extends upward to the arch. Anatomically, it is the weak area of the posterior inguinal wall, and it is in this area that direct and supravesical hernias are formed.

The myopectineal orifice of Fruchaud

Fruchaud believed that all groin hernias began in a single weak area within the groin, an area which he called the 'myopectineal orifice.'[17] The myopectineal orifice is bounded as follows: superiorly, the arch of the internal oblique muscle and the transversus abdominis muscle; laterally, the iliopsoas muscle; medially, the lateral border of the rectus abdominis muscle and its anterior lamina; and inferiorly, the pubic pectin. The inguinal ligament spans and divides this framework. The area is transversed by the spermatic cord and femoral vessels and is bridged on its inner surface by the transversalis fascia only.

Preperitoneal fat and space

Fat and other connective tissue, either thick or thin, lie within a space between the peritoneum and the transversalis fascia. Fibrous bands are present, and occasionally lipomata similar to those in the spermatic cord are found. The reflection of parietal peritoneum toward the iliac fossa before it reaches the pubic bone exposes the preperitoneal space.[9]

Peritoneum. The peritoneum is the innermost layer of the abdominal wall and, consequently, of the inguinal area. It is connected loosely with the transversalis fascia in most areas except at the internal ring, where the connection is stronger.

Fossae of the anterior abdominal wall

The posterior surface of the anterior abdominal wall above the inguinal ligament is divided into three shallow fossae. These fossae are located on either side of the midline and are marked by the obliterated embryonic urachus that extends from the dome of the bladder to the umbilicus (median umbilical ligament). Laterally, the fossae are separated by the medial umbilical ligaments (obliterated umbilical arteries) and the lateral umbilical ligaments (inferior or deep epigastric arteries), as shown in Fig. 6.

(1)   The lateral fossa, which is lateral to the inferioepigastric arteries, contains the internal inguinal ring. It is the site of indirect inguinal hernia.

(2)   The medial fossa, between the inferior epigastric arteries and the medial umbilical ligaments, is the site of direct inguinal hernia.

(3)   The supravesical fossa, between the medial and median umbilical ligaments, is the site of external supravesical hernia.

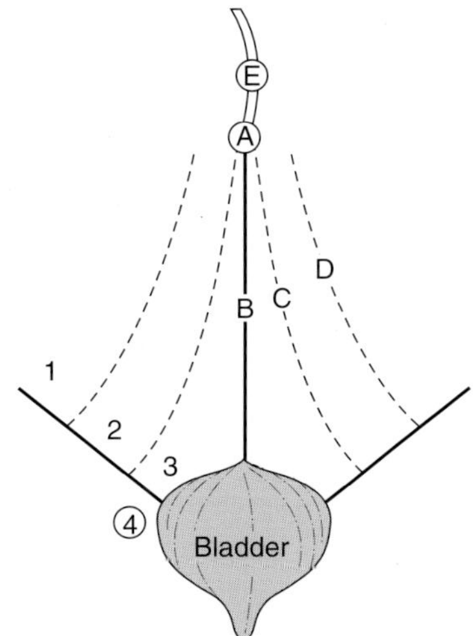

Figure 6. Diagram of the fossae of the anterior abdominal wall and their relation to the sites of groin herniae. A: Umbilicus. B: Median umbilical ligament (obliterated urachus). C: Medial umbilical ligament (obliterated umbilical arteries). D: Lateral umbilical ligament containing inferior (deep) epigastric arteries. E: Falciform ligament. Sites of possible herniae: 1: Lateral fossa (indirect inguinal hernia); 2: Medial fossa (direct inguinal hernia); 3: Supravesical fossa (supravesical hernia); 4: Femoral ring (femoral hernia)[18]

The supravesical fossa partially overlies Hesselbach's triangle so that the medial umbilical ligament lies within the triangle. Therefore, a hernia through either the medial or supravesical fossae is a direct inguinal hernia. One may also say that a direct hernia may be inguinal (in the medial fossa) or supravesical (in the supravesical fossa).

Hesselbach's triangle

Hesselbach's triangle is defined today as having the inferior (deep) epigastric vessels as its superior or lateral border, the rectus sheath as its medial border, and the inguinal ligament as its lateroinferior border. This area is smaller than the triangle originally described by Hesselbach in 1814.

It is in Hesselbach's triangle that most direct and external supravesical inguinal hernias occur. Only the medial border is suitable for hernia repair. The epigastric vessels above the triangle cannot be used. Many surgeons prefer to use the iliopubic tract or the pectineal ligament instead of the inguinal ligament.

The defective canal

A deficient posterior wall, found in 23–25% of patients, lacks the support of the aponeurosis of the transversus abdominis muscle (Fig. 7).[19]

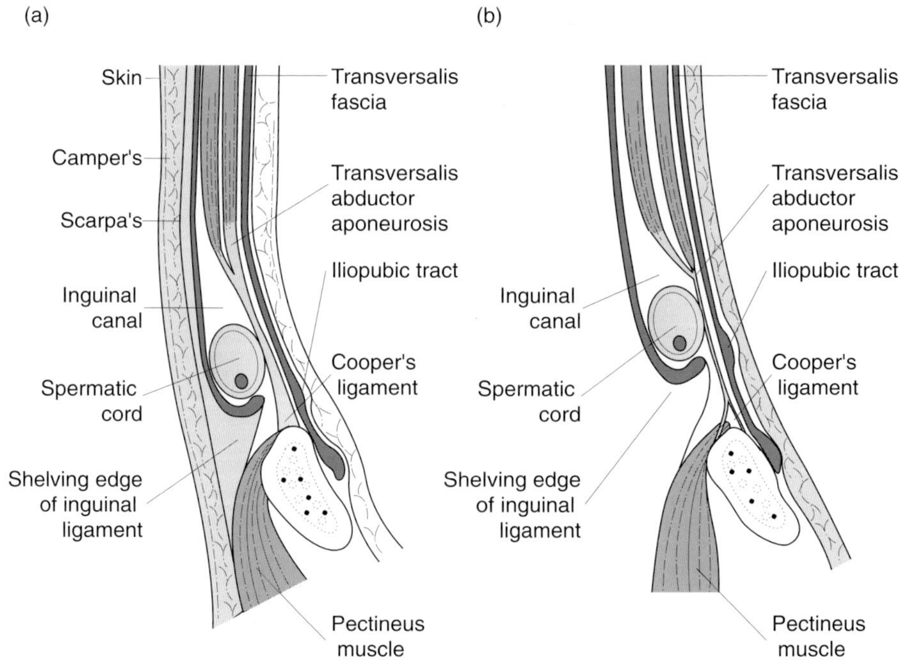

Figure 7. (a) Cross-section of a strong posterior canal wall. (b) Cross-section of a weak posterior canal wall[20]

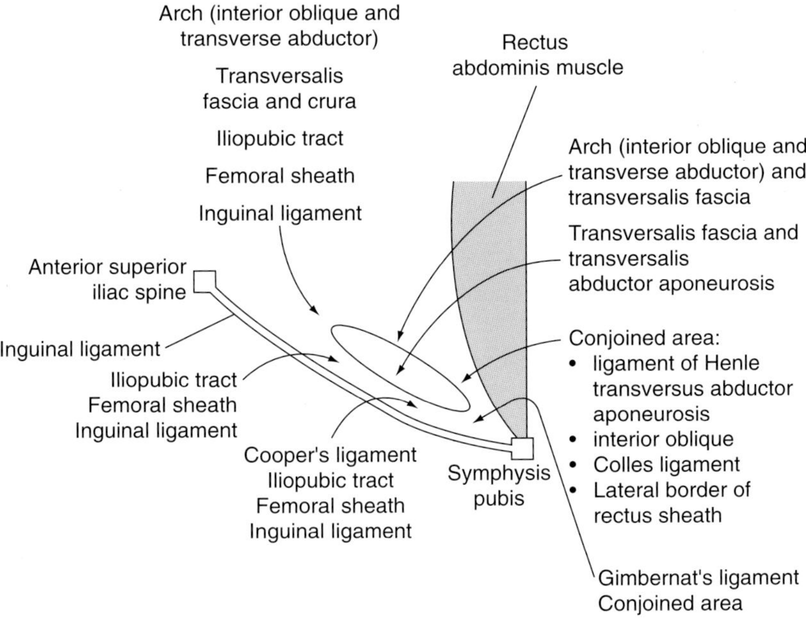

Figure 8. The surgical ellipse of the inguinal area[21]

The surgical ellipse

Upon incision of the aponeurosis of the external oblique muscle, the surgeon confronts several anatomic areas and entities which are incorporated into an elliptical area. The ellipse (Fig. 8) is created by the floor of the inguinal canal, a superior medial edge (above), an inferior lateral edge (below), a medial apex, and a lateral apex. Therefore, the following points must be considered:

- The floor (posterior wall) of the ellipse is formed by the fusion of the transversus abdominis aponeurosis and transversalis fascia. In direct hernias, the transversalis fascia and the transversus abdominis aponeurosis are attenuated to some degree. When the posterior wall is intact, none of the four types of inguinal hernias (indirect, direct, external supravesical, or femoral) will develop. However indirect inguinal hernias in newborns may exist even though there is a normal posterior wall.
- The superior medial edge (above) of the ellipse is formed by the conjoined area and the arch of internal oblique muscle and transversus abdominis muscle with their aponeuroses.
- The inferior lateral edge (below) is formed by the inguinal ligament, the iliopubic tract, the femoral sheath, and Cooper's ligament. Some or all of these structures are used for repair.

- The medial apex, close to the symphysis pubis, is formed by Gimbernat's ligament below and the conjoined area above.
- The lateral apex, at the internal ring, is formed by the arch of the internal oblique and transversus abdominis muscles and their aponeuroses, the transversalis fascia and crura, the iliopubic tract, the femoral sheath, and the inguinal ligament.

The space of Bogros

Bogros was a French anatomist and surgeon who described a triangular space in the iliac region with the following boundaries: laterally, the iliac fascia; anteriorly, the transversalis fascia; and medially, the parietal peritoneum.

According to Bendavid,[19] the space of Bogros is a lateral extension of the retropubic space of Retzius which may be explored by incising the transversalis fascia from the internal ring to the pubic crest. He reported that a venous network is frequently located at the lower anterior portion of the space of Bogros. The Bendavid 'venous circle' of veins is a variable venous network composed of the deep inferior epigastric vein, the iliopubic vein, the rectusial vein, the retropubic vein, and the communicating rectusioepigastric vein. The network is fixed to the anterior wall. Bendavid advised familiarity with this venous circle, particularly by those surgeons using prosthetic material.

Cooper's ligament

Almost 200 years ago (1804), Cooper[22] described the 'ligament' that now bears his name. The topographical anatomy is seen in Fig. 9; the scope of this paper does not permit a detailed discussion. A number of authors have, however, written very good statements concerning this ligament.[7,10,11,23–35]

For practical purposes Cooper's ligament consists of:
(1) the periosteum of the pectineal line; (2) the insertion of the iliopubic tract from above to the periosteum; (3) the insertion of the lacunar ligament from below to the periosteum; and (4) the insertion or origin of the pectineal fascia from below.

The femoral canal and the femoral sheath

Between the inguinal ligament and the linea terminalis (iliopectineal line) is a space organized into three compartments. The most lateral of these is the neuromuscular compartment, which contains the iliopsoas muscle, the femoral nerve, and the lateral femoral cutaneous nerve. Medial to the neuromuscular compartment is the vascular compartment, which is composed of the femoral artery and vein. Medial to the vascular compartment is the compartment of the femoral canal. The femoral canal is conical and approximately 1.25–2 cm long. At its apex is the fossa ovalis, the opening for the great saphenous vein. Thus, a femoral hernia may present as a bulge of the skin over the fossa ovalis.

The femoral sheath, an extension of the transversalis fascia of the abdomen, envelops the femoral artery, vein, and femoral canal.

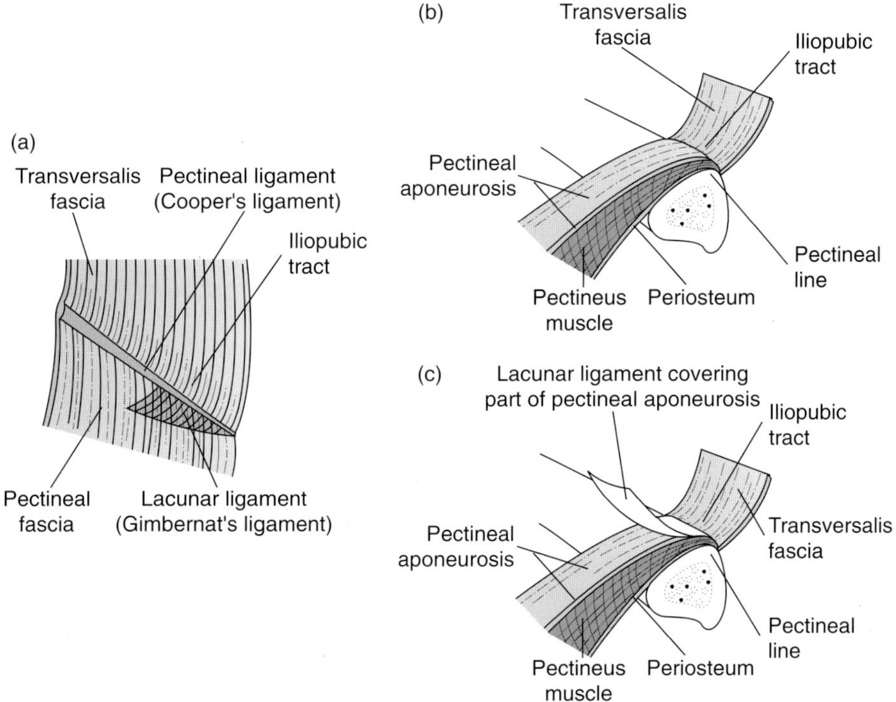

Figure 9.   (a) Diagram of some anatomical entities participating in the formation of the pectineal ligament (Cooper's). (b) Diagram demonstrating the insertion of the iliopubic tract into the ligament of Cooper and perhaps the origin of the pectineal aponeurosis. (c) Diagram showing that the lacunar ligament (Gimbernat's) partially covers the pectineal aponeurosis[15]

The femoral ring is inflexible. McVay[8] stated that the transverse diameter ranges from 8–27 mm and the anteroposterior diameter ranges from 9–10 mm, but that in 70% of patients these diameters are 10–14 mm and 12–16 mm, respectively. McVay[9] located the lacunar ligament at the medial margin of the femoral ring in only 8 of 362 subjects and stated that the aponeurosis of transversus abdominis is the usual boundary. Condon[8] reported that either the aponeurosis or the recurved iliopubic tract may form the medial boundary.

Surgical applications

I consider the following anatomical entities to be strong and dependable for open hernia repair: inguinal ligament, lacunar ligament, pectineal ligament, transversalis fascia (when fused with the transversus abdominis aponeurosis), iliopubic tract, anterior femoral sheath, transversalis fascia crura, conjoined area, and arch of the internal oblique and transversus abdominis muscles.

LAPAROSCOPIC ANATOMY

Understanding the anatomy is the most important and most difficult facet of laparoscopic herniorrhaphy (Fig. 10). There are several layers, fossae and potential spaces which must be recognized when performing laparoscopic hernia repair (Fig. 11 and

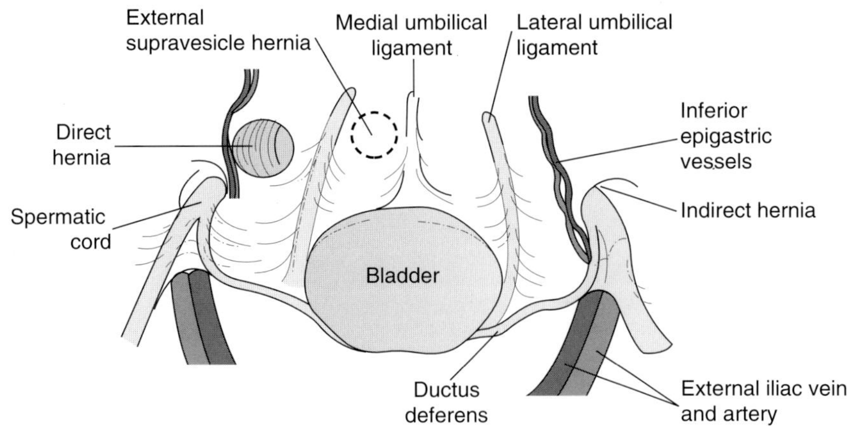

Figure 10. Laparoscopic topographic anatomy of the inguinal region. In men, the spermatic vessels join the vas deferens to form the spermatic cord. The presence of a fascial defect lateral or medial to the inferior epigastric vessels defines an indirect or a direct hernia, respectively[36]

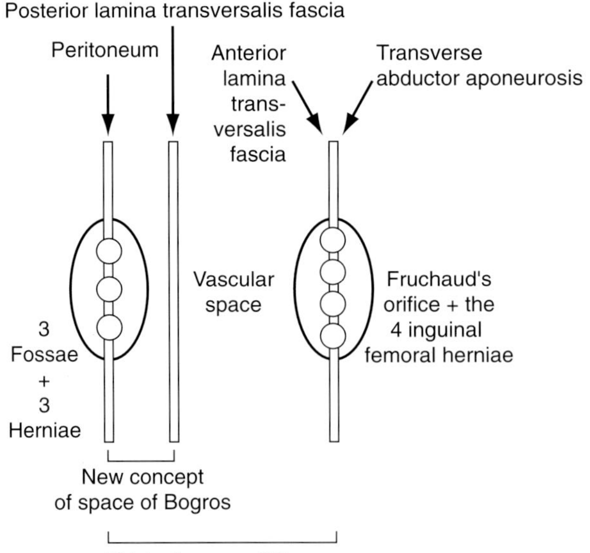

Figure 11. Diagram of laparoscopic anatomy of the inguinal area demonstrating layers, fossae, and spaces[36]

I. Three layers
   a. Peritoneum
   b. Transversalis fascia posterior
   c. Transversalis fascia anterior fused with transversus abdominis aponeurosis
II. Three fossae
   a. Lateral
   b. Medial
   c. Supravesical
III. Two spaces
   a. Space of Bogros
   b. Vascular space
IV. Myopectineal orifice of Fruchaud
V. Dangerous eye
   a. Arch (above)
   b. Iliopubic tract (below)
VI. Two potential triangles and one circle

Table 1. Laparoscopic peripatos of the inguinal area

Table 1). Figures 10–12 will be the basis of orientation for the study of anatomical entities, folds, and spaces with which the laparoscopist should be familiar.

Three layers of the abdominal wall

From a laparoscopic perspective, the peritoneum is the innermost layer of the inguinal area (Fig. 12). Just behind the peritoneum is another layer, the posterior lamina of the transversalis fascia. Further posterior is the anterior lamina of the transversalis fascia, which is fused with the transversus abdominis aponeurosis.

Three fossae

The supravesical, medial and lateral fossae are easily identified at laparoscopy. In many cases, with the peritoneum in place, the laparoscopist will also observe two underlying anatomical entities in the male: the gonadal vessels (bluish cordlike structures) and the ductus deferens (silver cordlike structure).

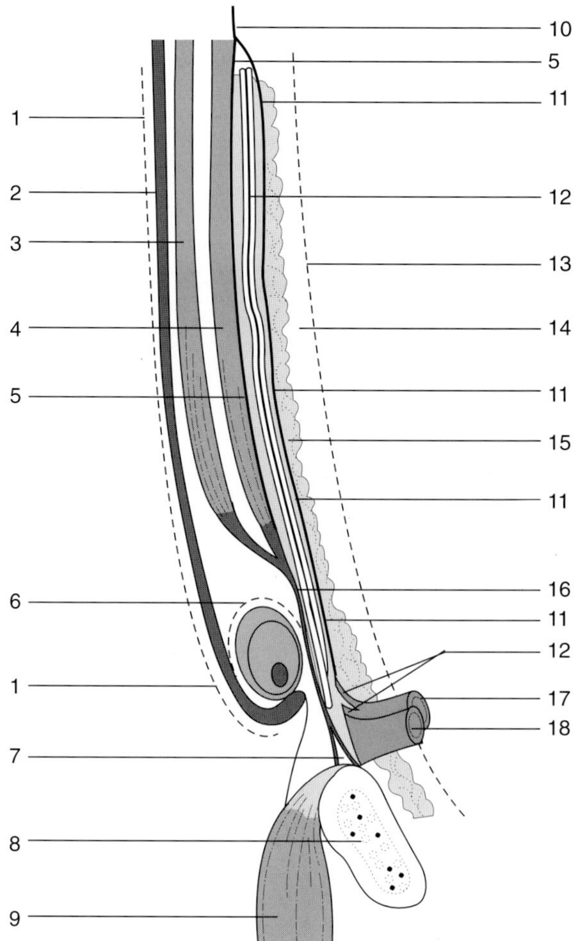

Figure 12. The space of Bogros. 1, innominate fascia; 2, external oblique aponeurosis; 3, internal oblique muscle; 4, transversus abdominis muscle; 5, transversalis fascia anterior; 6, external spermatic fascia; 7, Cooper's ligament; 8, pubic bone; 9, pectineus muscle; 10, transversalis fascia; 11, transversalis fascia posterior lamina; 12, vessels; 13, peritoneum; 14, home (space) of the prosthesis, space of Bogros; 15, preperitoneal fat; 16, transversus abdominis aponeurosis and anterior lamina of transversalis fascia; 17, femoral artery; 18, femoral vein[36]

Two spaces

Under the peritoneum and between the peritoneum and the posterior lamina of the transversalis fascia is the space of Bogros, which is filled with variable quantities of preperitoneal fat. This is the area in which the laparoscopist will insert the prosthesis.

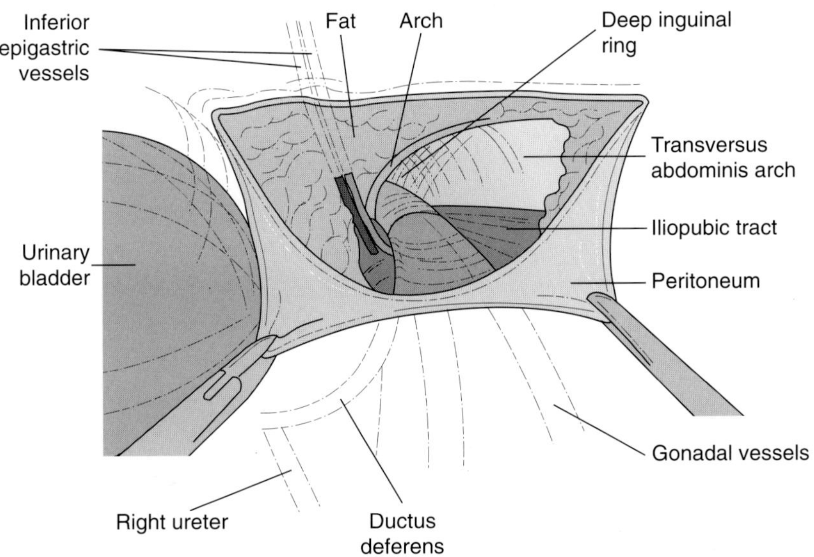

Figure 13. After incising and retracting the peritoneum, the inferior epigastric vessels (the most superficial anatomical entities) will be seen. The arch and the iliopubic tract may or may not be seen[36]

Another significant space is the area formed between the anterior and posterior laminae of the transversalis fascia; the inferior epigastric vessels are located within this area. Occasionally, the posterior lamina is very thin and unrecognizable. When this is the case, the space of Bogros extends to the anterior lamina of the transversalis fascia, which is the well-known 'transversalis fascia.' Within the lower part of the space of Bogros is the inguinal venous circle[19] which forms a venous network for several tributaries.

After the removal of fibrofatty tissues, the laparoscopist will see the most superficial anatomical entity, the inferior epigastric vessels (Fig. 13). With further cleaning, the transversus abdominis muscular arch and the iliopubic tract will be seen. Both are closely related to the internal ring; the arch forms the superior boundary, and the iliopubic tract forms the inferior boundary. Neither the inguinal ligament (Poupart's) nor the lacunar ligament (Gimbernat's) can be seen during laparoscopy. Cooper's ligament, however, will be seen at the pubic brim as a shiny white convex band on the brim of the minor (true) pelvis.

The external iliac artery and vein are located in a deeper plane within the triangle formed by the spermatic vessels and the ductus deferens. Distally, at the internal ring, these vessels lie to the right and left of the apex of the triangle, but, proximally in my dissections they were always within it. The origins of the inferior epigastric and deep circumflex iliac vessels are also within this area.

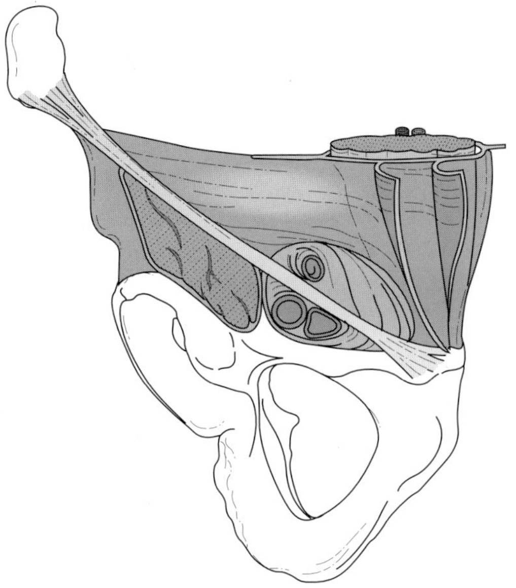

Figure 14. Anterior view of Fruchaud's myopectineal orifice[17]

The myopectineal orifice of Fruchaud

Another important area is the myopectineal orifice of Fruchaud (Fig. 14).

The dangerous eye

The iliopubic tract divides Fruchaud's orifice into two parts: above, the spermatic cord will be seen; below, the external iliac vessels, covered by the anterior lamina of the femoral sheath, are visible (Figs 15 and 16). Remember the anterior lamina of the transversalis fascia is fused with the transversus abdominis aponeurosis forming the floor or posterior wall of the inguinal canal. The overall anatomy of this area may be appreciated by Fig. 17. Characteristically, the nerves in this area are located lateral to the deep inguinal ring; the vessels are located below and medial to the ring (Fig. 18).

The most lateral nerve is the lateral femoral cutaneous nerve. Usually it leaves the iliac fossa just medial to the anterior superior iliac spine. Superficial to the external iliac artery is the genital branch of the genitofemoral nerve. Lateral to the external iliac artery is the femoral branch of the genitofemoral nerve. Further, but not far enough away to avoid injury, is the femoral nerve, which lies in the trough between the psoas and iliacus muscles (Fig. 19).

Several important vessels are medial to the ring: the venous circle, inferior epigastric artery and vein, internal and external iliac artery and vein, rectus vessels, suprapubic and retropubic vessels, and aberrant obturator artery and/or vein (present in 30–40% of cases).

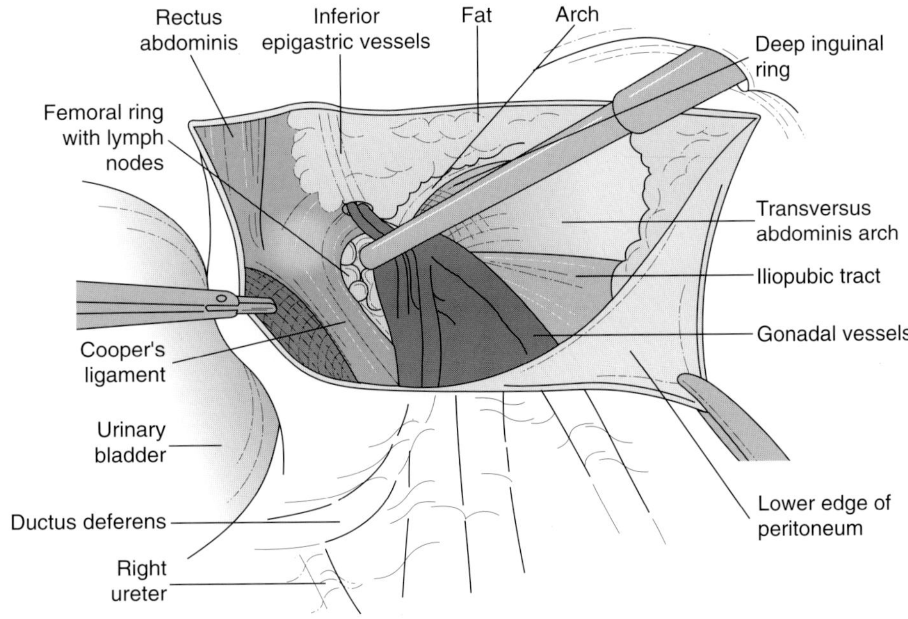

Figure 15. With more cleaning the arch, iliopubic tract, and ligament of Cooper can be seen[36]

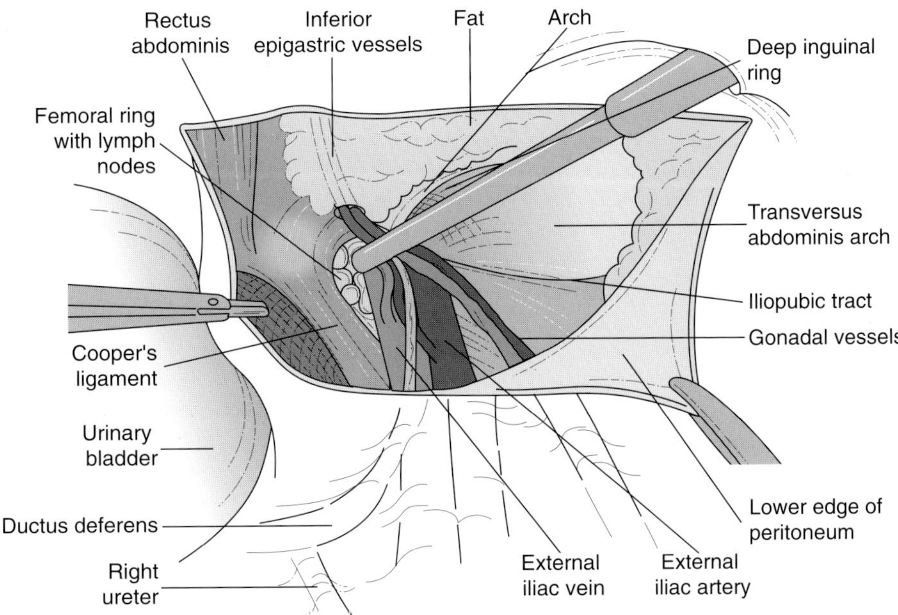

Figure 16. With further cleaning, more entities will be seen: the spermatic cord and the iliac vessels[36]

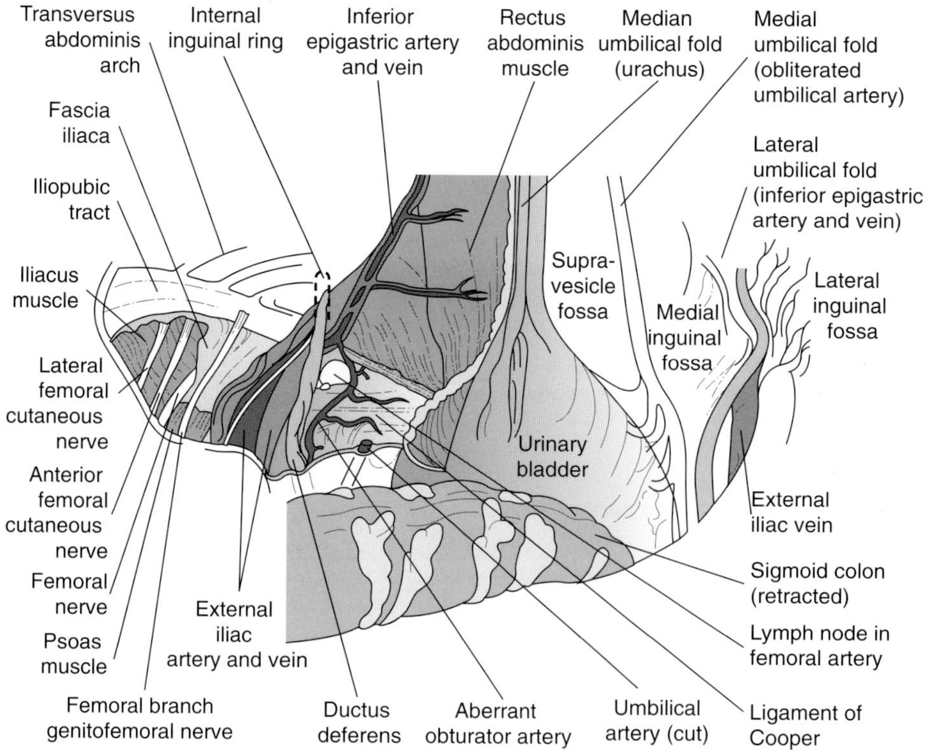

Figure 17. Panoramic laparoscopic view of the anatomical entities of the inguinal area[36]

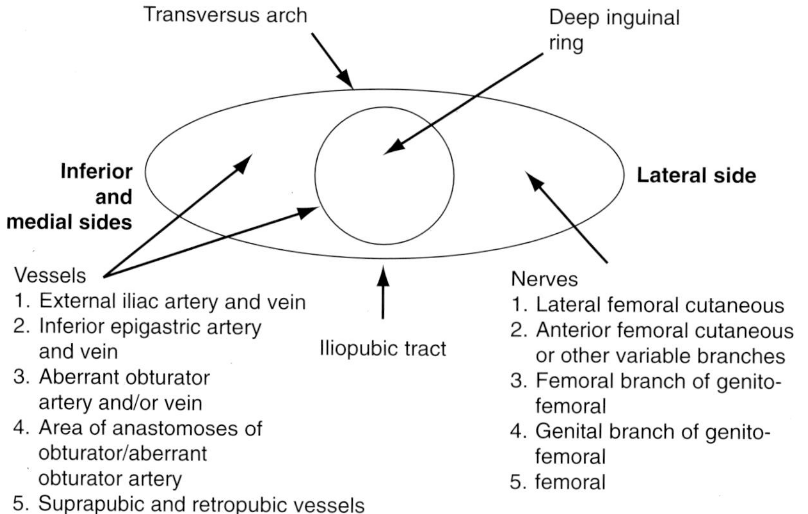

Figure 18. Diagram of the vessels and nerves related to the iliopubic tract[36]

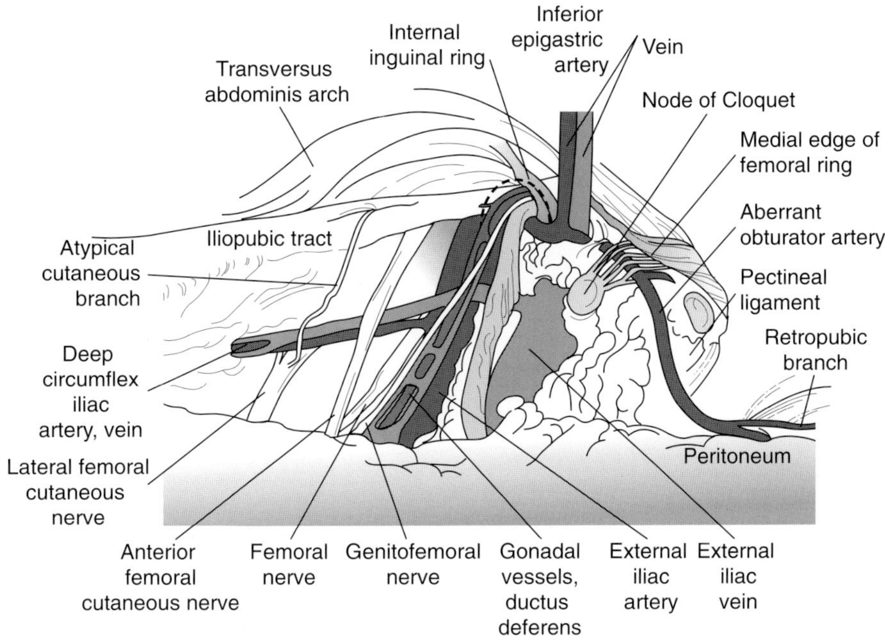

Figure 19. Another panoramic laparoscopic view of the anatomy of the inguinal area[37]

Two potential triangles and one circle

Three dangerous areas are the triangle of doom,[16] the triangle of pain[17] and the circle of death (unknown origin):

The triangle of doom (Fig. 20(a)) is formed by the gonadal vessels laterally and the ductus deferens medially. These anatomical entities meet at the deep inguinal ring. Within this triangle are: the external iliac vessels, deep circumflex iliac vein, genital branch of the genitofemoral nerve, and the femoral nerve (deeply).

The triangle of pain (Fig. 20(b)) is formed by the iliopubic tract inferolaterally and the gonadal vessels superomedially. The contents of this imaginary triangle include several nerves, such as femoral lateral cutaneous, femoral anterior cutaneous, femoral branch of genitofemoral, and femoral nerve.

The circle of death (Fig. 20(c)) is formed by an arterial network, the common iliac artery, internal and external iliac arteries, obturator artery, aberrant obturator artery, and inferior epigastric artery. The venous counterparts are similar in name, course, and position.

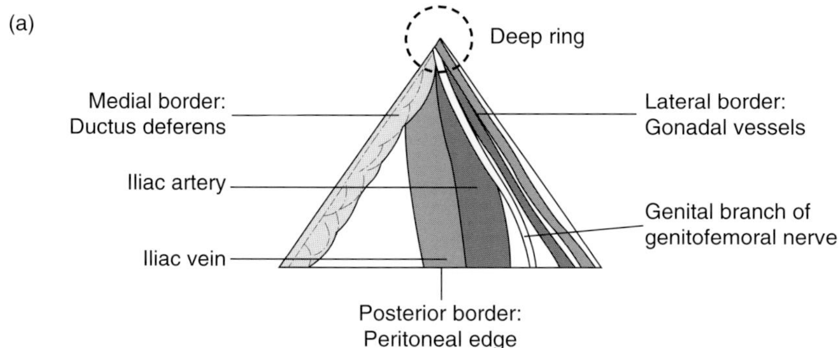

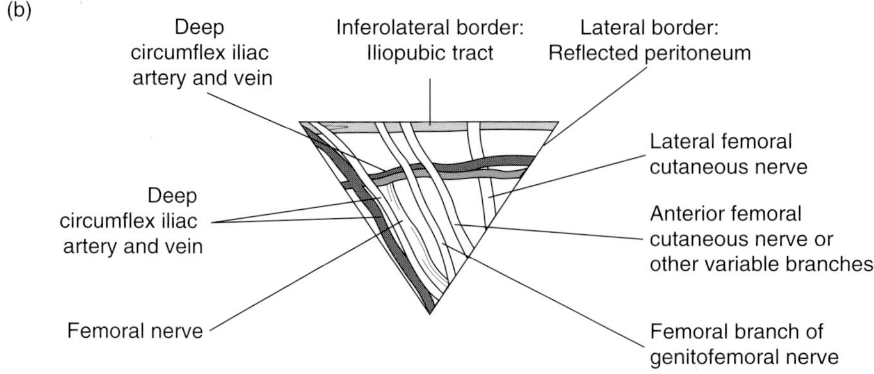

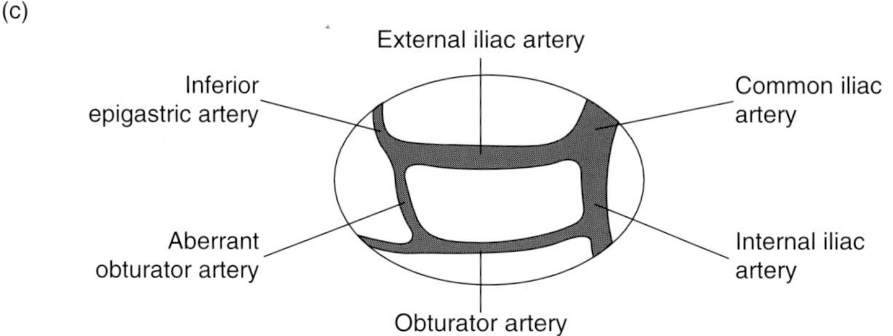

Figure 20.　(a) The triangle of doom. (b) The triangle of pain. (c) The circle of death[36]

REFERENCES

1　Rizk NN. A new description of the anterior abdominal wall in man and mammals. *J Anat* 1990; **131**(3):373–85.

2　Askar OM. Aponeurosis hernias: recent observations upon paraumbilical and epigastric hernias. *Surg Clin North Am* 1984; **64**: 315–33.

3 Askar OM. Surgical anatomy of the aponeurotic expansions of the anterior abdominal wall. *Ann R Coll Surg Engl* 1977; **59**:313–21.

4 Askar OM. A new concept of the aetiology and surgical repair of paraumbilical and epigastric hernias. *Ann R Coll Surg Engl* 1978; **60**:42–8.

5 Skandalakis JE, Colborn GL, Gray SW *et al.* The surgical anatomy of the inguinal area: part 1. *Contemp Surg* 1991; **38**(1):20–34.

6 Hoffman W. Who is Poupart? *Surgery* 1990; **170**:78–80.

7 Madden JL. *Abdominal wall hernias.* Philadelphia: WB Saunders 1989.

8 Condon RE. Surgical anatomy of the transversus abdominis and transversalis fascia. *Ann Surg* 1971; **173**:1.

9 McVay CB. *Surgical anatomy,* 6th edn. Philadelphia: WB Saunders 1984; 484–584.

10 Hollinshead WH. The abdominal wall and inguinal region. In Hollinshead WH, ed. *Anatomy for surgeons: the thorax, abdomen and pelvis,* vol. 2. New York: Paul B. Hoeber 1956; 217–68.

11 Condon RE. The anatomy of the inguinal region and its relation to groin hernia. In Nyhus LM, Condon RE, eds. *Hernia,* 4th edn. Philadelphia: JB Lippincott 1995; 16–72.

12 Gray SW, Skandalakis JE. *Atlas of surgical anatomy for general surgeons.* Baltimore: William & Wilkins 1985

13 Skandalakis JE, Colborn GL, Androulakis JA *et al.* Embryologic and anatomic basis of inguinal herniorrhaphy. *Surg Clin North Am* 1993; **73**(4):799–836.

14 Read RC. Cooper's posterior lamina of transversalis fascia. *Surg Gynecol Obstet* 1992; **174**:426–34.

15 Colborn GL, Skandalakis JE. Importance of the iliopubic, Cooper's, and Gimbernat's ligaments. *Prob Gen Surg* 1995; **12**(1):35–40.

16 Condon RE. The anterior iliopubic tract repair. In Nyhus LM, Condon RE, eds. *Hernia,* 4th edn. Philadelphia: JB Lippincott 1995; 136–52.

17 Wantz GE. *Atlas of hernia surgery.* New York: Raven Press 1991.

18 Rowe JS Jr, Skandalakis JE, Gray SW. Multiple bilateral inguinal hernias. *Am Surg* 1973; **39**(5):269–70.

19 Bendavid R. The space of Bogros and the deep inguinal venous circulation. *Surg Gynecol Obstet* 1992; **174**:355.

20 Nyhus LM, Condon RE, eds. *Hernia,* 4th edn. Philadelphia: JB Lippincott 1995.

21 Skandalakis JE, Colborn GL, Gray SW *et al.* The surgical anatomy of the inguinal area: part 2. *Contemp Surg* 1991; **38**(2):28–38.

22 Cooper A. *The anatomy and surgical treatment of abdominal hernia.* Philadelphia: Lea and Blanchard 1804; 26–7.

23 Spaw AT, Ennis BW, Spaw LP. Laparoscopic hernia repair: the anatomic basis. *J Laparoendosc Surg* 1991; **1**: 269–77.

24 Annibali R, Quinn T, Fitzgibbons RJ Jr. Avoiding nerve injury during laparoscopic hernia repair: critical areas for staple placement. In Arregui ME, Nagan RF, eds. *Inguinal hernia: advances or controversies?* Oxford: Radcliffe Medical Press 1994; 41–9.

25 Decker GAG, du Plessis DJ, eds. *Lee McGregor's synopsis of surgical anatomy.* Bristol: Wright, 1986.

26 Ellis H. *Clinical anatomy: a revision and applied anatomy for clinical students,* 6th edn. Oxford: Blackwell Scientific 1977; 257.

27 Gardner E, Gray DJ, O'Rahilly R. *Anatomy: a regional study of human structure.* Philadelphia: Saunders 1986; 364.

28 Grant JCB, Basmajian JV. *Grant's method of anatomy,* 7th edn. Baltimore: Williams & Wilkins 1965; 317.

29 Jones FW, ed. *Buchanan's manual of anatomy,* 8th edn. Baltimore: Williams & Wilkins 1950; 750.

30 Last RJ. *Anatomy: regional and applied.* Baltimore: Williams and Wilkins 1972; 213.

31 Lindner HH. *Clinical anatomy.* Norwalk: Appleton and Lange 1989; 288.

32 Lockhart RD. Myology. In Romanes GJ, ed. *Cunningham's Textbook of Anatomy,* 10th edn. London: Oxford University Press 1964; 302.

33 McVay CB. The anatomic basis for inguinal and femoral hernioplasty. *Surg Gynecol Obstet* 1974; **139**:931.

34 Neidhardt JPH. Surgical anatomy of the anterolateral and posterior abdominal walls and points of weakness. In Chevrel JP, ed. *Surgery of the abdominal wall.* Berlin: Springer-Verlag, 1987; 3–26.

35 Nyhus LM, Bombeck CT. Hernias. In Sabiston DC, ed. *Textbook of Surgery,* 13th edn. Philadelphia: WB Saunders 1986; 1231–52.

36 Colborn GL, Skandalakis JE. Laparoscopic cadaveric anatomy of the inguinal area. *Prob Gen Surg* 1995; **12**(1):13–20.

37 Brick WG, Colborn GL, Gadacz TR *et al.* Crucial anatomic lessons of the inguinal area. *Am Surg* 1995; **61**:172–7.

5 THE BASSINI OPERATION FOR INGUINAL HERNIA REPAIR

Oreste Terranova, Francesco Battocchio and Luigi De Santis

Edoardo Bassini, Professor of Surgery in the University of Padua at the end of last century, published his method for the treatment of inguinal hernias in 1889.[1] His operation involves the reconstruction of the posterior wall of the inguinal canal by a suture which includes the 'triple layer' (consisting of the internal oblique muscle, the transversus abdominis muscle and the transversalis fascia) superiorly and the inguinal ligament and the iliopubic tract (a thickening of the transversalis fascia) inferiorly. The spermatic cord is repositioned over the posterior wall and covered with the external oblique aponeurosis which is sutured over it (Fig. 1).[2]

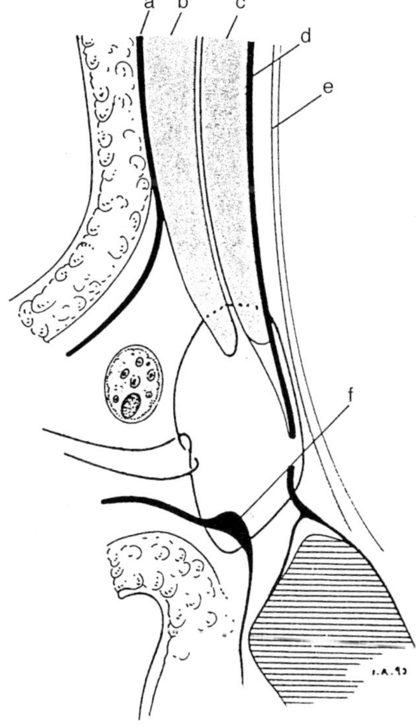

Figure 1. Diagram of a parasagittal section through the inguinal canal representing the Bassini operation. The suture includes the triple layer above (consisting of transversalis fascia, transversus abdominis muscle and oblique internal muscle) and the inguinal ligament and the iliopubic tract below.
(a) Aponeurosis of the external oblique muscle; (b) internal oblique muscle;
(c) transversus abdominis muscle;
(d) transversalis fascia; (e) peritoneum;
(f) inguinal ligament

The Bassini operation can easily be performed under local anaesthesia. It starts with a cutaneous incision extending 8–12 cm from the pubic tubercle (located immediately lateral to the pubic symphysis) towards the anterior superior iliac spine. When incising the subcutaneous tissue, one or two superficial epigastric veins are usually encountered; they should be divided and ligated. After incision of Scarpa's fascia and innominate fascia, the external oblique aponeurosis and the external inguinal ring, with its medial and lateral crura, come into view. The external oblique aponeurosis is opened by an incision along the direction of its fibres leaving a wide lower flap of fascia, which will be used later to reconstruct the anterior wall of the inguinal canal. A short scalpel incision of about 1 cm is made, the two margins grasped with clamps and the opening completed with scissors; particular care must be taken to avoid inadvertent division of the iliohypogastric and ilioinguinal nerves which run immediately underneath the external oblique aponeurosis. The cord is then separated by blunt dissection from the inguinal ligament and the margin of the internal oblique and the transversus abdominis muscles until it is completely detached from the posterior wall of the inguinal canal. Care must be taken at this stage not to injure the external spermatic vessels as they lie along the inferoposterior margin of the cord. A suspension tape is looped around the cord keeping together both the external spermatic vessels and the genital branch of the genitofemoral nerve.

If an indirect hernia is present, its sac remains with the cord, whereas the sac of a direct hernia remains part of the posterior wall of the canal, detached from the spermatic cord.

The cremaster muscle is grasped between two forceps and incised longitudinally over its entire length. The medial portion, being thin and poorly vascularized, can be cauterized and resected, while the lateral part should be ligated before division as it is thicker and more vascular.

After division of the cremaster muscle, the dissection of the spermatic cord continues by isolating and sectioning the cremaster artery and vein (also known as the external spermatic vessels), which emerge from the abdominal cavity medial to the elements of the cord at the level of the internal inguinal ring. Their division has no deleterious consequences as they supply only the tunica around the testicle. Division of the genital branch of the genitofemoral nerve has no unfavourable effects in men, though in women it can cause undesirable hypoaesthesia at the labia majora.

In cases of indirect hernia the sac is now isolated and separated from the spermatic cord up to and beyond the deep inguinal ring. Any lipoma is isolated, ligated at the base and resected. The sac is then opened and inspected. The herniated viscera are reduced after dividing any adhesions. The sac is then ligated with a transfixing suture in slowly absorbable material and resected.

In cases of sliding hernias, because the sac partly consists of a retroperitoneal organ (bladder, cecum or sigmoid colon) it should not be opened. The correct way to treat sliding hernias, whose diagnosis is usually intraoperative, is to isolate the sac from the cord and the abdominal wall and simply push it back into the abdominal cavity.

The transversalis fascia is now opened from beyond the deep inguinal ring to the pubic tubercle; the incision should run parallel to the inguinal ligament and 7–8 mm above it to leave an intact iliopubic tract. During this step care must be taken not to injure the inferior epigastric vessels which are near the deep inguinal ring. With a peanut sponge stick the preperitoneal fat of Bogros' space is bluntly dissected from the deep aspect of the transversalis fascia. In this way the rectus abdominis sheath and the transversus abdominis aponeurosis are revealed superiorly while, inferiorly, the iliopubic tract and Cooper's ligament come into view. After excision of any excess transversalis fascia at the site of the hernia, the hernial sac may be inverted with a continuous suture in slowly absorbable material. To prevent troublesome haemorrhages, the iliopubic veins, which run along the internal aspect of the iliopubic tract, should be coagulated before starting the suture.

The spermatic cord is lifted with two suspension tapes and displaced inferiorly beyond or below the inguinal ligament. The free margins of the external oblique aponeurosis are grasped with clamps so that the elements of the cord will not be in the opening field during the deep repair.

The reconstruction of the posterior wall of the inguinal canal starts with a suture which involves the triple layer superiorly and the iliopubic tract and inguinal ligament inferiorly.

The first suture takes in the medial part of the superior margin, incorporating the rectus sheath as well. To avoid inadvertent damage of the peritoneum or the bladder, the preperitoneal fat is moved away by pushing the handle of a forceps under the transversalis fascia (Fig. 2). (All the sutures except the final one have already been

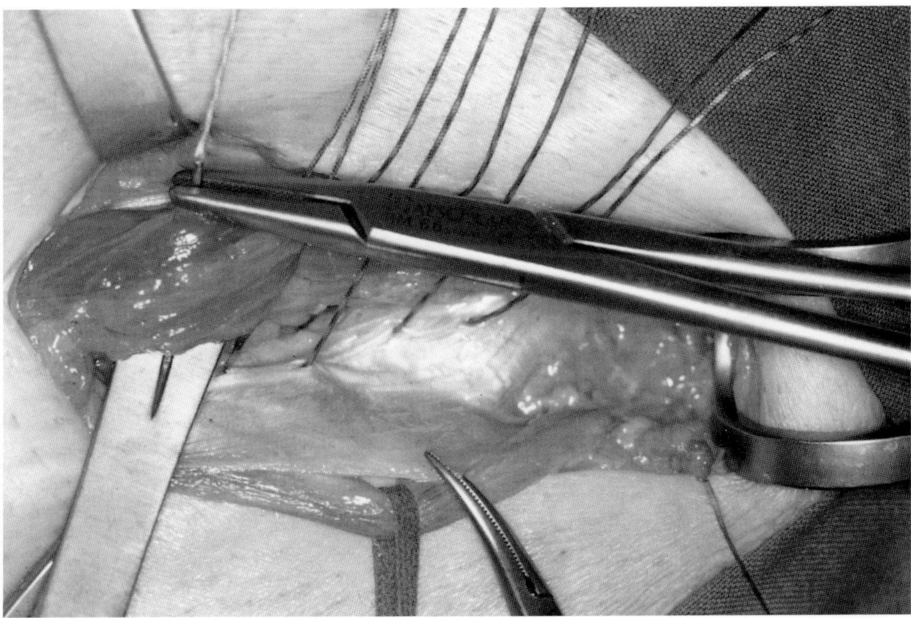

Figure 2. The reconstruction of the posterior wall of the right inguinal canal. Right: medial corner. Below: inferior edge. Insertion of the final suture taking in the triple layer (consisting of transversalis fascia, transversus abdominis muscle and oblique muscle). All sutures except the final one have been inserted but not tied. Reproduced with permission from F. Battocchio[3]

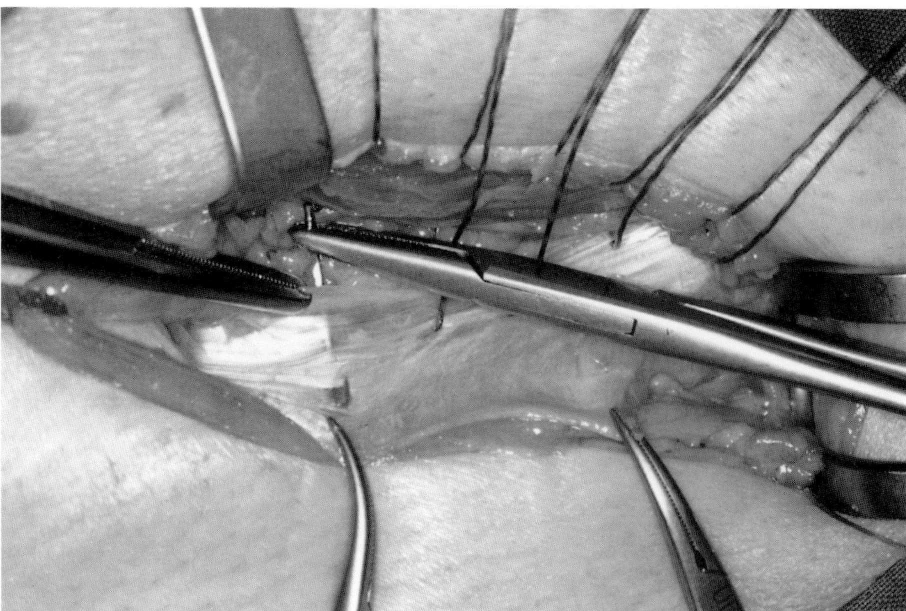

Figure 3. The reconstruction of the posterior wall of the right inguinal canal. Right: medial corner. Below: inferior edge. Insertion of the final suture is taking in the iliopubic tract and the inguinal ligament inferiorly. All sutures except the final one have been inserted but not tied. Reproduced with permission from F. Battocchio[3]

inserted.) Once the suture is passed through the upper part of the abdominal wall, a retractor is used to move the triple layer and the underlying structures upwards, making it easy to insert the first suture in the lower part of the public tubercle (Fig. 3). The following sutures take in the triple layer at about 3 cm from its free edge. They are placed 1 cm apart (this is the optimum distance) to avoid leaving a weak area or causing ischaemia. The handle of the forceps should protect the underlying structures (Figs 2–4). Care must be taken not to incorporate the iliohypogastric nerve and to leave a margin of external oblique aponeurosis wide enough for the subsequent reconstruction of the superficial plane. Usually the number of stitches varies from six to eight, depending on the length of the inguinal canal. The deep inguinal ring is reconstructed leaving enough space to insert the tip of the forceps inside the ring. The repair is done with slowly absorbable material to avoid septic complications with granulomas and fistulization (these òccurred in 2–3% of cases when nonabsorbable material was used).

This technique has two weak points: (1) the inguinal ligament is drawn upwards in this repair, thereby weakening the underlying femoral region; and (2) interrupted sutures may leave weak areas between the stitches so that recurrent hernias may develop in these areas in time. To avoid these possible causes of failure we usually make some modifications to the classical Bassini technique, which, in our experience, have markedly improved the results. With the second and third stitches we take in, inferiorly, not only

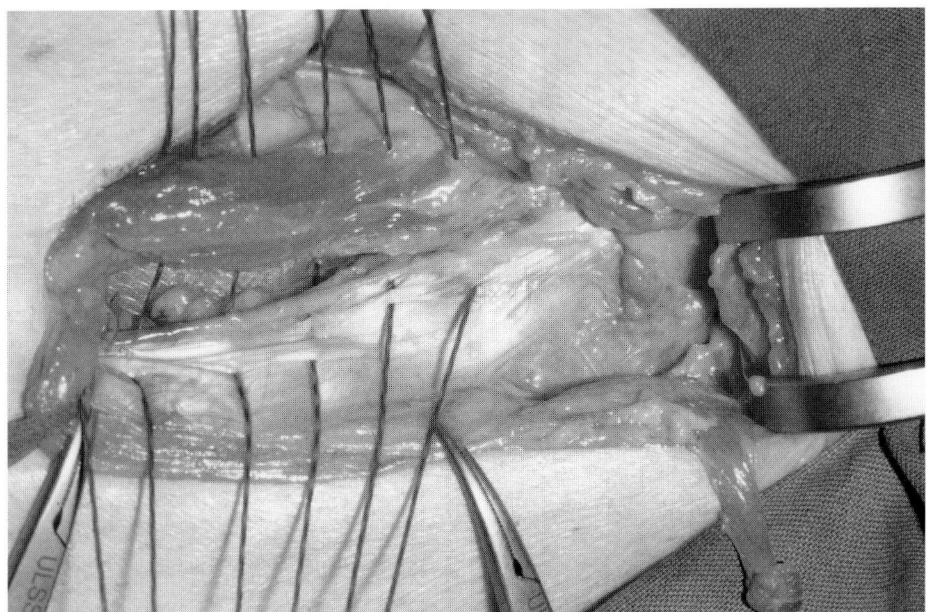

Figure 4. Each stitch has been inserted 1 cm apart. Usually the number of stitches varies from six to eight, according to the length of the inguinal canal. All sutures except the final one have been inserted but not tied. Reproduced with permission from F. Battocchio[3]

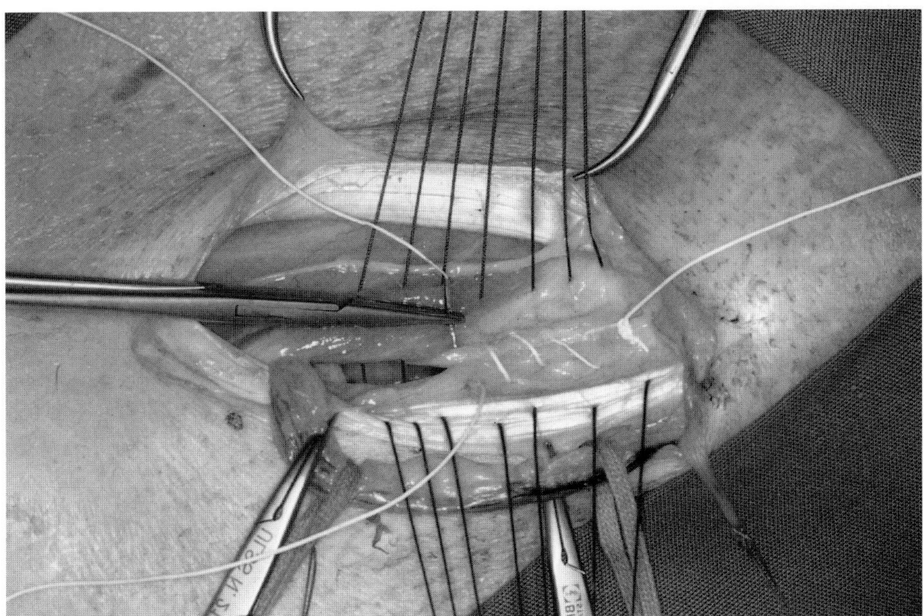

Figure 5. Right inguinal canal. Right: medial corner. Below: inferior edge. Before tying the Bassini stitches we insert a continuous 00 polypropylene suture through the iliopubic tract, the transversalis fascia and transversus abdominis muscle. Reproduced with permission from F. Battocchio[3]

the iliopubic tract and the inguinal ligament, but also Cooper's ligament, thus reinforcing the femoral region.[2,4] After inserting all the stitches, but before tying them, we insert a continuous 00 polypropylene suture through the iliopubic tract, transversalis fascia and transversus abdominis muscle (Fig. 5). This eliminates the weak areas between the previous stitches which are now tied.[5]

Once the spermatic cord is placed in position, the anterior wall of the inguinal canal is closed through a continuous suture of the external oblique aponeurosis. To avoid undue descent of the testicle, the distal stump of the cremaster muscle may be fixed to the external oblique aponeurosis at the newly formed external inguinal ring. The subcutaneous tissue is closed with slowly absorbable interrupted sutures, so as to leave no dead space. The skin is closed with an intradermal continuous suture.[2,4]

REFERENCES

1 Bassini E. *Nuovo metodo per la cura radicale dell'ernia inguinale.* Padova: Prosperini 1889.
2 Catterina A. *L'operazione di Bassini per la cura radicale dell'ernia inguinale.* Bolgna: L. Cappelli 1932.
3 Battocchio F. *Testo atlante di chirurgia delle ernie.* Torino: UTET 1994.
4 Terranova O, Battocchio F. *La chirurgia delle ernie della regione inguinale e crurale.* Padova: La Garangola 1988.
5 Terranova O, Battocchio F, Nistri R *et al.* Ernioplastica secondo Bassini modificata. *Chirurgia* 1991; 4:197–8.

6 LOCAL ANAESTHESIA IN GROIN HERNIA REPAIR

Nick Barwell

> Almost all cases of hernia, with the possible exception of those in young children, could undoubtedly be subjected to the radical operation under similar local methods...
>
> Harvey Cushing, *Annals of Surgery* (1900)

HISTORICAL PERSPECTIVE

Despite this classic observation,[1] many surgeons have been slow to appreciate the benefits to patients of surgery to groin hernias under local anaesthetic. Cushing reported on 49 of 233 operations under 'regionary' anaesthesia on cases unfit for general anaesthesia. These cases were often severe and strangulated and represented contemporary problems at the Johns Hopkins Hospital 100 years ago. Many severe elective cases had to endure a period of recumbency in the ward before surgery to ensure they could urinate in this position. The prospective patients therefore had a chance to observe the recovery of others. Cushing concluded:

- many individuals awaiting elective operation choose to have cocaine rather than ether for themselves;
- the patient can assist with testing the operation;
- almost all cases of hernia are suitable for the radical operation under local anaesthesia;
- when a general anaesthetic can safely be administered it is much to be preferred by both patient and operator.

In an interesting late addition to this paper he commented that they were so impressed with the results on unfit patients that they operated on some 24 young men using cocaine or eucaine B and local anaesthesia became the method of choice in their department.

Presumably advances in anaesthetic techniques and more sophisticated monitoring were thought to make general, spinal and epidural anaesthesia preferable. It seems likely that the natural reluctance of surgeons to inflict any pain or discomfort on patients together with increasing numbers of skilled anaesthetists caused a reduction in popularity of local anaesthesia for hernia surgery.

During World War II, 72 recruits in Toronto required elective hernia repairs in order to enter the army. Dr Earle Shouldice, with financial support from an entrepreneur, reduced costs by using surgeon-administered local anaesthesia; using his batman as a surgical assistant and encouraging early ambulation and discharge.

This approach was so successful that he had a waiting list of hernia sufferers at the end of the war, but few facilities were made available to him because of his eccentric behaviour. He therefore started his hernia surgery clinic in a small duplex building which was later transferred and expanded to the Shouldice Hospital of today, and which now services about 7400 cases a year. Most cases are groin hernias, and 97% of these are operated on under local infiltration anaesthesia.[2]

It was reported that the average volume of 1% procaine administered was 150 ml. The percentage would be lowered in the elderly or unfit but still caused consternation amongst anaesthetists and pharmacologists. This dosage should have been a considerable overdose but the patients came to no harm. Later studies of plasma levels of procaine in these cases at the Shouldice Hospital were reported to be within safe limits and the jibe that their heavy premedication was to prevent fits could be withdrawn!

A more recent study has shown that serial plasma lignocaine concentrations reached using the recommended maximum dose of 7 mg/kg lignocaine with adrenaline were always less than one-fifth of the toxic dose.[3] This confirms the considerable dose latitude available when using local infiltration anaesthesia in the groin, in contrast to more vascular areas.

Improved effectiveness of hernia surgery, reduction in hospital stay, early ambulation and speedy return to work are all helped by local anaesthesia, either alone or as an adjunct to general anaesthesia. Reduction in thrombotic complications, urinary retention and post-operative analgesic requirement have all been reported by enthusiasts for local anaesthesia. More pleasing still is the ready acceptance by most patients, with some 85% preferring to have local anaesthetic after a previous experience with general, spinal or epidural anaesthetics. An extra bonus is the reduction in subsequent analgesia needed with a minimal tension repair of Shouldice or other type. Operating under local anaesthetic demands a gentle, tissue-caring technique.

The author's traditional early training included some bad and unsupervised experiences with local anaesthetic (LA). It required demonstration at the Shouldice Hospital together with vigorous encouragement by satisfied previous patients to convert him. Local anaesthetic remains my method of choice for routine inguinofemoral hernia repair in adults 23 years later.

PRACTICAL CONSIDERATIONS

Patient preparation

Initial consultation with explanation of the anaesthetic and operative technique usually results in a confident patient who readily accepts LA (Fig. 1). The best advocate is a

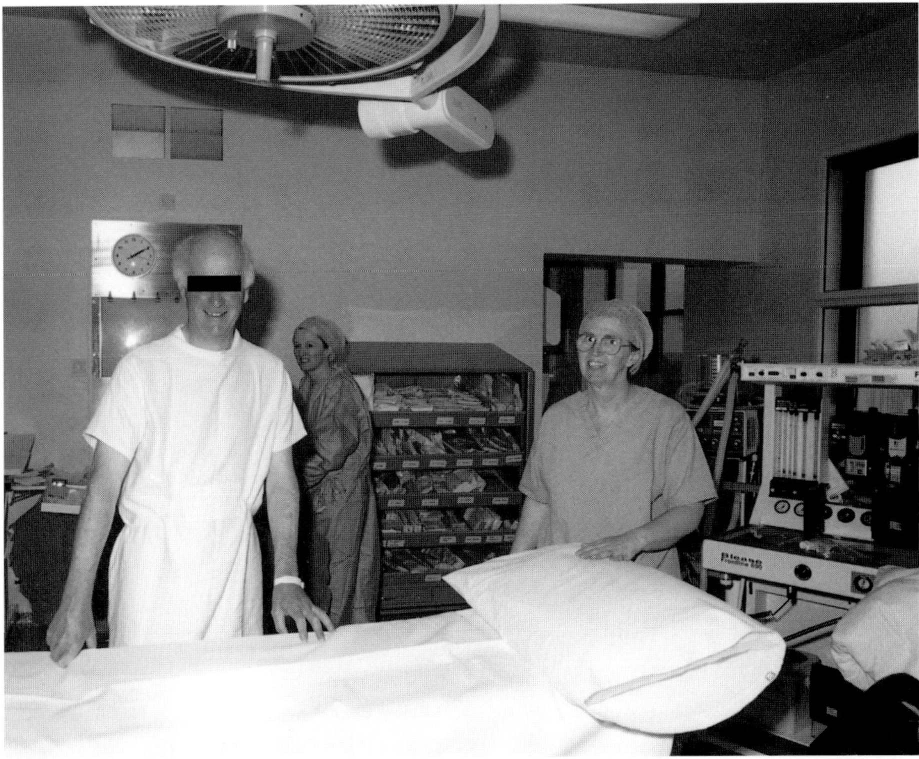

Figure 1. Local anaesthetic groin hernia repair. Patient about to step onto the operating table. Note the time – 2.10 pm

satisfied, recent patient, though an over enthusiastic patient who 'never felt a twinge before, during or after surgery' is not helpful. Some centres use sedation routinely pre- and peri-operatively. Unless there is a chance of needing conversion to general anaesthesia, the patients may eat and drink in moderation until the operation. They may even drink a little during it (Cushing used to supply whisky after the first few minutes). A 100 mg diclofenac suppository is given 45 min before surgery to give background analgesia which lasts many hours after surgery.

Variation in techniques of local anaesthesia

Various choices can be made when using LA:

- infiltration vs. field block
- xylocaine vs. bupivacaine

- use of adrenaline
- use of sodium bicarbonate

Infiltration has gradually supplanted the field block, and the type of anaesthetic is an individual choice. Although I prefer 0.5% lignocaine without adrenaline, the use of adrenaline is routine in some clinics. Surgeons who have used bicarbonate to neutralize the acidity of local anaesthesia and reduce the discomfort of the infiltration comment on its benefits: 1 ml of 8.4% bicarbonate is added to each 9 ml of local anaesthetic.

Local anaesthetic administration

The patient is placed supine with head down tilt; the skin is prepared with warmed antiseptic and draped.

I use a 20-ml syringe filled with 0.5% lignocaine and a 22-gauge spinal needle (Fig. 2). This avoids frequent needle changes and readily allows generous infiltration of tissues. The 22-gauge needle is stiff enough to be sensitive to the perforating pop through the external oblique (Fig. 3). Provided the initial infiltration is subcuticular, the anaesthetic effect of lignocaine is so fast that the surgeon may incise as soon as the initial infiltration is completed (Fig. 4). We were unable to demonstrate any increased duration of anaesthesia with bupivacaine, though the latter does take longer to act.

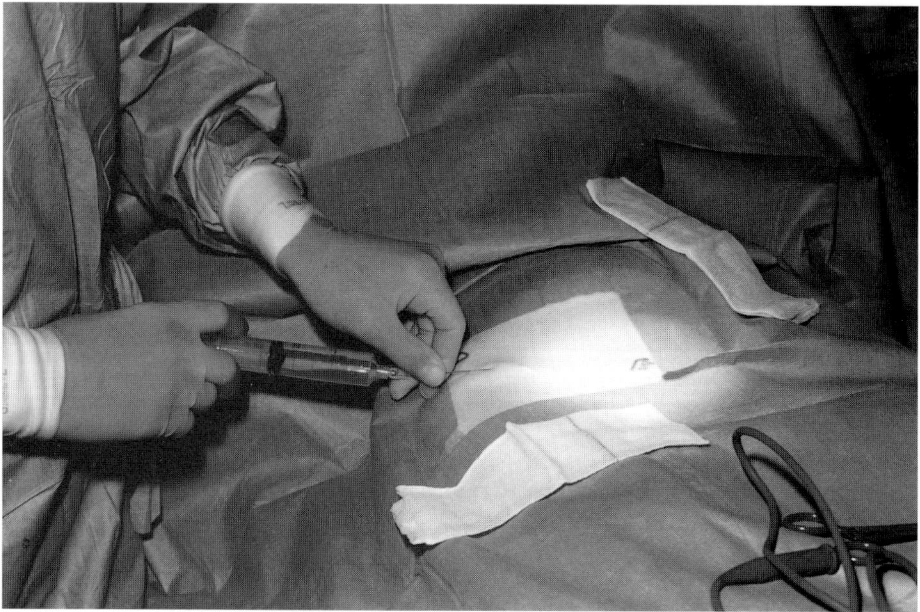

Figure 2. Start of local anaesthetic infiltration. The anterior superior iliac spine and pubis have been marked on the skin

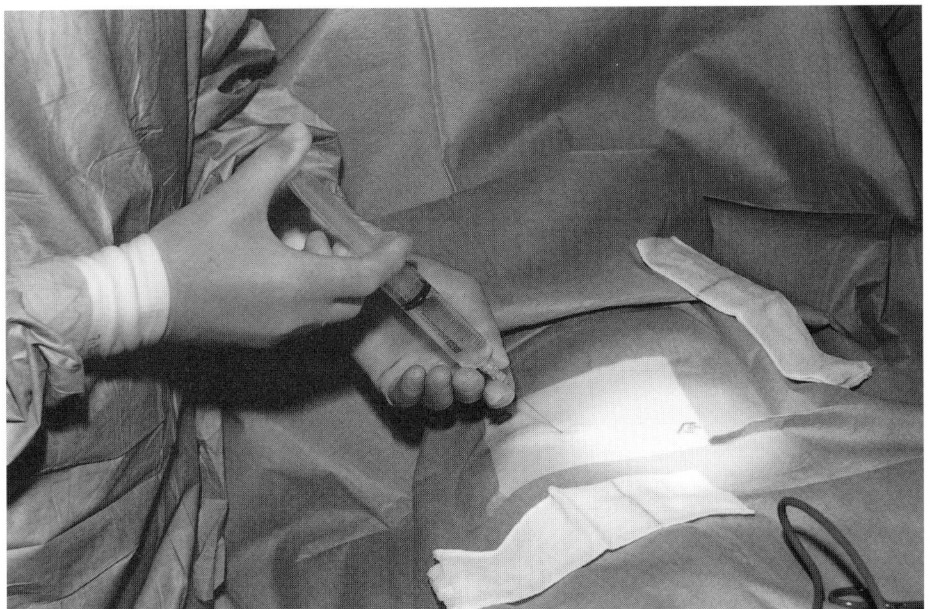

Figure 3. Deeper infiltration with the needle more vertical, inserted at 2-cm intervals along the proposed line of the incision

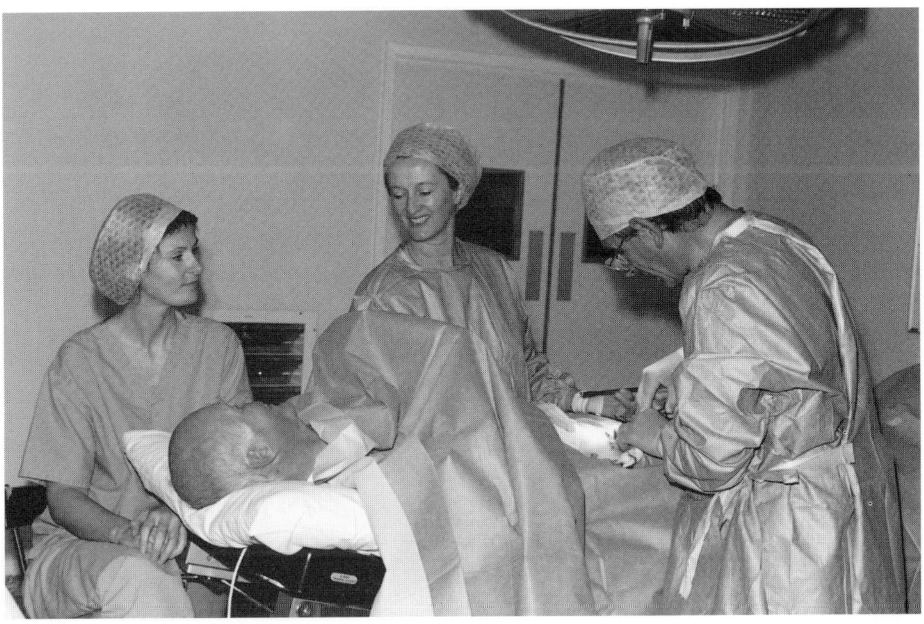

Figure 4. Intra-operative scene. Relaxed awake patient with surgeon, scrub nurse/assistant and nurse/runner 'monitoring' the patient

Summary of local anaesthetic repair (Figs 5–10)

The following steps are taken:

- a subcuticular wheal about 1-cm wide is made along the line of the incision;
- generous infiltration throughout the length of the incision down to external oblique;
- incision made down to the external oblique without delay;
- distension injection under external oblique to include any visible nerves;
- incision of external oblique and exposure of spermatic cord;
- further injection at the medial end of the inguinal canal (perforating or cross-over nerve);
- injections around the neck of any indirect sac especially around the vas;
- injections around the emerging genital branch of genitofemoral nerve;
- dissection and repair may proceed according to surgical choice;
- for the Shouldice dissection and repair preferred by the author:
    — local anaesthetic is infiltrated behind the posterior inguinal wall;
    — posterior wall is split throughout, followed by Shouldice repair.

At the end of the repair the patient is asked to strain and lift head and shoulders off the operating table to check the integrity of the repair.

Femoral hernias

For femoral hernias my preferred route is to approach and reduce the hernia from above, through the divided posterior inguinal wall. Gut resection, if necessary, is then possible through this incision as well as repair, without further dissection. In addition to the steps listed above local anaesthesia must also be infiltrated into Cooper's ligament. The excellent anatomical view means that the femoral canal can be darned easily from above. This approach has been incorporated at the Shouldice Hospital as a 'complete groin' repair. An alternative is to do a unilateral giant prosthetic reinforcement of the visceral sac repair under local anaesthetic (see Chapter 17).

Intraoperative supervision and monitoring

Throughout the operation, a nurse sits at the head end of the operating table and can reassure or entertain the patient as necessary, and also observe and communicate any changes in measurements from the pulse oximeter or blood pressure to the surgeon. It is seldom that an anaesthetist is required to be present and the operation is therefore suitable for smaller hospitals and day-case units. An assistant other than a scrub nurse is a luxury except for education.

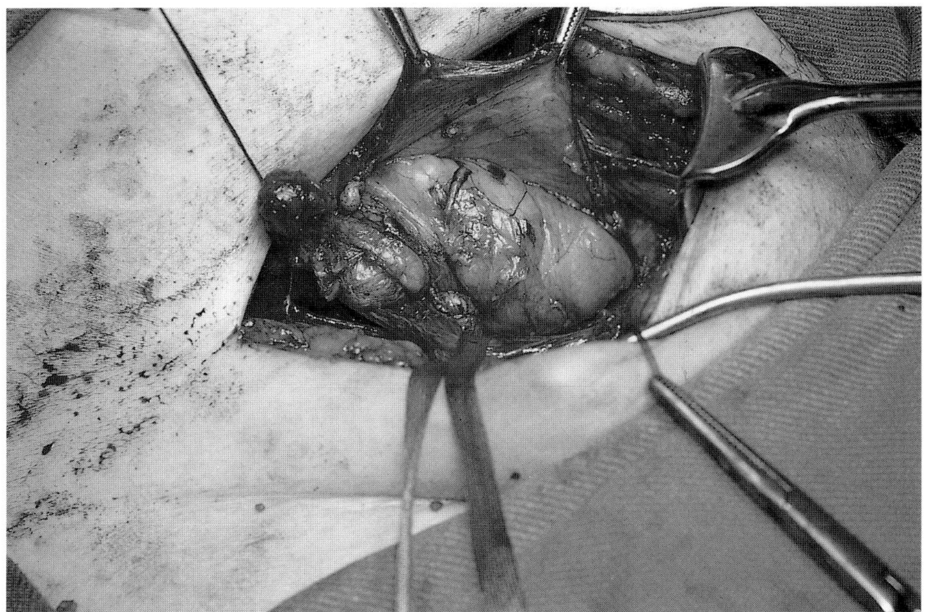

Figure 5. Right inguinal hernia, Shouldice repair. The posterior wall of the inguinal canal has been opened and both upper and lower leaves of transversalis fascia developed. The upper leaf of the transversalis fascia is held up revealing the bulging preperitoneal fat. The ligated stump of an indirect sac is seen to the left of the picture, and the spermatic cord is retracted inferiorly using a tape sling

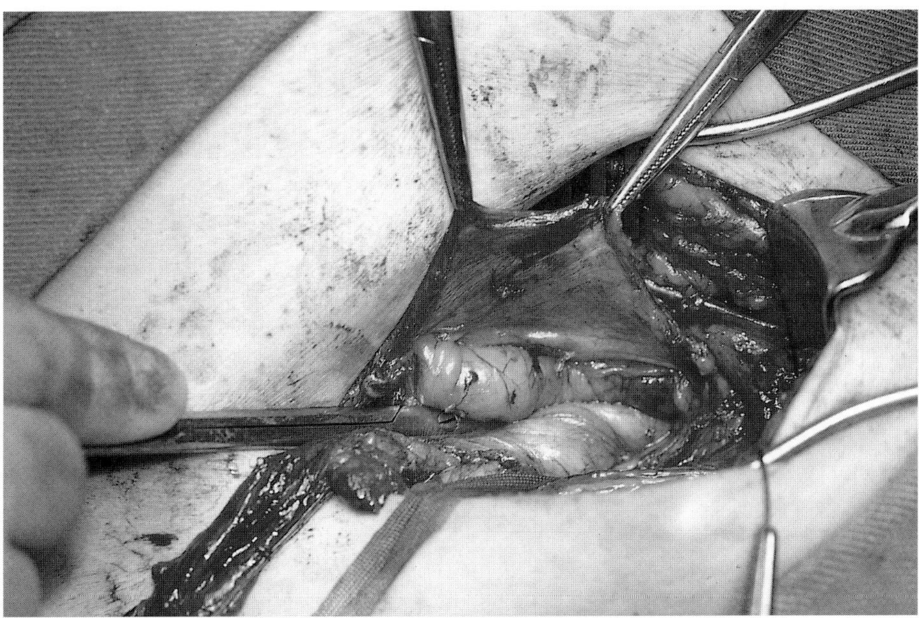

Figure 6. Preperitoneal fat pushed back prior to starting the first row of sutures

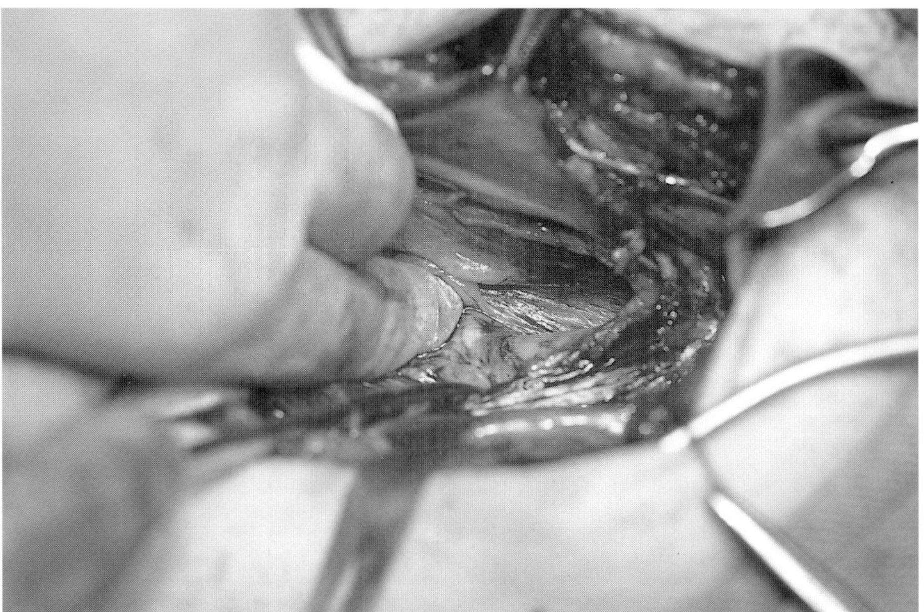

Figure 7. Preperitoneal fat pushed back prior to starting the first row of sutures

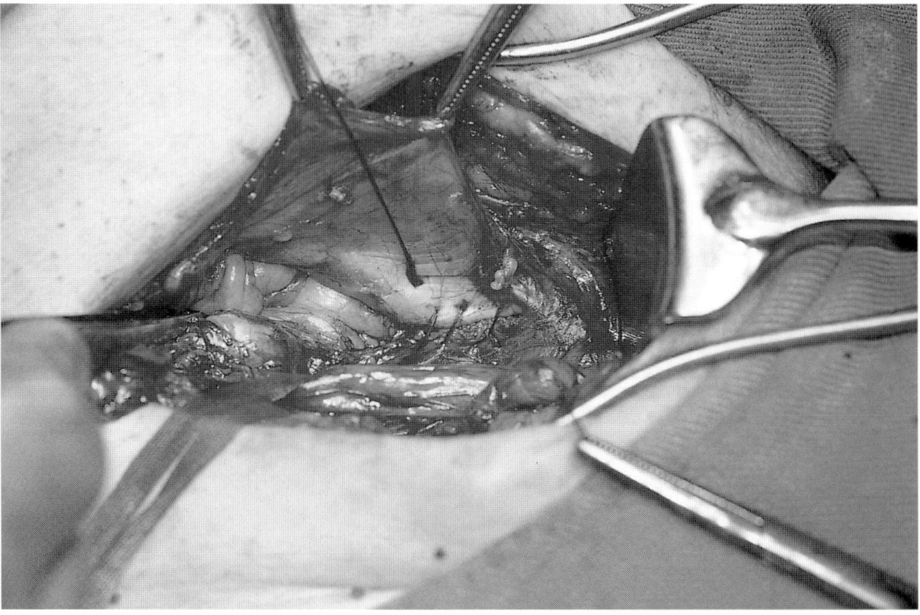

Figure 8. First row – suturing the inner aspect of the upper leaf of the transversalis fascia to the cut edge of the lower leaf, from medial to lateral

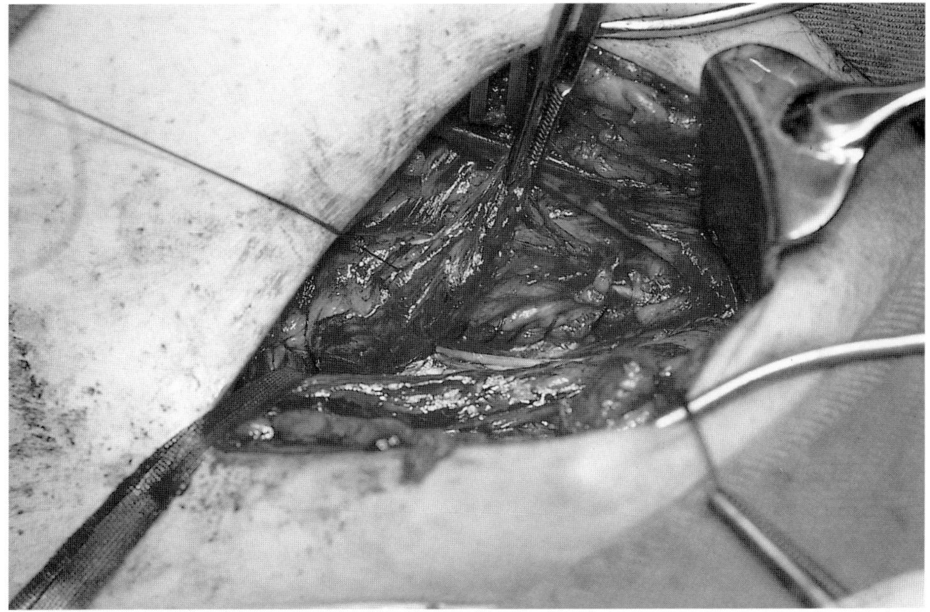

Figure 9. Completed first row of sutures. Free superior edge of transversalis held up

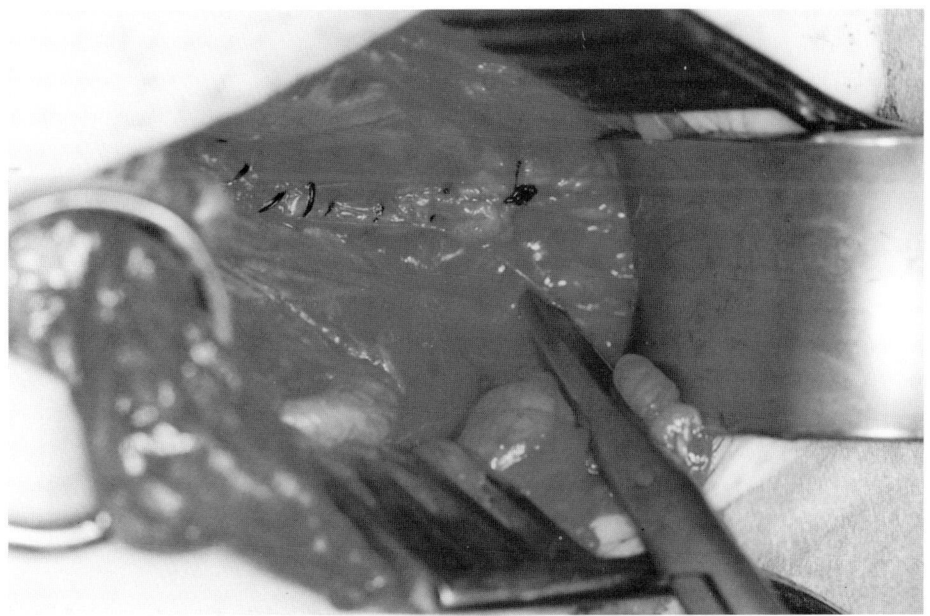

Figure 10. Completed second row of sutures

Postoperative care

After the operation the patient walks to the recovery area (Fig. 11) where vital signs are rechecked, and can soon return to the ward, dress, drink, eat and return home the same day providing there is appropriate social support. It is very unusual for a patient to be less happy in his own environment.

There is no need for any physical restriction in activity. Many patients drive the next day and are encouraged to be active and energetic. Regular paracetamol orally and/or Voltarol suppositories should be used as required and are all the analgesia necessary for most patients.

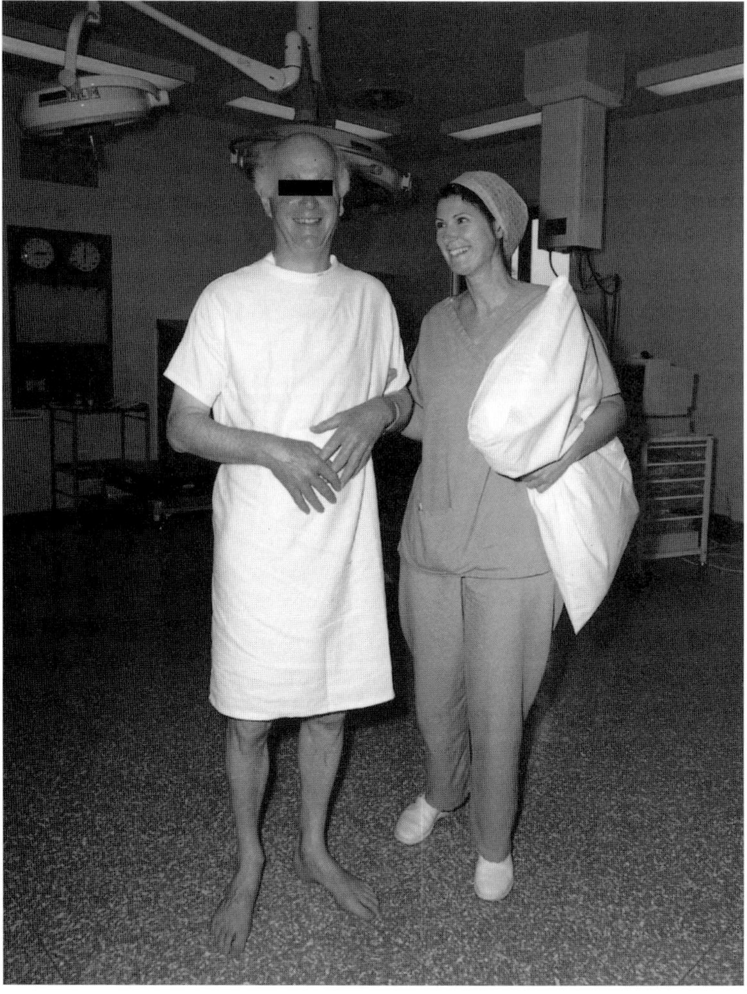

Figure 11. Patient leaving the operating room. Note the time – 3.15 pm

Unsuitability for local anaesthetic

Hernias may be unsuitable for repair under LA if the patient requires another procedure at the same time, such as transurethral resection of the prostate or open prostatectomy. In addition, patients may prefer or request general anaesthesia because of anxiety or unsuitability for LA. Children and patients with mental subnormality or mental instability are unsuitable for LA repair because co-operation is essential.

Nine out of approximately 4000 of my patients needed conversion to general anaesthesia. The reasons are as follows (number in parenthesis is number of cases).

- restlessness and anxiety (4)
- error in selection (mentally subnormal and violent reaction to sedation) (2)
- no LA available in operating theatre (1)
- unexpected carcinoma in sliding hernia of colon. (Home in 4 days after resection despite unprepared bowel) (1)
- to speed up operating list (1)

Contraindications

Contraindications include:

- patient refusal
- requirements of other operation
- unsuitability (children, mentally subnormal and mentally unstable)
- adverse reaction to previous LA

Training requirements

Kingsnorth and colleagues suggested that working with LA might inhibit inexperienced hernia surgeons and therefore explain increased recurrence rates.[5] It was observed that results were improved after six cases, though this was using the nylon darn technique of Moloney, Gill and Barclay.

It is perhaps more difficult to persuade senior surgeons to use LA or get them to change their long-established techniques rather than their more junior colleagues. We have found no difficulty using LA even on training courses, with the simple technique described.

Shouldice surgeons require their new appointees to assist with 100 cases and be assisted with 50 cases before operating alone. This is to ensure rigidity of technique for the repair, not for the anaesthesia.

Glassow in the report of his Hunterian lecture 'Inguinal Hernia Repair using Local Anaesthesia' concentrated on the Shouldice technique and results.[4] Welsh and Alexander reported that 97% of groin hernia repairs are carried out under local anaesthesia at the Shouldice Hospital.[2] This experience will therefore number some 220 000 cases, with remarkable technical success.

Schumpelick studied the availability and acceptability of local anaesthesia in German clinics after being converted to the desirability and advantages of local anaesthetic in his own clinic in Aachen.[6] He found that:

- Only 5.1% of German clinics offered choice LA
- LA is acceptable in 96% of patients
- intraoperative testing of repair increases confidence for patient and surgeon
- the technique resulted in less pain and less need for postoperative analgesia
- LA hernia repairs had fewer complications
- LA repair permitted earlier discharge.

WHEN SHOULD WE USE LOCAL ANAESTHESIA?

- Method of choice in many major hernia clinics.
- Suitable for primary and recurrent inguinal hernias.
- Emergency or strangulated hernias?

With the more complicated emergency and strangulated hernias, an anaesthetist should always be present. The peri-operative care is more complicated and the need for a naso-gastric tube and intravenous fluids as well as additional sedation all require specialist advice and the availability of another uncommitted doctor in the operating theatre. There is no reason why a patient should not have a definitive repair at the time of the emergency surgery unless there is really gross sepsis present. Even then, nylon suturing carried out correctly seldom results in sinus formation. It is, of course, well recognised that gut resection is virtually painless provided traction on the mesentry is avoided. We should remember that Cushing's cases were often strangulated and this was where we started.[1]

Perhaps the most important message for those hernia surgeons who do not like to use or even consider local anaesthetic is not to listen to surgeons who enthuse about local anaesthetic. They should instead look at the recovery times and listen to patients who have had experience of both local anaesthetic and general anaesthetic. These are the real advocates for local anaesthesia in groin hernia repair and were the ones who demanded that we make it available to all hernia surgery patients.

Nearly 100 years after Cushing's report on local infiltration anaesthesia it remains the anaesthetic of choice on grounds of economy, safety and acceptability for patients and surgeons despite the enormous advances in general anaesthesia.

REFERENCES

1   Cushing H. The employment of local anesthesia in the radical cure of certain cases of hernia, with a note upon the nervous anatomy of the inguinal region. *Ann Surg* 1900; **31**:1–34.

2   Welsh DRJ, Alexander MAJ. The Shouldice repair. *Surg Clin North Am* 1993; **73**:451–69.
3   Karatassas A, Morris RG, Walsh D *et al.* Evaluation of the safety of inguinal hernia repair in the elderly using lignocaine infiltration anaesthesia. *Aust N Z J Surg* 1993; **63**:266–9.
4   Glassow F. The Shouldice repair for inguinal hernia. *Ann R Coll Surg* 1984; **66**:382–7.
5   Kingsnorth AN, Britton BJ, Morris PJ. Recurrent inguinal hernia after local anaesthetic repair. *Br J Surg* 1981; **68**:27–275.
6   Peiper C, Tons C, Schippers E, Busch F *et al.* Local versus general anaesthesia for Shouldice repair of the inguinal hernia. *World J Surg* 1994; **18**:912–16.

Robert Bendavid

7 PROSTHESES AND HERNIORRHAPHIES

INTRODUCTION

The evolution of hernia surgery has been carefully recorded: firstly, there was the *anatomical period* when the architecture of the inguinal canal was identified (by such men as Bogros, Poupart, Hesselbach, Gimbernat, Cooper, Thomson, Cloquet and Scarpa); secondly, a *surgical period* involved the definition and classification of the anatomy and pathology of hernias (enriched by the contributions of Narath, Lotheissen, Bassini, Marcy, Halsted, Ferguson, McVay, Lucas-Championniere and Shouldice); and currently, a third era which will probably become known as the *prosthetic period,* is still being defined as several operative procedures are attempted, tried, tested and evaluated (names that will mark this period will be Aquaviva, Zagdoun, Natta, Usher, Lichtenstein, Rives, Stoppa and others).

PROSTHESES

The search for an ideal tissue replacement was stimulated by Billroth's statement that: 'if an adequate tissue replacement could be found, the problem of hernia would no longer exist'. This search led to metallic prostheses such as steel, which were used as early as the 1920s, their use popularized by Abel and Hunt[1] as well as Babcock;[2] Preston and Richards reported a series of 2000 patients in 1973.[3] However, although steel tended to fragment, fray and migrate, its main advantage was that it did not require removal during infection. It is still being used in Paris (France) by Duron who recently reported a series of 198 patients studied from 1963 to 1991.[4]

Silver filigrees were used by Goepel[5] and Witzel[6] as reported by Throckmorton.[7] The objections to their use were rigidity, discomfort, aversion to foreign bodies and persistent sinus tract formation.

Tantalum gauze became popular after the reports of Throckmorton,[7] Koontz,[8] Douglas[9] and Lam *et al.*[10] Long-term follow-up by Burton[11] and Adler[12] revealed major

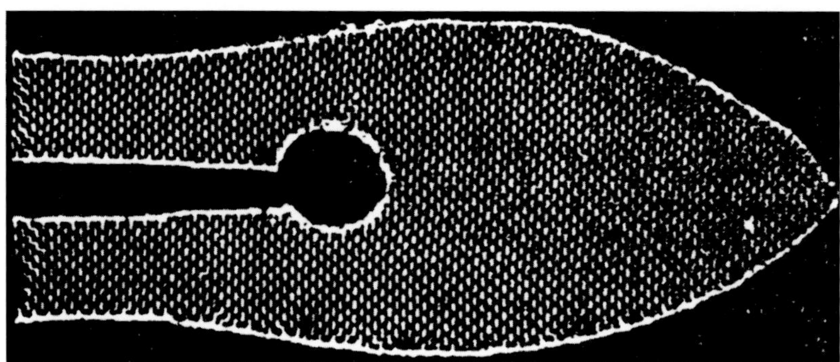

Figure 1. Prosthesis made of nylon, used by Aquaviva in 1944 and subsequently by Zagdoun and Sordinas in 1953

drawbacks such as fracture of the 'fatigued' prosthesis with recurrent herniation through the fracture sites and transmigration of the mesh into viscera. Other alternative prostheses include: heterografts such as porcine dermal collagen, ox fascial grafts and kangaroo tendons reported by McArthur,[13] Koontz[14] and Horsley.[15] Homografts such as dehydrated human fascia lata, aorta and dura mater required rehydration prior to use and tended to form seromas, were eventually replaced by fibrous tissue, and tended to bulge and break down. In addition, there is the risk of transmission of viral diseases (Hep C, Hep B, HIV, Jakob–Creutzfeld).

In the late 1940s new synthetic prostheses were introduced including Fortisan (a regenerated cellulose fabric), polyvinyl sponge (a polymer of polyvinyl alcohol and formaldehyde), nylon (dicarboxylic acid and diamine), Teflon (polytetrafluoroethylene) and carbon fiber (filamentous carbon fiber).

The first corroborated record of the use of a synthetic (nylon) prosthesis in hernia surgery was by Aquaviva in Marseille (France) in 1944.[16] Zagdoun and Sordinas of France, carrying out the same procedure, reported the first large series of tension-free repairs of 200 cases in 1954.[17] Figure 1 shows their nylon pattern which has come to be a common picture in publications by more recent authors.

This chapter discusses the three most important synthetic prostheses that have gained popularity: polyester (Dacron), polypropylene (Prolene, Marlex) and polytetrafluoroethylene (e-PTFE). The resorbable synthetics polyglycolic acid (Dexon) and polyglactin (Vicryl) are not of interest in the permanent repair of hernias, and their primary use should be reserved for temporary measures in clinical situations associated with abdominal trauma where contamination and visceral edema present problems of abdominal wall closure.

POLYESTER MESH (DACRON, MERSILENE)

Developed in 1939 and introduced in the US in 1946, this synthetic polyester polymer was developed from ethylene glycol and terephthalic acid. Among the first reports of its use were those of Wolstenholme in 1956 (19 cases),[18] Adler in 1962 (45 cases)[12] and Bellis in 1969 (3000 cases).[19] Dacron has many of the qualities sought in the ideal prosthesis: it is strong, pliable, durable, moderately elastic and can be autoclaved; it has interstices which become 'inhabited' by fibroblasts and collagen and need not necessarily be removed should infection supervene.

As the first synthetic to be introduced, it has been extensively used in North America by Wantz, Adloff and Arnaud and in Europe by Stoppa and Flament (France), Van Damme (Belgium) and Trivellini (Italy). Dacron has been used for incisional hernias as onlays, inlays and intraperitoneally. However the latter position should be avoided unless the surgical situation leaves no other option, since visceral adhesions, fistula formation and transmigration have all been reported.[20,21]

POLYPROPYLENE MESH (MARLEX, PROLENE, TRELEX)

Polypropylene was introduced in 1954 and consists of ethylene with an added methyl molecule. The earliest experimental studies were reported by Usher and colleagues in 1958.[22,23,24] Polypropylene showed all the advantages of Dacron but stimulated less foreign body reaction and had less tendency to sinus tract formation, qualities which may be because it is a monofilament (unlike Dacron). Usher was instrumental in the growing popularity of polypropylene and described several techniques that have been superseded by tension-free repairs and transversalis fascia replacements.

Polypropylene has become the most widely used synthetic prosthesis in North America, with an extensive literature. Like polyester, polypropylene mesh contains interstices through which fibroblasts and collagen penetrate to incorporate the mesh and make it part of the abdominal wall; it is also reasonably priced. The literature on the use of polypropylene mesh includes work by Gilbert,[25] Lichtenstein,[26] Rutkow,[27] Nyhus[28] and many others.

e-PTFE

Polytetrafluoroethylene is a fluorinated polymer which was accidentally discovered by R. J. Plunket in 1938 and became known as Teflon. Though chemically a most inert substance, Teflon mesh was associated with infection and sinus tract formation. A process of 'expanding' PTFE was described in the 1960s by S. Oshige[29] in Japan which resulted in a uniform, fibrous, smooth, microporous material (the pore size is 20–25 µm) which has the appearance of a smooth non-woven sheet to the naked eye.

e-PTFE is the most controversial of the synthetic prostheses. The manufacturers and Elliott and Juler,[30] reported complete incorporation of the e-PTFE patch, but it is commonly known by surgeons that the patch can easily be removed – literally peeled from its bed – whenever subsequent surgery requires its removal. The manufacturers also claim a tensile strength which is superior to polypropylene, but snapping a prolene suture driven through e-PTFE will enlarge the hole made in the patch by the needle.

An e-PTFE patch can become infected – dictating its removal – because bacteria, e.g. staphylococci (1 μm), can enter the pores (20–25 μm), but heterophilic leucocytes (9–15 μm) and macrophages (18–35 μm) cannot reach them for phagocytosis to occur.

To improve incorporation of the e-PTFE patch, the manufacturers have introduced other products such as 'Mycromesh' with macropores, and 'Dual mesh', which has micropores of 22 μm on one side and micropores of 3 μm on the other.

e-PTFE is expensive and its only indication, in my view, is in incisional hernias where an extraperitoneal space cannot be created and hence the prosthesis will come in contact with viscera. I have nevertheless observed adhesions between large bowel, small bowel and e-PTFE, though such adhesions were easy to lyse.

The qualities displayed by the three prosthetic materials discussed above go a long way towards satisfying the criteria listed by Cumberland,[31] Scales,[32] and Ponka.[33] The ideal prosthesis would incorporate all the following properties:

- strength
- flexibility
- tissue tolerance
- durability
- ease of handling
- easy sterilization
- resistance to infection and, if infected, will respond to appropriate antimicrobial treatment
- nonallergenic
- no adhesion formation
- no transmigration
- low cost.

THE USE OF PROSTHESES AT THE SHOULDICE HOSPITAL

The modern surgeon who needs to use a prosthesis has three options:

- the tension-free onlay repair
- the preperitoneal transversalis fascia replacement
- one of the laparoscopic approach methods.

At the Shouldice Hospital all the laparoscopic techniques have been rejected for various reasons detailed elsewhere[34–36] including the nature and severity of the potential complications, limitation of the techniques to a particular class of patients, (e.g. exclusion of patients who are unfit for or unsuitable for general anesthesia) and, not least, cost.

The tension-free repair and 'plug technique' represent only a partial solution, which ignores the nature of the 'hernia disease' and the concept of 'metastatic emphysema' of Read.[37] Experience with thousands of recurrences (1300 a year on average) at the Shouldice Hospital reveals that onlay mesh and plugs do get dislodged or detached. There is no doubt that the operations are easier and perhaps less traumatic, than other techniques, but, physiologically and anatomically, the proper site of insertion of a prosthesis is the preperitoneal space, which requires a more sophisticated dissection.

At the Shouldice Hospital prostheses were introduced in 1983, though the surgeons still rely on the Shouldice pure tissue repair for most cases (97.75%) and still obtain results that not only compare favorably with other methods, but have set standards in terms of recurrence rate, return to normal activities and a lesser incidence of complications. Two techniques have been used at the Shouldice Hospital: the transversalis fascia replacement and the umbrella.

Table 1 summarized our statistics in the use of prostheses from 1983 to 1995 on 2059 patients out of a series of 93 958 patients. Tables 2 and 3 provide an accurate

| Procedures | Primary | Recurrences | | | | | Total |
		1	2	3	4	5	
Inguinal	37	121	129	71	36	20	414
Femoral	96	148	80	33	10	4	371
Incisional	347	159	65	29	13	13	626
Inguinofemoral	4	48	72	38	13	8	183
Indirect-direct-femoral	117	59	26	5	3	3	213
Paravascular	7	9	5	3	1	1	26
Umbilical	12	11	9	1	1	0	34
Epigastric	25	13	4	0	0	0	42
Interstitial	13	0	3	2	0	0	18
Spigelian	5	1	0	0	0	0	6
Umbilical-epigastric	21	11	3	1	0	0	36
Other	10	47	21	6	5	1	90
Total							2059

The header "Hernia type (no.)" spans the columns from Primary through Total.

Table 1. Types of hernia requiring a prosthesis

Hernia type	No. requiring mesh/total	Percentage
All	154/7529	2
Groin	98/7085	1.4
Direct inguinal	26/2890	0.9
Indirect inguinal	4/4028	0.1
Femoral	48/144	33.3
Inguinofemoral	21/23	91.3
Nongroin	56/444	12.6

Table 2. Need for mesh in hernia repairs (primaries) (7529 patients)

Hernia type	No. requiring mesh/total	Percentage
Indirect inguinal	3/316	0.95
Direct inguinal	25/537	4.70
Femoral	38/60	63.33
Inguinofemoral	20/22	91.00
Nongroin	40/105	38.00

Table 3. Need for mesh (on recurrences)

Hernia type	Total no. of operations	Repaired with mesh	Percentage
Indirect inguinal	42976	114	0.26
Direct inguinal	29332	374	1.3
Femoral	1459	256	17
Interstitial	367	22	6
Inguinofemoral	172	172	100

Table 4. Review of cases done between 1 April 1985 and 31 March 1996

record of the number of operations done in 1989 which required a mesh. With reference to the inguinal region, the use of prostheses has been recorded largely for femoral and inguinofemoral hernias where the need has been demonstrated. Mesh was required most often when there was a femoral component to the problem at hand. Table 4 provides further information, encompassing 10 years (1985–96); again, the highest incidence of the use of prostheses is seen when a femoral component is present.

Transversalis fascia replacement

This technique has been used whenever there has been destruction of the inguinal ligament due to repeated previous procedures and the defect may be an indirect, direct or inguinofemoral hernia. The essential step after dissection is completed is to demonstrate Cooper's ligament (Fig. 9.2). A piece of polypropylene mesh (Marlex, Trelex, Prolene) measuring 12×10 cm or larger is then anchored to Cooper's ligament (four to seven sutures) as laterally as possible without impinging on the femoral vein. Superolaterally the mesh is inserted deep to the transversus, and anchored through the full abdominal wall thickness (Figs 2–4). The mesh is not cut to allow passage of the spermatic cord; instead the cord is lateralized, as is done in the Stoppa procedure. Medially, the mesh is inserted deep to the rectus abdominis and the transversalis fascia, almost to the midline. The prosthesis must be lax.

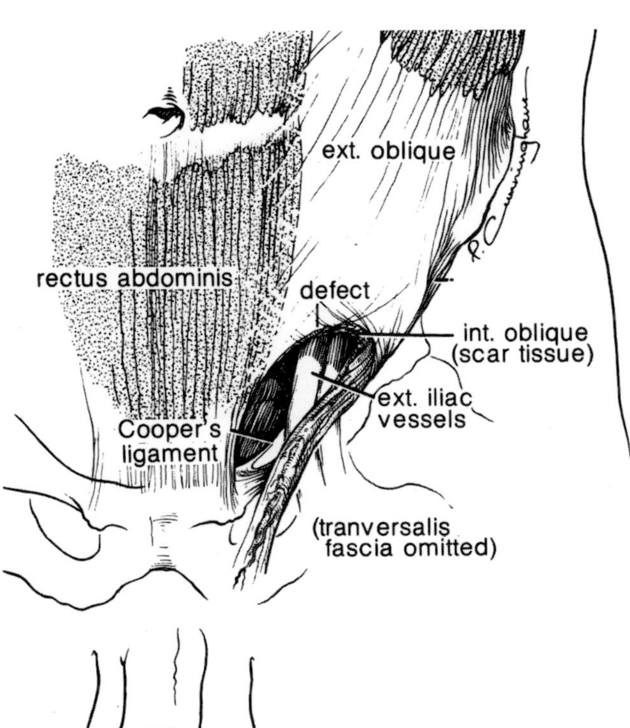

Figure 2. In the absence of a substantial portion of the inguinal ligament, dissection must reveal Cooper's ligament to which a prosthesis will be anchored. (With permission: Bendavid R. New techniques in hernia repair. *World J Surg* 1989; **13**:524–5)

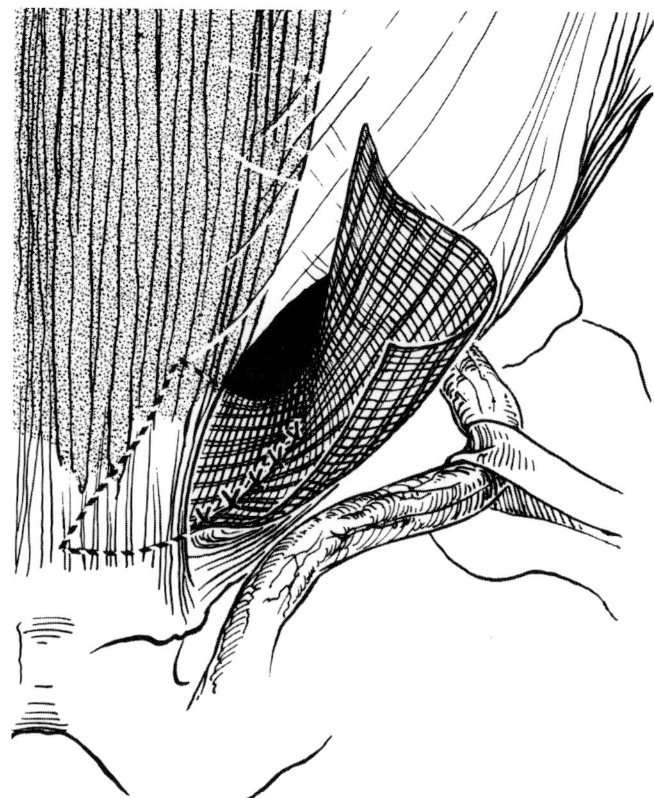

Figure 3. Insertion of a prosthesis. The prolene sutures are first inserted in Cooper's ligament. The free ends of the suture are then threaded through the mesh. (With permission: Bendavid R. New techniques in hernia repair. *World J Surg* 1989; **13**:524–5)

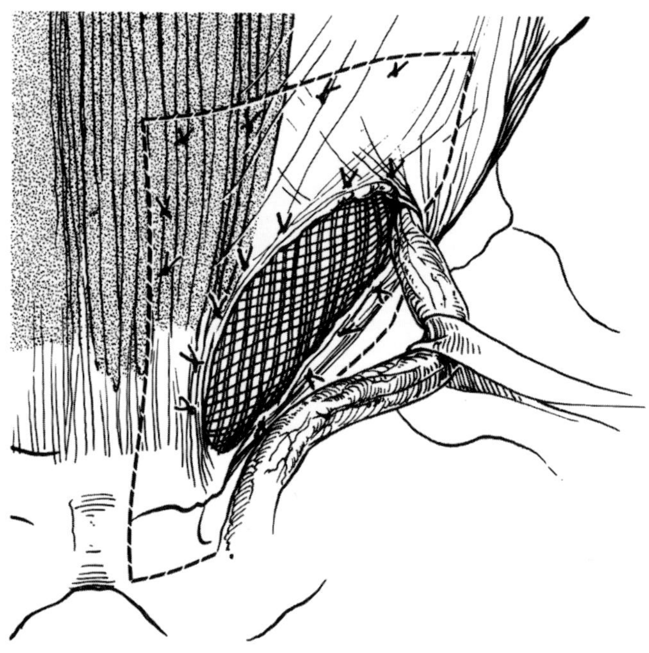

Figure 4. The prosthesis anchored in place. Note that no slit is created in the mesh for the egress of the spermatic cord, which is lateralized instead. The prosthesis must always be generously larger than the defect. (With permission: Bendavid R. New techniques in hernia repair. *World J Surg* 1989; **13**:524–5)

The umbrella

Femoral hernias have traditionally yielded the poorest results of all abdominal wall hernia repairs. The magnitude of this failure has always escaped notice because femoral hernias have always made up a very small percentage (2–5% at most) of all groin hernias. Their follow-up is often lost within a group of inguinal hernias and the average general surgeon would only see one to two cases a year, which accounts for the small and inaccurate series for study. The largest femoral hernia study report[38] has identified 508 femoral herniorrhaphies with a recurrence rate of 6.1% for primaries varying between 11% and 75% for recurrent repairs, depending on the number of previous attempts. This group of hernias represents one surgical condition where the introduction of prostheses has made a remarkable difference.

The umbrella used for femoral hernia repairs consists of a disc of polypropylene, 8 cm in diameter (Fig. 5). A prolene suture is threaded through the center of the disc

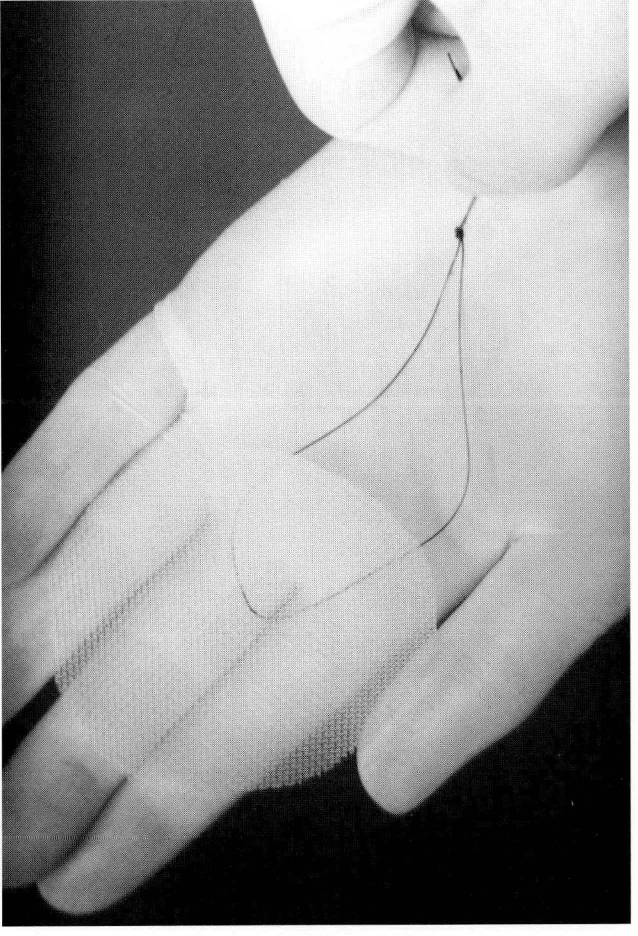

Figure 5. An umbrella can easily be fashioned from a polypropylene mesh (8 cm in diameter)

for easy handling and will eventually be cut away. The repair can be done from below or from above the inguinal ligament.

If done from below, one must be able to identify Cooper's ligament so that two or three sutures may be inserted safely. The disc of mesh is then slid on to the sutures by threading their ends through the interstices of the mesh. The knots are tied so that the disc is anchored posteriorly. Additional sutures are inserted medially through the lacunar ligament, anteriorly through the iliopubic and inguinal ligaments (two to three sutures). Laterally the umbrella is allowed to lie generously over the femoral vein and a single suture inserted beneath the disc approximating the femoral sheath to the mesh. If the umbrella is used through an inguinal preperitoneal approach, a pair of Kelly forceps is introduced into the femoral defect from below the inguinal ligament. The prolene suture which forms the stem of the umbrella is then grasped and pulled down, allowing the umbrella to overlie the defect. Sutures are inserted as described above (Fig. 6).

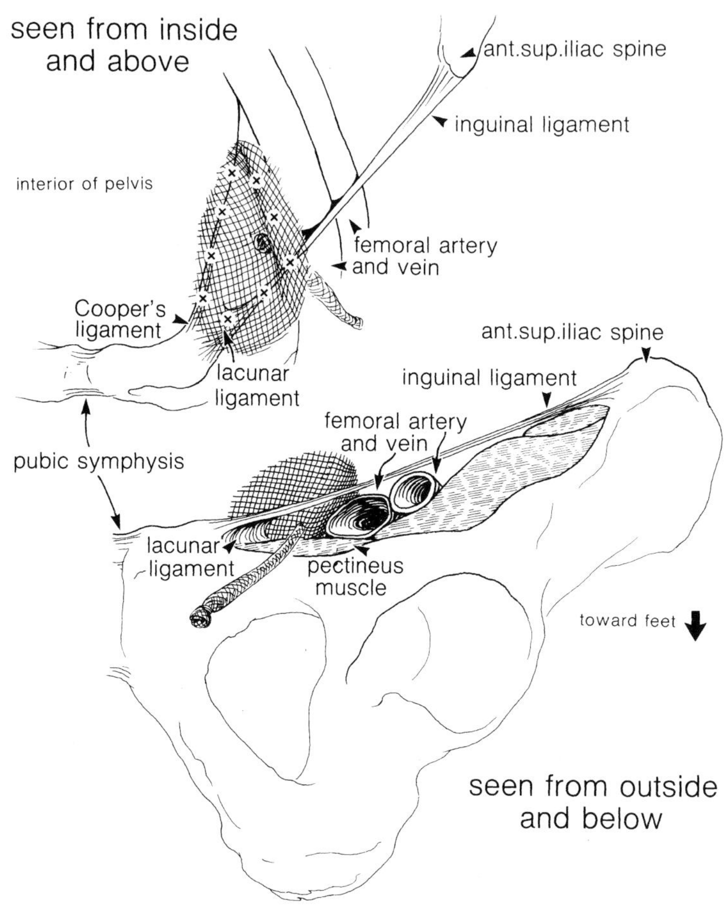

Figure 6. Final position of the umbrella which is held secured with prolene sutures. (With permission: Bendavid R. A femoral 'umbrella' for femoral hernia repair. *Surg Gynecol Obstet* 1987; **165**:155; now known as *J Am Coll Surg*)

Results

A transversalis fascia replacement was carried out on 828 patients. Eight recurrences have been identified (recurrence rate, 0.97%). The causes of these failures have been identified at surgery and were due to torn Cooper's ligament sutures (two cases), the appearance of a prevascular hernia (one case), reherniation as an interstitial hernia lateral to the internal ring (four cases) and a true direct hernia through the midportion of the posterial inguinal wall, likely due to detachment of the mesh medially (one case). Where umbrellas were inserted (397 cases), five recurrences have been recorded (failure incidence, 1.26%). These failures were subsequently identified at surgery and consisted of four direct inguinal hernias following femoral mesh repair, all of them occuring just lateral to the public crest; and one femoral hernia recurring as a femoral hernia, probably because of the sutures tearing off Cooper's ligament.

CONCLUSION

A major problem with the use of prostheses is the belief that it will supplant the knowledge of anatomy and do away with the necessity of an accurate dissection. Nothing can be further from the truth, and this observation has been firmly substantiated by the publication of Obney and Chan[39] who reported on 1057 recurrent inguinal hernias in 964 patients who came to the Shouldice Hospital. Their findings revealed that the aetiology of the recurrent hernias was as follows:

- Indirect inguinal hernias, 37%, a technical error which should never occur
- Femoral hernias, 8%, which can be classified as missed hernias
- Two or more hernias, 10%
- Direct inguinal hernias, 45%, a very high incidence of recurrence which implies that the hernias were either overlooked or the repair was based on imbrication of the posterior wall of the canal, an inadequate procedure.

Prostheses have become important adjuncts in the treatment of complicated groin hernias. Prostheses however, cannot supplant a thorough knowledge and understanding of the anatomy, physiology and pathology of the inguinal region.

REFERENCES

1   Abel AL, Hunt AH. Stainless steel wire for closing abdominal incisions and for the repair of herniae. *BMJ* 1948; **2**:379.
2   Babcock WW. The range of usefulness of commercial steel cloths in general and special forms of surgical practice. *Ann W Med Surg* 1952; **6**:15.
3   Preston DJ, Richards C. Use of wire mesh prostheses in the treatment of hernia. *Surg Clin North Am* 1973; **53**:549.

4   Duron JJ. Stainless steel mesh in the treatment of hernias. In Bendavid R, ed. *Prostheses and abdominal wall hernias.* Austin, Texas: RG Landes Co 1994; 265–7.

5   Goepel R. Weber die verschliessung von bruchpforten durch einheilung geflochtener fertiger silberdrahnetze (Silberdrah Pelotten). *Verh Dtsch Ges Chir* 1900; **19**:174.

6   Witzel O. Ueber den verschluss von bauchwunden und bruchpforten durch versenkte silberdrahntnetze. *Centralbl F Chir Leipz* 1900; **27**:257.

7   Throckmorton TD. Tantalum gauze in the repair of hernias complicated by tissue deficiency. *Surgery* 1948; **23**:32.

8   Koontz AR. Preliminary report on the use of Tantalum mesh in the repair of ventral hernias. *Ann Surg* 1948; **127**:1079.

9   Douglas DM. Repair of large hernia with Tantalum gauze. *Lancet* 1948; **i**:936.

10 Lam CR, Szilagyid E, Puppendahl M. Tantalum gauze in the repair of large postoperative ventral hernias. *Arch Surg* 1948; 57:234.

11 Burton CC. Facia lata, cutis and Tantalum grafts in repair of massive abdominal incisional hernias. *Surg Gyn Obst* 1959; **109**:621.

12 Adler RH. An evaluation of surgical mesh in the repair of hernias and tissue defects. *Arch Surg* 1962; **85**:156.

13 McArthur DL. Autoplastic suture in hernia and other diseases: preliminary report. *JAMA* 1901; **37**:1162.

14 Koontz AR. Dead (preserved) fascia grafts for hernia repair. *JAMA* 1927; **89**:1230.

15 Horsley GW. The behavior of alcohol preserved fascia lata of the ox, autogenous fascia and chromicized kangaroo tendon in dog and in man. *Ann Surg* 1931; **94**:410.

16 Aquaviva, quoted by Zagdoun J, Sordhas A. L'utilisation des plaques de nylon dans la chirurgie des hernies inguinales. *Academie de Chirurgie.* Seance du 25 Nov 1959, pp 747–54.

17 Zagdoun J Sordinas A. L'utilisation des plaques de nylon dans la chirurgie des hernies inguinales. *Academie de Chirurgie.* Seance du 25 Nov 1959, pp 747–54.

18 Wolstenholme JT. Use of commerical Dacron fabric in the repair of inguinal hernias and abdominal wall defects. *Ann Surg* 1956; **73**:1004.

19 Bellis CJ. Immediate unrestricted activity after inguinal herniorrhaphy. *Int Surg* 1969; **52**:107.

20 Annibali R, Fitzgibbons RJ Jr. Prosthetic materials and adhesion formation. In Arregui MA, Nagan RF, eds. *Inguinal hernia: advances or controversies.* Oxford: Radcliffe Medical Press 1994; pp 115–24.

21 Dufilho A. Les complications des protheses en tulle de Dacron. A propos de 414 observations. Thesis, Paris 1981.

22 Usher FC, Wallace SA. Tissue reaction to plastics; comparison of Nylon, Orlon, Dacron and Teflon. *Arch Surg* 1958; **76**:997.

23 Usher FC, Gannon JP. Marlex mesh: a new plastic mesh for replacing tissue defects; experimental studies. *Arch Surg* 1959; **78**:131.

24 Usher FC, Ochsner J, Tuttle LLD. Use of Marlex mesh in repair of incisional hernias. *Am Surgeon* 1958; **24**:969.

25 Gilbert A. Tension free repair. In Bendavid R, ed. *Prostheses and abdominal wall hernias.* Austin, Texas: RG Landes Co 1994; pp 375–9.

26 Lichtenstein I. Hernioplasty. In Bendavid R, ed. *Prostheses and abdominal wall hernias.* Austin, Texas: RG Landes Co 1994; pp 389–94.

27 Rutkow I. Tension free repair. In Bendavid R, ed. *Prostheses and abdominal wall hernias.* Austin, Texas: RG Landes Co 1994; pp 383–8.

28 Nyhus LM. The inlay prosthetic buttress for repair of inguinal hernias. In Bendavid R, ed. *Prostheses and abdominal wall hernias.* Austin, Texas: RG Landes Co 1994; pp 443–5.

29 Oshige S. Japanese patent no 42-13560 (67/13560) August 1967.

30 Elliott MP, Juler GL. Comparison of Marlex mesh and Teflon sheets when used for hernia repair in the experimental animal. *Am J Surg* 1979; **137**:342.

31 Cumberland VH. A preliminary report on the use of prefabricated nylon weave in the repair of ventral hernia. *Med J Aust* 1952; **1**:143–4.

32 Scales FT. Discussion on metals and synthetic materials in relation to soft tissues. Tissue reaction to synthetic materials. *Proc R Soc Med* 1953; **46**:647.

33 Ponka JL. Desirable qualities in prosthetic materials (Table 26–1). In *Hernias of the abdominal wall.* Philadelphia: WB Saunders 1980; 535.

34 Bendavid R. The merits of the Shouldice repair. *Probl Gen Surg* 1995; **12**:105–9.

35 Gilbert AI, Graham MF. Technical and scientific objections to laparoscopic herniorrhaphy. *Probl Gen Surg* 1995; **12**:209–14.

36 Amid P, Shulman AG, Lichtenstein IL. The goals of modern hernia surgery. How to achieve them: open or laparoscopic repair? *Probl Gen Surg* 1995; **12**:165–71.

37 Read RC. The role of protease-antiprotease imbalance in the pathogenesis of herniation and abdominal aortic aneurysms in certain smokers. *Postgrad Gen Surg* 1992; **4**:161–5.

38 Bendavid R. Femoral hernias: primary vs recurrence. *Int Surg* 1989; **74**:99–100.

39 Obney N, Chan CK. Repair of multiple time recurrent inguinal hernias with reference to common causes of recurrence. *Contemp Surg* 1984; **25**, Dec:25–32.

8 THE SHOULDICE OPERATION AND TRANSINGUINAL PREPERITONEAL (TIPP) MESH REPAIR

Volker Schumpelick and Georg Arlt

The laparoscopic approach to surgery was estimated to become the procedure of choice in inguinal hernioplasty within a few years of its introduction. Following the proposals of the McKinsey Company (USA), the percentage of groin hernias done laparoscopically should have increased to about 50% of the total from 1993 to 1995. Today the reality looks quite different. For example, in Nordrhein in the most western part of Germany (where the Technical University of Aachen is located), the percentage of laparoscopic hernioplasties carried out in 1995 was about 7% of a total of 21 000 groin hernia operations. The most common technique used was the Shouldice procedure (57%) followed by the Bassini repair (about 30%) and other techniques. About 10–13% of the procedures were for a recurrence, and in 2.5% of all cases the hernia was operated on in the presence of an incarceration. These figures show that all other techniques of repair apart from the Shouldice operation are a long way from becoming the procedure of choice in Germany today.

In spite of the widespread use of the Shouldice technique, which is reported as showing an exceptionally low recurrence rate, there is still a recurrence rate of about 10%; a figure that is in accordance with the current experience in the UK, USA, Sweden and other western countries and that is undoubtedly much too high. The unacceptably high recurrence rate might be due to inappropriate technique, questions of indication, or both. Looking at technique, many individual modifications have been applied to the Shouldice technique, but virtually none of them have been evaluated in clinical studies. In Germany, for example, a so-called Shouldice–Bassini technique is done by 10% of surgeons and another 18% use a Kirschner modification (epifascial displacement of the cord) in primary Shouldice repairs. In recurrent hernias, the epifascial displacement of the cord is the preferred method in more than 35% of clinics. Other obvious advantages on techniques in hernia surgery, such as local anaesthesia and short-stay surgery, which were proposed at the same time as the Shouldice technique, are rarely used.[1]

TECHNICAL PRINCIPLES OF SHOULDICE REPAIR

Our technique of Shouldice repair is closely related to the original method proposed by surgeons from the Shouldice Hospital in Thornhill, Ontario, Canada. The principles are as follows:

- horizontal incision of the skin
- identification and preservation of the ilioinguinal nerve and the genital branch of the genitofemoral nerve
- resection of the cremasteric muscle
- incision of the transversalis fascia
- a two-layer overlapping repair of the transversalis fascia using a running non-absorbable suture (polypropylene 0)
- attachment of the conjoint tendon to the inguinal ligament with a double row of running suture (polypropylene 0)
- no subcutaneous displacement of the cord
- no subcutaneous drain.

RESULTS OF SHOULDICE REPAIR

From January 1986 until December 1995 a total of 3236 Shouldice repairs were carried out at the Surgical University Clinic of Aachen. There were 2307 primary repairs and 929 Shouldice procedures for recurrent hernia (range: first to eighth recurrence). Details of early and late (1 year) postoperative complications are given in Table 1.

Nearly half of the operations were done by the author personally. Of the rest of the procedures, 19.2% were performed by senior surgeons ($n = 10$), 47.1% by assistants ($n = 12$) with more than 3 years of surgical experience and 33.7% by younger assistants ($n = 23$). Mean operating time was 40 min ($\pm$10 min) for a primary and 60 min ($\pm$30 min) for a recurrent repair. Using local anaesthesia, the patients' mean total time in the operating suite was reduced from 115$\pm$38 min to 92$\pm$25 min.

LOCAL ANAESTHESIA

The anaesthetic policy in our clinic was changed in 1992. From January 1986 until January 1992, general anaesthesia was routinely used in hernia surgery. Local anaesthesia was used only in respiratory or cardiac high risk patients, or for patients who

Complication	Hernia	
	Primary (%)	Recurrent (%)
Seroma	1.9	2.4
Haematoma	2.3	3.2
Infection	0.9	2.1
Ischaemic orchitis	1.2	1.4
Thrombosis	0.5	0.6
Testicular atrophy	0.6	0.9
Chronic inguinal pain	1.4	2.9

Table 1. Early and late postoperative complications in 3236 Shouldice repairs for primary and recurrent hernias at the Surgical University Clinic of Aachen 1986–95

asked for this type of anaesthesia. Since February 1992, local anaesthesia has become the routine anaesthetic method and it is currently used in 92% of primary hernia repairs and 62% of recurrent repairs. With increasing experience the conversion rate to general anaesthetic is now extremely low at 0.26%.

Comparing the intra- and postoperative course under general and local anaesthesia several advantages of the latter were found:

- patients' total time in the operating suite was reduced from 115±38 min to 92±25 min
- the rate of nonspecific postoperative complaints (nausea and vomiting, urinary retention, headache) decreased three- to four-fold
- postoperative inguinal pain was reduced and immediate postoperative mobilization was achieved.

Apart from these advantages, the rate of early and late postoperative complications was not affected by the type of anaesthesia. Approximately 96% of our patients would choose local anaesthesia for a second hernia repair.

RECURRENCE RATE

Data on our recurrence rates are available up to 5 years postoperatively. The 10-year follow-up of patients operated on in 1986 is currently under evaluation. Follow-up consists of clinical examination and ultrasonography. The 5-year examination rate is 85% in primary repairs and 83% in recurrent repairs; 11 recurrences were found in

| | Recurrence rate (%) | | | | | |
| | Primary hernia | | | Recurrent hernia | | |
Type[1]	I	II	III	I	II	III
L	0	0	0.2	0	0	1.9
M	0	1.0	1.9	0	1.6	2.4
Mc		0.6	0.6		2.6	7.7

[1]L, Lateral; M, medial; Mc, combined.

Table 2. Recurrence rate of Shouldice repair in primary and recurrent hernia using the Aachen classification

each group giving recurrence rates of 1.4% (11/786) and 3.8% (11/293) respectively. Similar figures have been reported by others.[2,3] Even clinics which do not specialize in hernia surgery achieve quite low recurrence rates with the Shouldice technique in primary repairs. For example, Mückter *et al.* from Germany reported a rate of 2.6% recurrences in 195 primary repairs after a 4-year follow-up.[4]

In contrast, the figures after a recurrent repair are not always as good. Wantz[5] found an overall recurrence rate of 7.2% and Petersen[6] found further recurrences exceeding 10%. Several factors might influence the rate of failures, such as an inappropriate surgical technique or a problem with the suture material, but the main contributory factor is probably the diverse nature of the hernias themselves.

DEVELOPMENT AND EVALUATION OF THE TIPP TECHNIQUE

Re-evaluation of the results of the Shouldice repair using the Aachen classification of groin hernias[7] shows the distribution of the recurrences (Table 2). All primary lateral (L I–III) and small medial (M II) hernias achieved a recurrence rate of no more than 1%. Only in large primary direct hernias (M III) did the rate rise above 1% to 1.9%. After a recurrent repair the rate exceeded the 2% margin in M III type and combined hernias (Mc II–III). The recurrence rate was unacceptably high (7.7%) in the huge combined hernias (Mc III) with a defect of the entire posterior wall. Consequently, in

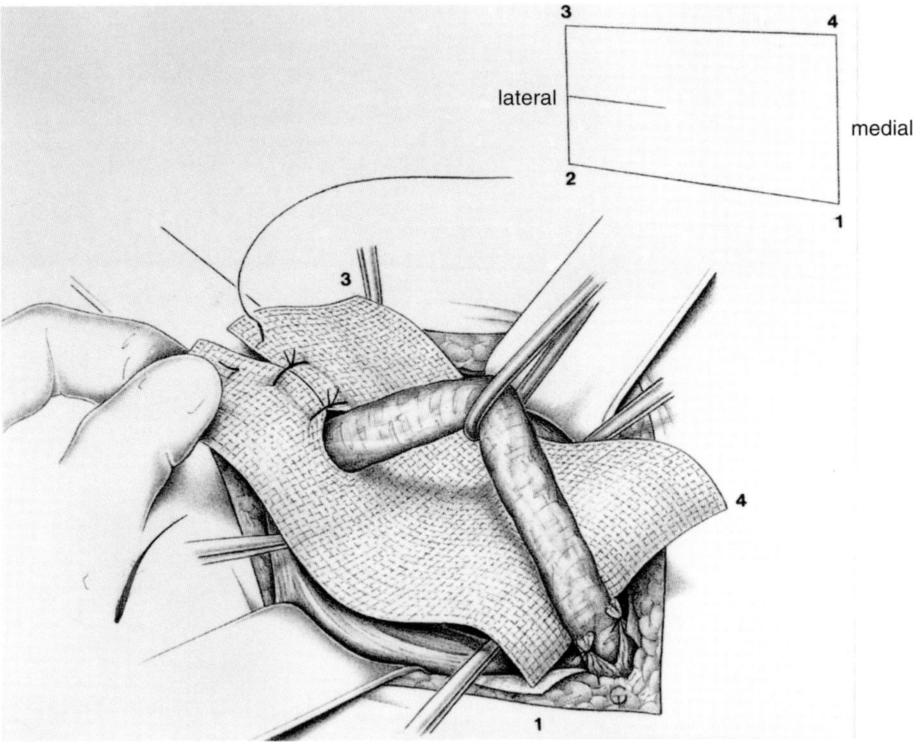

Figure 1. Transinguinal preperitoneal prosthesis repair: creation of a new internal ring by closure of the lateral slit with interrupted sutures

large or combined recurrent hernias the additional placement of a preperitoneal polypropylene prosthesis has been under evaluation since January 1994.

In the so-called TIPP (transinguinal preperitoneal prosthesis) technique, the initial approach is the same as in the Shouldice repair with preparation of the hernia done by an open transinguinal approach under local anaesthesia. The decision whether to use a conventional Shouldice repair or a TIPP procedure depends on the intraoperative classification of the hernial defect. In general, the TIPP technique is indicated in all recurrent hernias with a medial defect of more than 3 cm diameter (M III) and in cases of a combined recurrence with a medium (1.5–3 cm, Mc II) or large (>3 cm, Mc III) hernial orifice.

After classification of the defect, the posterior wall is completely opened and the preperitoneal fat is widely dissected away from the transversalis fascia. A polypropylene mesh of 15 × 10 cm with a lateral slit, two-thirds above and one-third below, is placed in the preperitoneal space. A new internal ring is created by closing the slit laterally to the spermatic cord with interrupted polypropylene sutures (Fig. 1). The medial lower edge

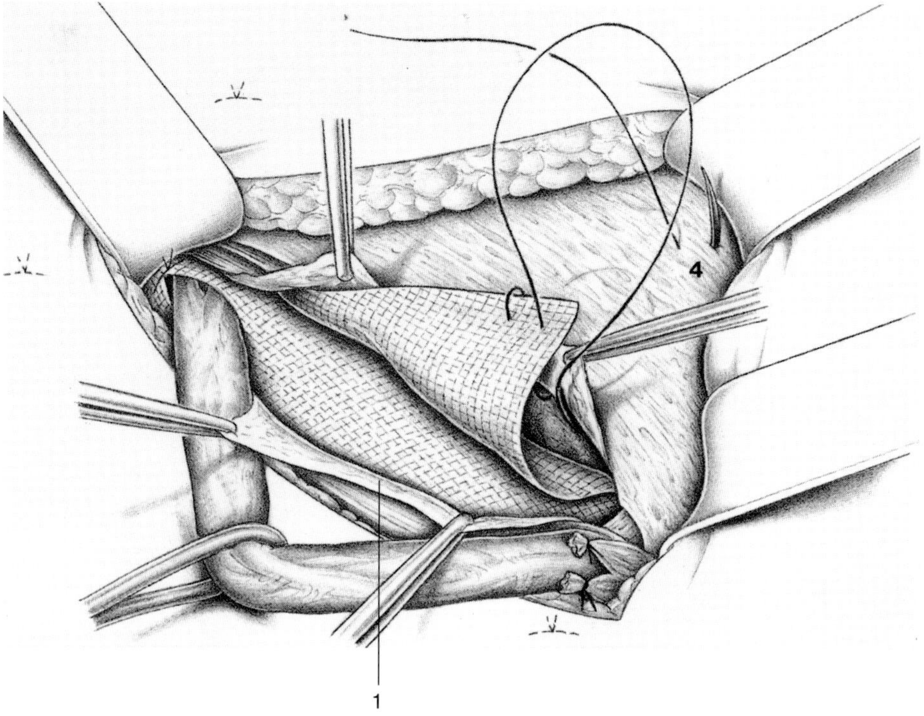

Figure 2. Transinguinal preperitoneal prosthesis repair: placement of the mesh in the preperitoneal space and transfacial–transmuscular fixation

1 transversalis fascia (inferior edge)

of the mesh is sutured to Cooper's ligament. The upper edges are fixed transfascially and transmuscularly to the ventral abdominal wall (Fig. 2). The procedure is completed by reconstruction of the posterior wall using a classical Shouldice technique (Fig. 3).

From January 1994 through December 1995, 58 TIPP procedures were performed. The indication for a TIPP repair was thus limited to 8.4% of all inguinal hernias, and about 23% of all recurrent repairs. The additional operation time was 5–8 min during routine use. Conversion of the anaesthesia from local to general anaesthesia was not necessary in any case. Early postoperative complications were one haematoma and one subcutaneous infection. Up to October 1996 there has been no recurrence detected during follow-up by clinical examination and ultrasound.

COMMENTS

The results of follow-up studies abdicate that the Shouldice repair remains the superior technique. No other technique has been evaluated so often and in such large and long-

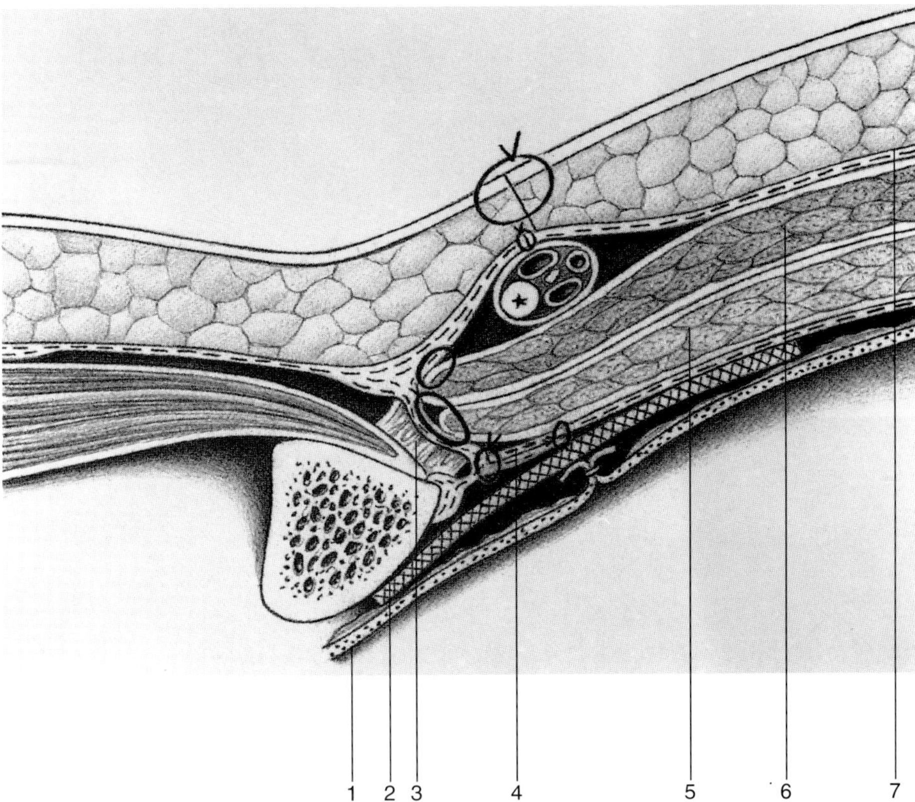

Figure 3. Transinguinal preperitoneal prosthesis repair: cross-section through the inguinal canal showing the mesh positioned beneath the reconstructed floor (transversalis fascia) of the inguinal canal

1 peritoneum
2 mesh
3 conjoint tendon
4 transversalis fascia
5 transversus abdominis muscle
6 internal oblique muscle
7 external oblique aponeurosis

term clinical studies.[8] In primary repairs the recurrence rate rarely exceeds 2%; consequently, the Shouldice repair is recommended as the procedure of choice in primary hernias of the groin by us[8] and others.[5,9–11]

In addition, the routine use of local anaesthesia offers several advantages such as intraoperative demonstration of the hernia and testing of the repair, safe anaesthesia for the elderly and those with cardiac or pulmonary disease, a decrease in the rate of urinary retention even in the age group prone to prostate problems, reduction of time spent in the operating suite, immediate postoperative mobilization and a reduction of hospital costs.[12]

Our detailed analysis of the recurrence rate after recurrent repair showed unsatisfactory and unacceptable results in certain types of inguinal hernias. While most of the lateral and small medial recurrences can be cured using the Shouldice technique, large medial or combined recurrences require an additional reinforcement of the posterior wall. Thus a classification-related intraoperative decision is made on whether or not additional support is necessary, and whether TIPP placement is indicated.[13] Using this policy, the use of prosthetic mesh can be restricted to those cases that really need it.

REFERENCES

1 Töns Ch, Muck-Töns A, Schumpelick V. Leistenhernienchirurgie in Deutschland 1992: Ergebnis einer Umfrage an 1656 deutschen Kliniken. *Chirurg* 1993; **64**:204.

2 Berliner SD. An approach to groin hernia. *Surg Clin North Am* 1984; **64**:197–213.

3 Glassow F. Inguinal hernia repair using local anaesthesia. *Ann R Coll Surg Engl* 1984; **66**:382.

4 Mückter H, Reuters G, Vogel W. Leistenhernienreparation nach Bassini und nach Shouldice. *Chirurg* 1994; **65**:121–6.

5 Wantz GE. The Canadian repair: personal observations. *World J Surg* 1989; **13**:516–21.

6 Petersen P. Die Versorgung des Leistenhernienrezidivs unter Verwendung der Reparationsmethode nach Shouldice. *Akt Chir* 1989; **24**:106–8.

7 Schumpelick V, Treutner K-H, Arlt G. Klassifikation von Inguinal-Hernien. *Chirurg* 1994; **65**:877–9.

8 Schumpelick V, Treutner K-H, Arlt G. Inguinal hernia repair in adults. *Lancet* 1994; **344**:375–9.

9 Barwell NJ. The technique of Shouldice repair in Great Britain. In Schumpelick V, Wantz GE, eds. *Inguinal hernia repair*. Basel: Karger 1995; 135–8.

10 Bendavid R. The Shouldice repair. In Schumpelick V, Wantz GE, eds. *Inguinal hernia repair*. Basel: Karger 1995; 122–34.

11 Welsh DJR, Alexander MAJ. The Shouldice repair. *Surg Clin North Am* 1993; **73**:451–69.

12 Peiper Ch, Töns Ch, Schippers E, Busch F, Schumpelick V. Local versus general anesthesia for Shouldice repair of the inguinal hernia. *World J Surg* 1994; **18**:912–16.

13 Schumpelick V, Arlt G. Transinguinale präperitoneale Netzplastik (TIPP) beim Leistenbruch in Lokalanästhesie. *Chirurg* 1996; **67**:419–24.

9 PROSTHETIC MESH REPAIR USING LOCAL ANAESTHESIA

Allan E Kark, Martin Kurzer and Philip A Belsham

Operative treatment of inguinal hernias has undergone a dramatic change in the last 15 years. It has progressed from being a procedure carried out in hospital under general anaesthesia to an out-patient one using local anaesthesia, followed by immediate mobilization and return to work as soon as the patient wishes. It has become a low-cost operation with minimal complications and no need for complex technology (Fig. 1).

In this chapter the evolution of prosthetic replacement, the technique used at the British Hernia Centre, and the many criteria that need to be considered in assessing the choice and success of inguinal hernia operations are described. The role of specialist units is also discussed.

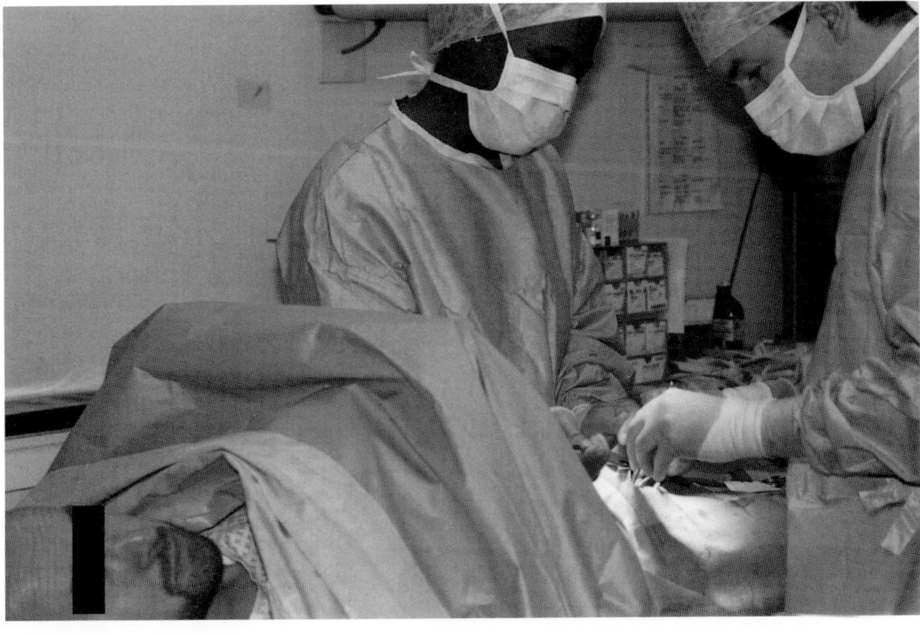

Figure 1.   The surgeon, scrub-nurse/assistant and a second nurse are all the staff required for local anaesthetic hernia repair

EVOLUTION

Bassini's technique[1] was universally followed in Europe from the turn of the twentieth century. His innovative operation consisted of excision of the sac after tying the neck, removal of the cremaster muscle and opening the length of the transversalis fascia. This latter was regarded as essential to allow for placement of interrupted nonabsorbable sutures to unite the inguinal ligament to the three-fold layer of internal oblique, transversus muscle and transversalis fascia. With modifications by Halstedt, this soon became the predominant operation in the USA.

As early as 1909 McGavin,[2] working in the Seamans' Hospital, London, noted the high rates of recurrence following the Bassini repair and developed the concept of reinforcement of the posterior inguinal canal by a prosthesis made of silver filigree. Ball[3] in Melbourne subsequently reported over 400 such repairs with the filigree placed under the transversalis, followed by a modified Bassini repair. However, these pioneering attempts as well as others using stainless steel filigree or polyethylene plastic inserts[4] generally failed because of the slow disintegration of the material.

In 1948 Shouldice in Toronto introduced his method[5] of a 4-layer repair under local anaesthesia. The results are widely recognised and applauded, and the low recurrence rates have generally been regarded as the standard to which to aspire.

Ten years later Usher[6] described the use of polypropylene mesh in repair of hernias and thus opened up the modern era of prosthetic repair. Within a few years Lichtenstein[7] introduced the concept of a 'tension free' repair, a method radically different from that of Bassini. Instead of repairing the posterior wall by suturing muscle to ligament, he reinforced it with a large piece of mesh secured only at its periphery without any tension. The results have been highly successful and the method has been developed and attested to by many others, including a series of reports by Shulman et al.[8] The use of mesh in hernia repair was given a further boost by the pioneering work of Stoppa[9] and Rives[10] in France and Gilbert[11] and Wantz[12] in the USA.

THE BRITISH HERNIA CENTRE EXPERIENCE

We adopted the tension-free mesh technique in 1992. Having previously used the Shouldice repair, we found that, although excellent in most cases, it was often technically difficult, particularly in obese people and those with large posterior wall defects. We visited several specialized hernia surgeons including Gilbert in Miami, Shulman at the Lichtenstein Clinic, Stoppa in Amiens, Wantz in New York and Kingsnorth in Liverpool and decided to adopt the tension-free method of repair. The initial experience was very favourable and received high patient acceptance.[13]

We have continued its use for all cases and here report the results of 4376 primary elective inguinal hernia repairs in a 5-year period. Apart from small asymptomatic direct hernias in very elderly men and four patients with huge, longstanding, irreducible scrotal hernias (Fig. 2) where the right of abdominal domain had been lost, no other patient was excluded for any reason, neither age (Fig. 3), physical infirmity

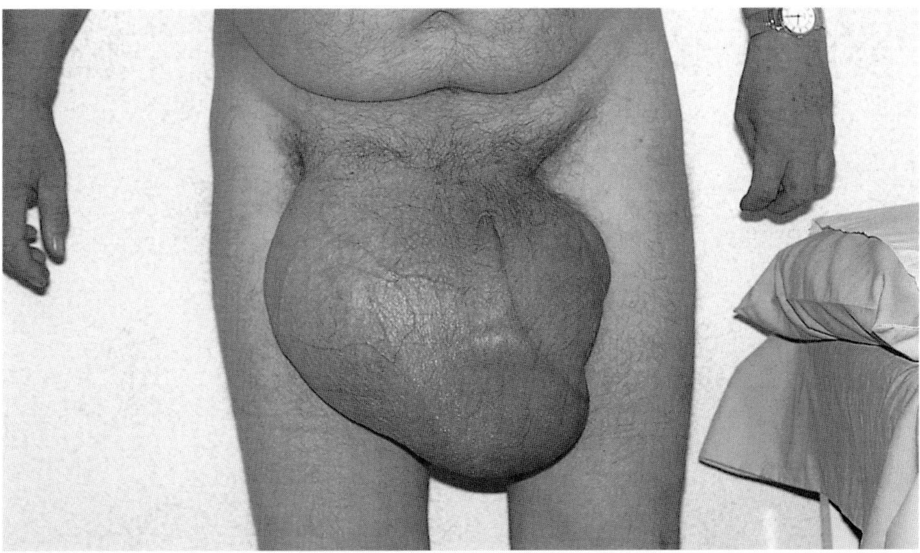

Figure 2. Massive long-standing irreducible inguinal hernia, an absolute contraindication to local anaesthetic. The age of the patient and the technical difficulty of the procedure often mitigate against attempting repair even under general anaesthetic

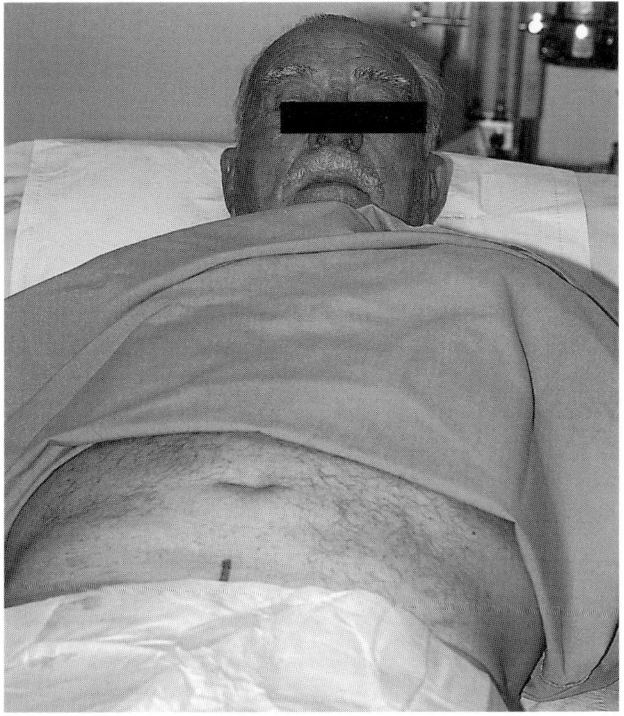

Figure 3. An elderly patient preparing for inguinal hernia repair under local anaesthetic

		%	No.
Age	16–92 years		
	over 80 years	2.9	(125)
Sex	98% men	2	(60) women
High risk	Post stroke/cardiopulmonary	7.9	(335)
Occupation	Manual	37	
	Office	31	
	Retired	32	
Type	Indirect 62%, Direct 38%		
	Bilateral 8.7% (380)		

Local anaesthesia, 99.3%; Day case, 99.5%; Exclusions: 30 patients (0.7%) had general anaesthesia for obesity, anxiety, irreducibility; 4 patients inoperable

Table 1. 4376 primary inguinal hernia repairs (1992–7 at the British Hernia Centre)

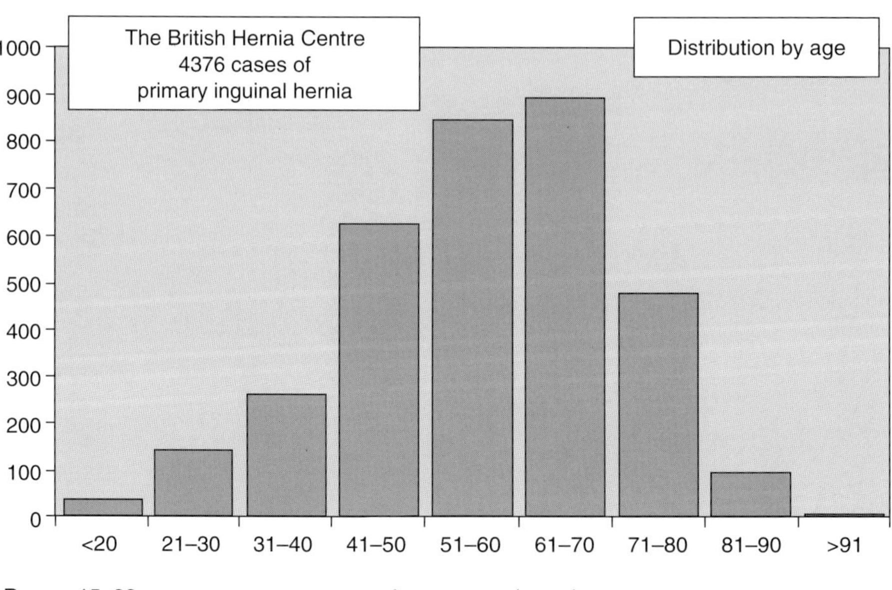

Figure 4. Distribution by age of 4376 cases of primary inguinal hernia at the British Hernia Centre

nor prostatic symptoms. The operations were done under local anaesthesia (99.3%) and as day cases (99.5%) (Table 1); 125 patients (2.9%) were over 80 years of age and 98% were men. 380 patients (8.7%) had bilateral hernias and 95% of these were repaired at the same time. The age range was 15–92 years and the age distribution is shown in Fig. 4.

TECHNIQUE

Patients were permitted a light meal up to 2 h before operation. The patient was shaved by the nurse, and monitored by pulse oximetry. A consultant anaesthetist supervised sedation in patients over 70 and in all patients with a history of cardiopulmonary disease or cerebrovascular disease (335 patients, 7.9%). No antibiotics have been administered in the last 2000 cases.

Local anaesthesia was supplemented by intravenous medication (midazolam 1 mg/ml, 2–12 ml). The anaesthetic solution consisted of 25 ml of 0.5% lignocaine and 25 ml of 0.25% bupivacaine, both without adrenaline, together with 5 ml of 8.4% sodium bicarbonate to neutralize the solution. Administration was by local layer infiltration (see Chapter 10) (Fig. 5).

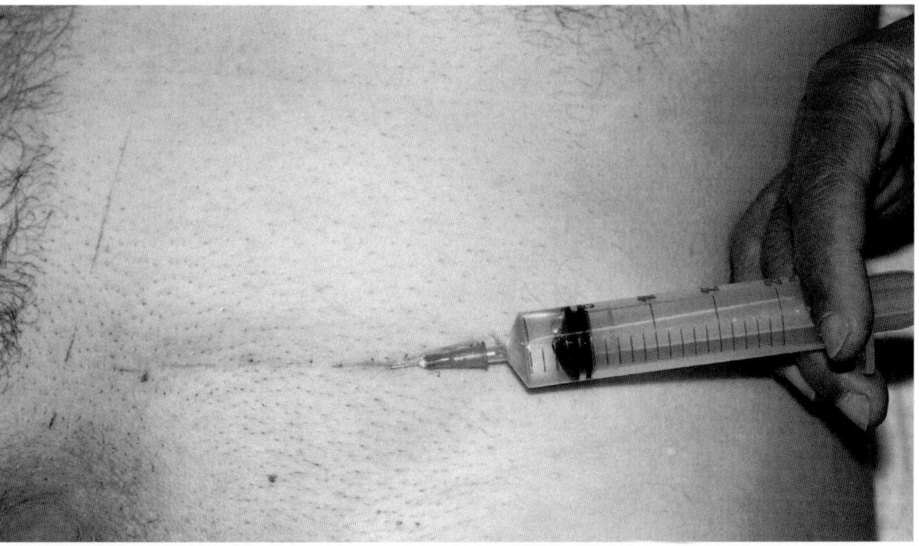

Figure 5. The line of the wound is infiltrated with local anaesthetic prior to the surgeon scrubbing and before the patient is 'towelled up'

Some of the key steps of the operation are shown in Figs 6–19. Indirect inguinal hernial sacs were dissected to expose extraperitoneal fat and either transfixed or simply inverted. Large scrotal sacs were transected in the canal leaving the distal portion undissected but widely open. If the deep ring was not dilated and closed itself over the reduced or ligated stump, no ring narrowing or occlusion was deemed necessary. If the deep ring was more than 3 cm in diameter a cone of mesh was inserted and anchored to the margin of the ring by three to four nonabsorbable sutures. Direct sacs were inverted and imbricated using a loose nonabsorbable suture to flatten the posterior wall.

The posterior wall was covered by an onlay of polypropylene mesh anchored immediately medial to the pubic tubercle. The mesh was then attached circumferentially using a loose running prolene suture. The mesh was cut at the lateral edge into a one-third lower leaf and a two-thirds upper leaf, fitted to surround the cord and the two flaps sutured laterally to the cord to form a snug ring. Both external oblique and subcutaneous tissues were closed with interrupted or continuous absorbable sutures and the skin by a subcuticular absorbable suture.

A diclofenac suppository was inserted at the end of the procedure, unless medically contraindicated.

Patients were discharged 1–2 h after operation, having emptied their bladder first. If living beyond 75 miles of the clinic, they stayed locally, returning home the following day by car or train. Patients were provided with a supply of oral analgesics, and given detailed

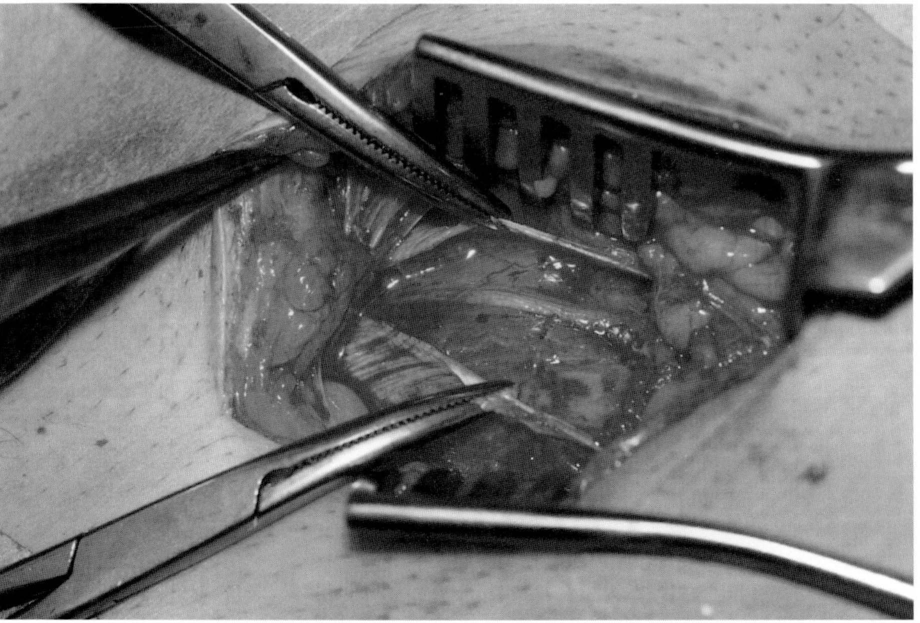

Figure 6. Left inguinal hernia view from the left and inferiorly. The inguinal canal has been opened and the ilio-inguinal nerve can be seen lying on the spermatic cord

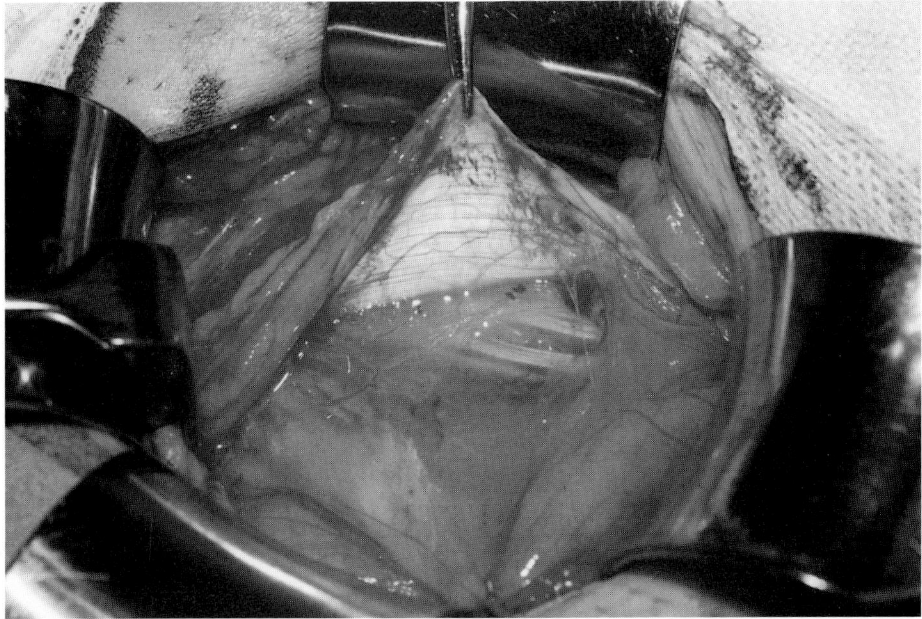

Figure 7. The upper leaf of the external oblique aponeurosis retracted superiorly. This is an avascular plane. Note the appearance of the tissues when local anaesthetic has been infiltrated.

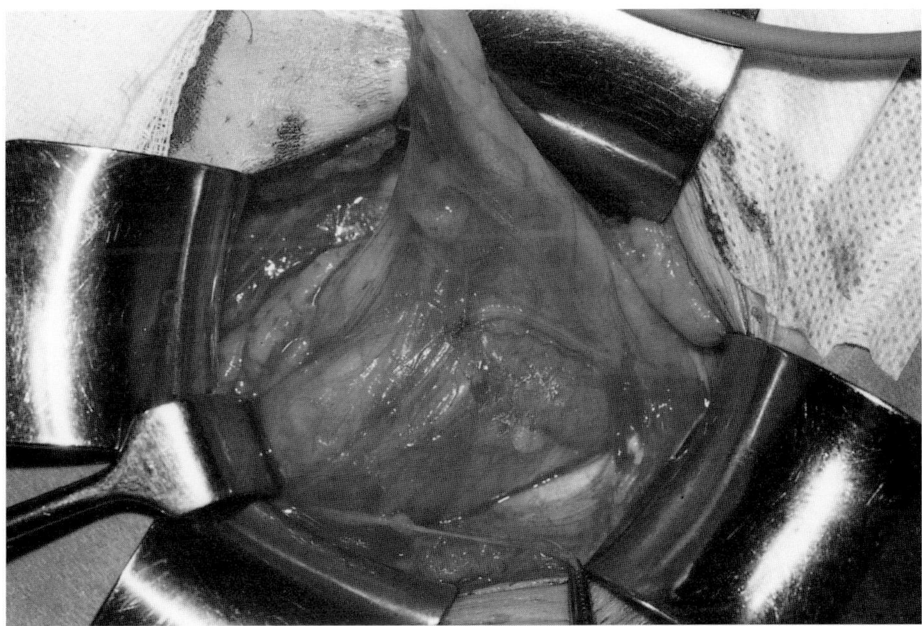

Figure 8. The inguinal canal is widely open and Poupart's ligament is seen inferiorly. The ilio-inguinal nerve can be seen lying on the spermatic cord

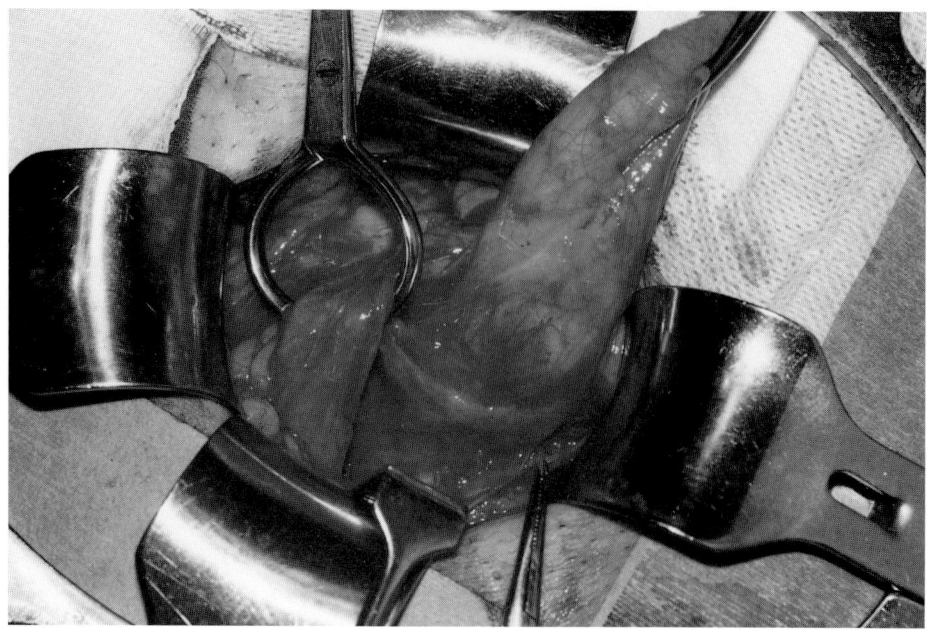

Figure 9. Fatty indirect sac emerging from the deep ring

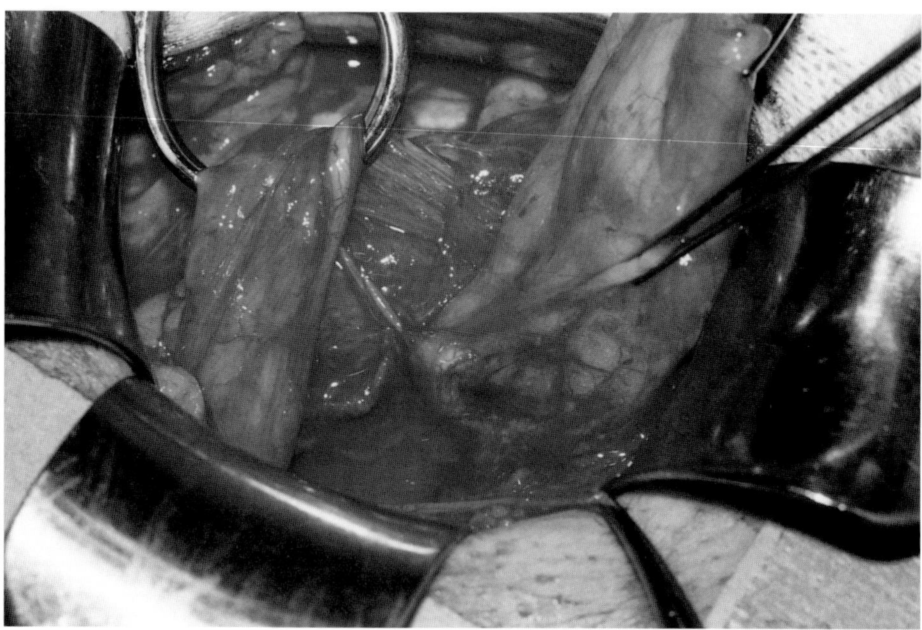

Figure 10. Indirect sac: the inferior epigastric artery can be seen at the medial edge of the deep ring, giving off the cremasteric artery

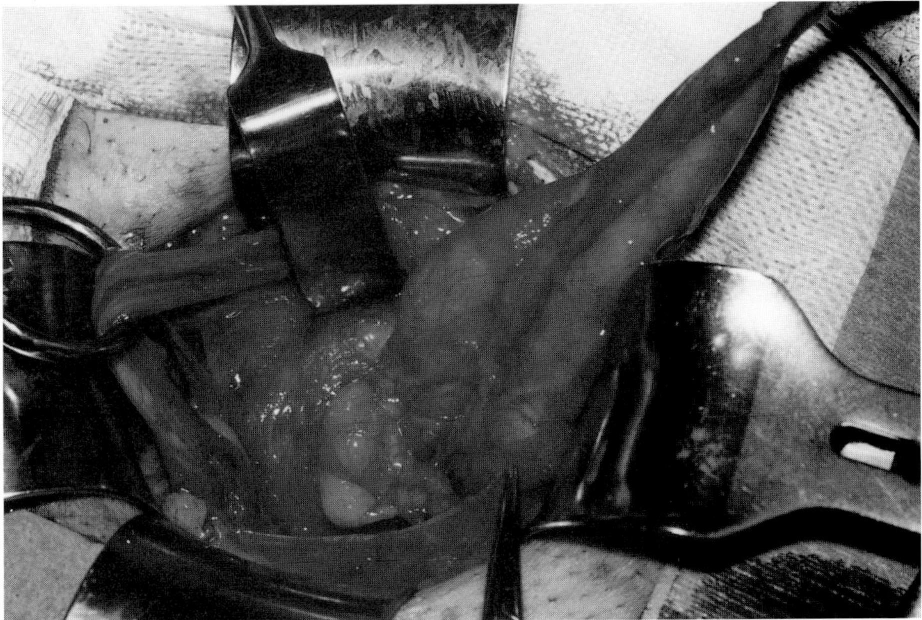

Figure 11. The spermatic cord is raised in a 'ring' retractor, and the vas can be seen clearly

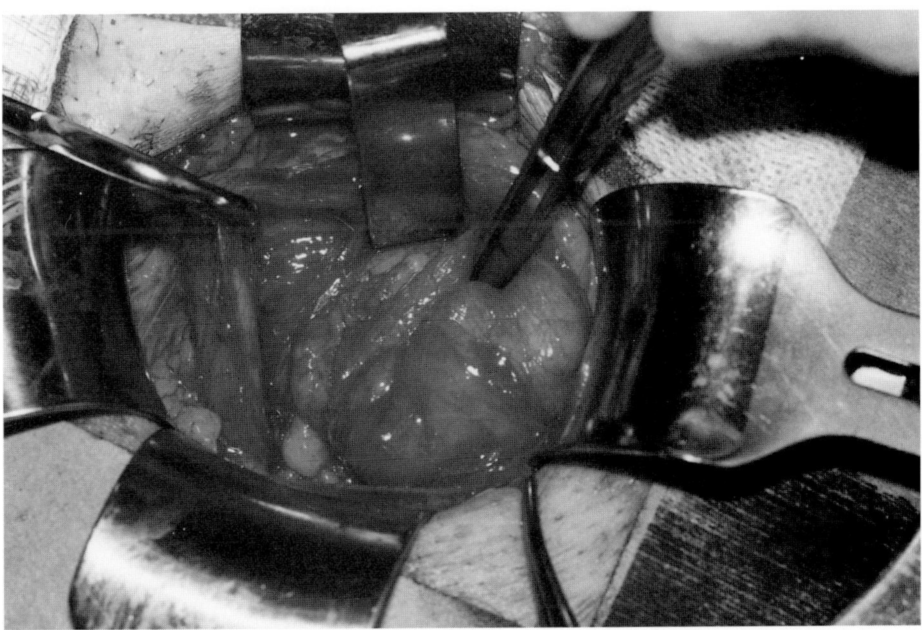

Figure 12. The indirect sac has been inverted by simply pushing it back through the deep ring with a pair of forceps

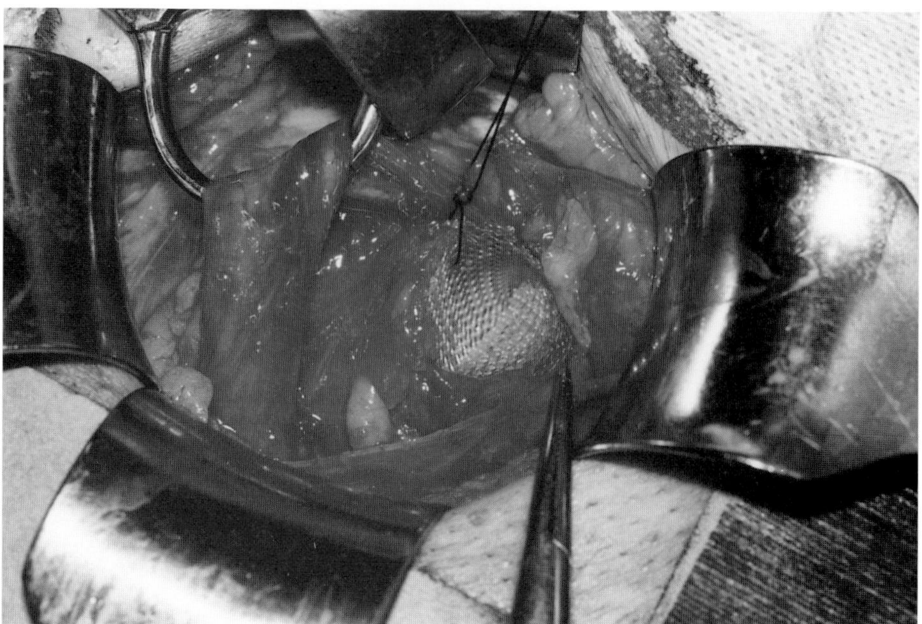

Figure 13. A cone of mesh has been inserted into the deep ring and prevents the indirect sac from emerging. A non-absorbable suture has been inserted at the superior margin

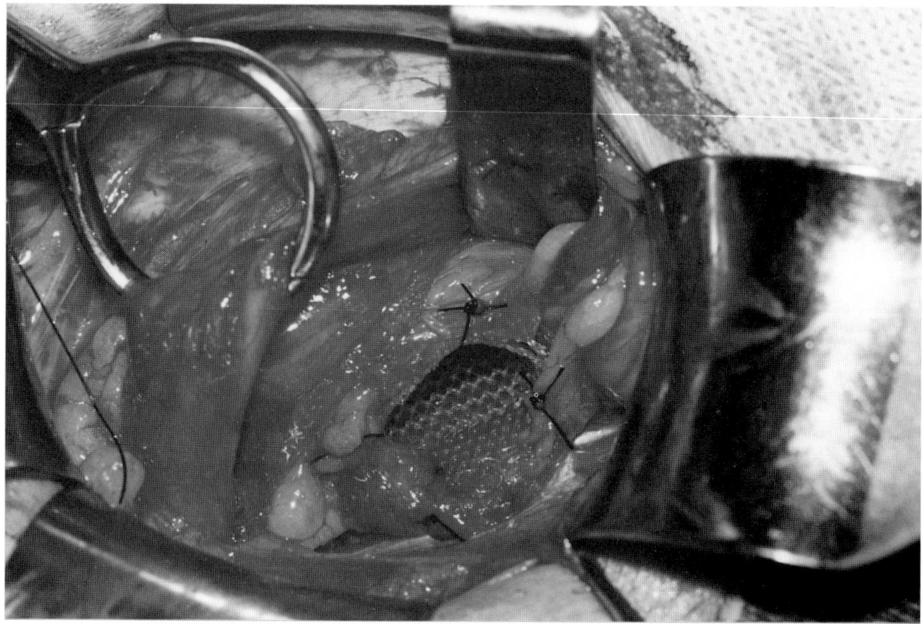

Figure 14. The mesh cone held in place by four interrupted sutures at its edge. The indirect sac has been controlled, and there is no tension at the margins of the deep ring

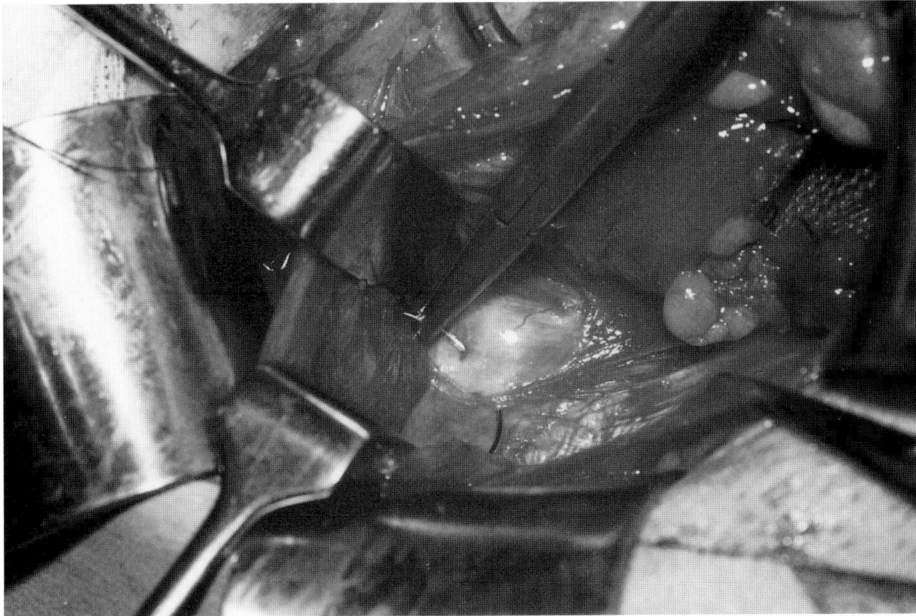

Figure 15. The needle is inserted into the soft tissue overlying the pubic tubercle. It is not necessary to place the suture through the periosteum. It is, however, important to ensure that this point is as far medial (towards the mid line) as possible

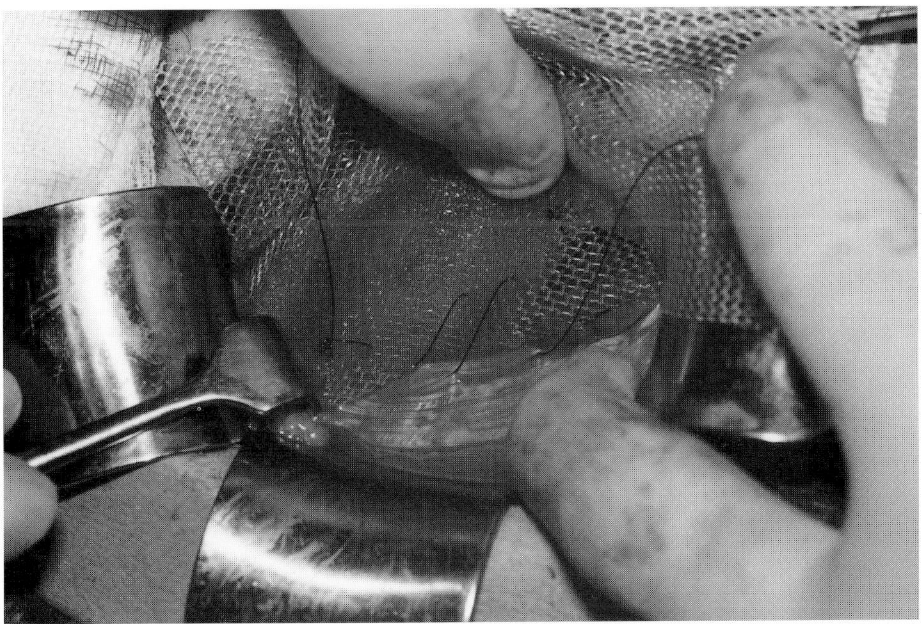

Figure 16. The inferior edge of the mesh sutured loosely to Poupart's ligament

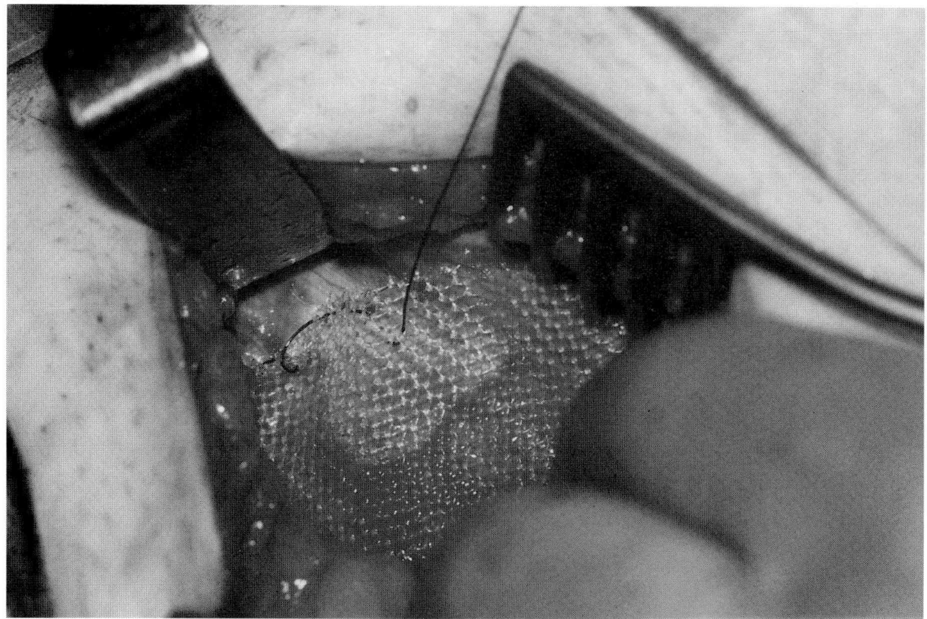

Figure 17. The upper edge of the mesh is similarly attached with a loose continuous suture

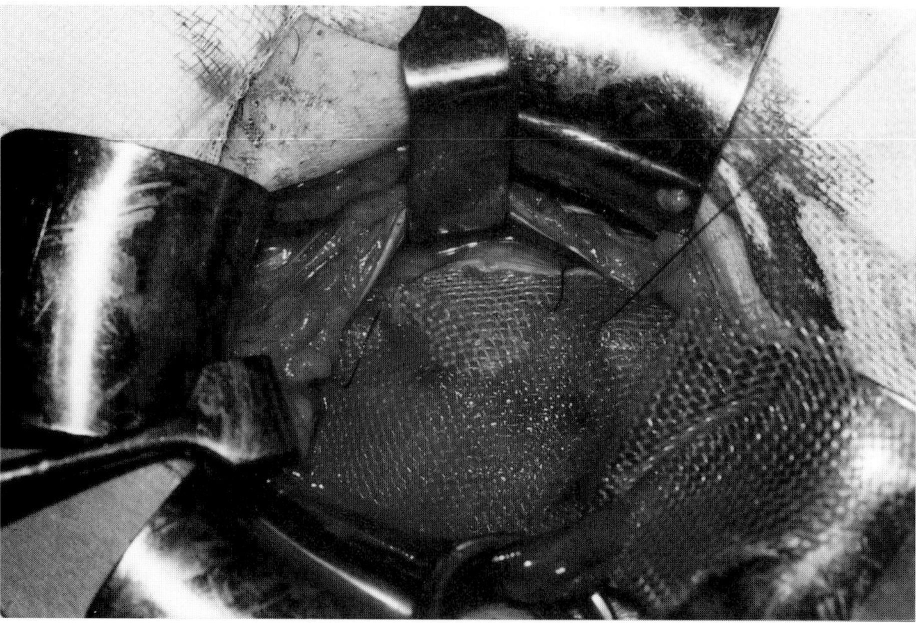

Figure 18. The loose continuous suture attaches the mesh to the internal oblique with the upper flap of the external oblique aponeurosis retracted firmly upwards and medially

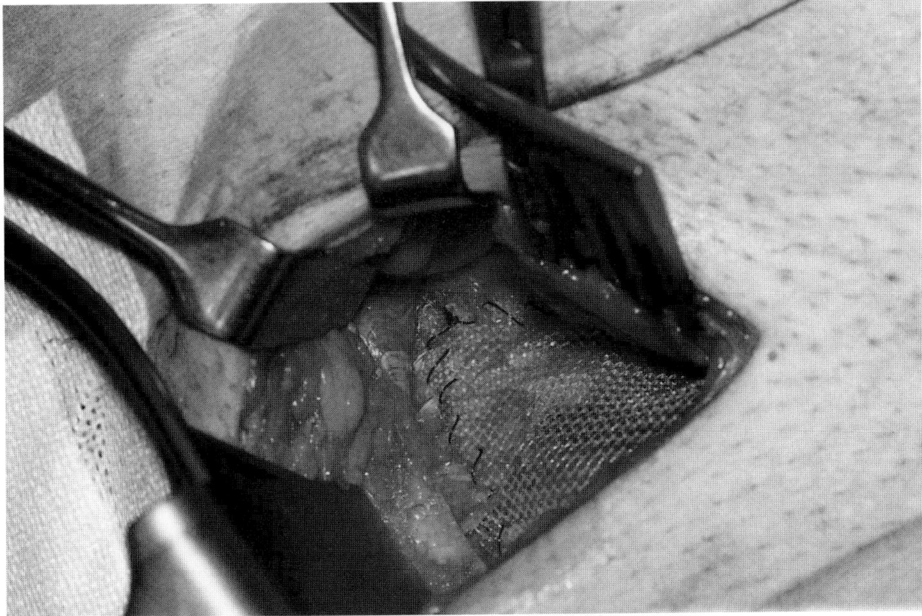

Figure 19. Completed placement of the medial corner of the mesh, overlapping the pubic tubercle and showing the superior and inferior rows of suture

written postoperative instructions reinforced by a senior nurse. These included strong recommendations to walk up to a mile the following day, and to increase activities accordingly thereafter. Driving was the only physical activity to be avoided immediately, until the brake pedal could be applied easily and quickly, practised first in a stationary vehicle.

All patients were telephoned the day after operation and were asked after 2 weeks to complete a detailed questionnaire with special emphasis on levels of postoperative discomfort and time of resumption of normal activities. In addition patients were encouraged to telephone with any immediate concern rather than have the problem foisted on to their general practitioner. In fact 20% of patients did telephone with questions concerning analgesia or blood staining of the dressing. Patients were either examined within 1 month of operation (88%) or were contacted by letter or telephone. Further follow-up was repeated at yearly intervals.

Postoperative problems

Within the first month (Table 2)

1   Two patients while still in the recovery area required immediate evacuation of an enlarging haematoma.

	No.	%
Mortality	Nil	0
Urinary retention	Nil	0
Haematoma	76	1.7
Venous thrombosis	3	0.1
Testicular pain/swelling	42	1
Infection: subcutaneous	44	1
deep	10	0.2

Table 2. Early complications (<1 month) of primary inguinal hernia in 4376 mesh repairs (local anaesthesia)

2 Urinary retention did not occur in any patient although a third of all patients were retired and mostly over 60 years old, and most had varying degrees of prostatism. As every patient was telephoned the day following operation any urinary complications would have been reported.

3 Haematomas were seen in 76 (2%) cases. Although they cause swelling and pain, often with cord thickening and testicular swelling and pain, haematomas almost all absorb in 1–2 weeks. In two cases evacuation of the haematoma was necessary under local anaesthesia and in one further case the haematoma became infected and required drainage and antibiotic chemotherapy.

4 Infection is a much discussed hazard of a foreign body left in any part of the body, and this fear has been exposed in the case of prosthetic hernia repair. In our experience, supporting that of the Lichtenstein Clinic, this has not been the case. Deep infection with pain, redness, swelling and fever occurred in 10 cases (0.2%). In three of these incision and drainage were required while the remainder settled with antibiotic chemotherapy. The incidence of infection following various methods of hernia repair has ranged from 0.5% to 8%.[13–14] Medina et al[14] in a controlled prospective trial investigating a range of possible causes of postoperative infection following hernia repair, observed that the two most important factors are the length of operation time and the experience of the surgeon. In our series the operating time ranged between 30 and 50 min. No case of sinus formation occurred and in only one patient was removal of the mesh undertaken by a surgeon elsewhere, despite our advice to persist with antibiotic treatment.

5 Thromboembolic problems have been strikingly rare. Three patients reported having had calf pain in the first few days after operation, but were asymptomatic when seen 10–14 days after operation.

Late complications (occurring after one month)

No cases of testicular atrophy have occurred. Both Reid and Devlin[15] and Wantz[16] have discussed this distressing complication in detail and perhaps no other sequel to hernia surgery is the cause of so much litigation and ill-feeling by the aggrieved patient. Wantz has provided much evidence that venous congestion and thrombosis are the main causes of testicular damage; the avoidance of extensive distal sac dissection, particularly in large longstanding inguinoscrotal hernias, is a significant surgical manoeuvre to help minimize this serious complication.

Postoperative pain is not easy to assess objectively. Three criteria have been used in this series: the subjective response by patients, the amount of analgesia used, and the time before return to normal activities (e.g. office routines, gardening, golf and manual work). Subjective patient assessment based on a mild, moderate or severe scale demonstrated that 20% of patients had no pain or mild discomfort for 1–2 days, and 13% had severe pain for up to 10 days. The majority, 67%, complained of a moderate but quite tolerable degree of pain for an average of 6 days requiring 4–6 co-proxamol tablets daily. Nevertheless almost all patients were able to walk 1–2 miles daily and resume ordinary household work from the first postoperative day. Standing and bending were usually described as the cause of discomfort in the early postoperative period. Older patients, those over 65 years, were less likely to have marked pain, nearly 40% of these complaining of mild discomfort, whereas younger men more frequently suffer more discomfort.

Pain persisted in 36 patients (1%) for up to 2 months. Whether this is due to stretching of branches of the ilioinguinal or genitofemoral nerves or to incorporation in a stitch is not known. In a few, 13 (0.4%), pain continued although with lessening severity for up to 1 year.

Return to work

This is influenced by multiple factors; doctors' advice, ingrained attitudes of family or friends who have had hernia repairs, social and economic pressures, degree and tolerance of discomfort, the type of repair, the extent of insurance cover, patient age, type of work and individual motivation. Doctors' advice has overwhelmingly been to 'take it easy' for 8–12 weeks, and delay a return to any lifting, exercise or manual labour for at least that length of time and sometimes even longer. Ingrained in generations of patients is the perception that too early a return to full activities is a factor in causing the need for further operation; this is bolstered by a documented long-term recurrence rate of 10–20% following Bassini type repairs, widely recognized by prospective patients.

Muscle–tendon suturing depends on firm apposition of these structures and in the first 10–14 days after the traditional sutured type of repair all movements creating tension or pulling on the suture line such as coughing, turning, sitting upright and even walking cause a degree of pain ranging from moderate to 'agonizing.' A measure of this is reflected in the median time of return to work reported variously as 49,[17] 45[18] and

28[19] days. This compares with the tension-free mesh repair reported by Amid et al[20] of 50% of manual workers resuming work in 7 days and 90% by 14 days.

Patients covered by insurance are more liable to prolong convalescence. Salcedo-Wasicke and Thirlby[21] compared those patients who received workmens' compensation with a group who had commercial insurance and observed that the former had pain for 27 days and returned to work after 36 days, while the latter had pain for 7.5 days and returned to work in 8.5 days.

We have noted in this series a time of return to work similar to the Lichtenstein Clinic. The total number of repairs was divided into four successive groups of 1100 patients each in the 5-year study period. Each of these was divided into office, manual and retired groups. In the first 1100 operations office workers returned to work in a mean of 10 days, which by the third and fourth groups had reduced to 6.5 days. Similarly manual workers returned in 16.2 days in the first group and this was reduced to 9–10.5 days in the last two groups.

This reduction in time of return to work in successive series by the same surgeons is due in part to improved technical skill and also because of active encouragement of patients. Moreover both patients' and general practitioners' attitudes are slowly changing and the long-held belief and expectation of considerable pain and avoidance of physical effort is being slowly replaced by the realization that the tension-free method offers dramatic improvements and economic advantages.

Laparoscopic hernia repair has been promoted in the belief that it is relatively pain free and permits an early return to work. The first aspect is undoubtedly true where a 'significant benefit' has been shown in the first 7 days postoperatively.[22] However, the time of return to work is very little different, if any, from the anterior approach. Brough and Royston[23] reported a return to normal activities (driving a car) in 5 days after unilateral and 7 days after bilateral repair; but the median time for return to work was 13 days and 14 days following unilateral and bilateral repairs. Kald et al[24] similarly observed a return to work in 2 weeks in 75% of laparoscopic repairs; Lawrence and McWhinnie[22] noted only small differences in return to work times between open and laparoscopic repairs with social class rather than type of operation explaining more of the variance.

RESULTS OF HERNIA REPAIRS

Rutkow[25] deserves credit for exposing the often blinkered thinking concerning assessment of the results of hernia surgery. He cites the leading surgeons of the last 100 years who have judged the success of hernia operations *solely* in terms of recurrence rates. With the very low rates of recurrences achieved in many specialized hernia clinics it is increasingly clear that other factors need to be entered into the equation to assess the choice of operation (Table 3). Nevertheless the incidence of recurrence after any method of hernia repair remains the main criterion for assessing its worth, and recurrence of the hernia represents a failure of the operation. It was precisely because so many Bassini-type repairs failed that

	Laparo-scopic	Open suture	Open non-tension mesh
Learning curve	Slow	Medium	Rapid
Anaesthetic risk	Present	Very low (if LA)	Very low
Risk of serious morbidity	Yes	No	No
Postoperative complications	Variable	Variable	Variable
Postoperative pain	Low	Moderate to high	Low to moderate
Return to work	1–2 weeks	>2 weeks	1–2 weeks
Aged & post-cardiac/ stroke	No	Only if LA	Yes
Recurrence risk	Low? (Unknown)	Low to Medium	Low
Cost	High	Low (if LA)	Low

Table 3. Choice of hernia repair based upon multiple factors

caused many surgeons to introduce modifications to try to reduce an unacceptably high rate of failure. The Cooper ligament repair by Halverson and McVay,[26] the Moloney darn[27] and the Shouldice method[5] are three of the most popular and enduring. The recurrence rate following the Bassini and Cooper ligament repair has been reported to range between 5% and 21%. The Shouldice technique has resulted in a remarkably low recurrence rate in that Clinic's hands, but not so in those perhaps less experienced.[28]

The recurrence rate following the muscle–ligament suture technique depends on many factors chief among which are:

(a)   the length of follow-up; Halverson and McVay[26] have forcefully pointed out that 'hernias keep recurring over many years,' and in their series doubled in a second 11-year period;

(b)   surgeons' experience and skill; not unexpectedly operations performed by relatively inexperienced junior surgeons have a significantly higher recurrence rate than those performed by experienced more senior surgeons[15];

(c)   high recurrence-risk patients; e.g. those with obesity and longstanding scrotal hernias.

Halverson and McVay[26] pointed out that the reason 'hernias keep recurring over many years' is that in any suture repair using the patient's own tissues, the inevitable effect of wear and tear over several decades will result in an increasing number of repairs breaking down. However, the repair by an onlay of prosthetic mesh produces completely different circumstances whereby reinforcement of the posterior wall of the inguinal canal by a nonabsorbable permanent material eliminates this time-related factor. Although a small percentage of recurrences will occur in patients who have had prosthetic mesh repair, they will occur relatively early (say within 1 or 2 years) and will be related to technical factors. Our experience of operating on an admittedly small number of recurrent inguinal hernias following mesh repair has identified only two causes:

(a) using too small a piece of mesh so that it pulls away from the margin of the defect; this is particularly true inferomedially over the pubic tubercle; Shulman et al[8] maintained that there is always a 20% shrinkage of the mesh, and the Lichtenstein technique lays great store on a wide overlap of the posterior wall on to the internal oblique and at least 2 cm past the pubic tubercle medially;

(b) a 'missed' indirect sac; our three cases of a 'recurrent' indirect inguinal hernia occurred in patients who had primary direct inguinal hernias repaired and in whom a small indirect sac had not been identified at the first operation.

If this contention is true then the recurrences seen at 2 years following mesh onlay repair may well represent the total of those that will occur. This can only be confirmed by assiduous long-term follow-up. The outstanding feature of the tension-free mesh repair is the exceedingly low recurrence rate now being widely reported between 0.1% and 0.7%.[8,13,21] The large series from specialized hernia centres with up to 5-year follow-up are as excellent as those reported from the Shouldice Clinic. In our series there were 14 (0.4%) recurrences with a 1–4 year follow-up in 3175 repairs. In our first 1098 repairs with a minimum of 4 years follow-up, there were 4 (0.3%) recurrences.[13]

FACTORS THAT SHOULD BE CONSIDERED IN THE CHOICE OF PRIMARY HERNIA REPAIR

These are listed in Table 3.

The *learning curve* of the operation is important in what is the commonest operation in surgery. While we strongly advocate the establishment of specialist hernia clinics, the sheer number of operations required (about 2000 per million population per year) will still leave young surgeons in training continuing to perform a large number, probably the majority of repairs worldwide. The non-tension mesh repair is less complicated and more quickly learned by junior staff than the Shouldice method and far less demanding than laparoscopic technique.

The type of *anaesthesia* is important in terms of both safety and the type of repair. General anaesthesia is the easiest option for surgeons but not without some small risk of both death and morbidity, as well as requiring a skilled anaesthetist. A significant minority of patients are averse to general anaesthesia, which additionally requires more staff, time and cost. Spinal or epidural anaesthesia is effective and has many of the advantages of local but these too require an anaesthetic specialist. Local anaesthesia is much the best method available. It poses almost no risk, is highly effective and provides much patient satisfaction during the operation. In addition patient co-operation by coughing and straining during the operation accurately defines the hernia. Above all local anaesthetic permits immediate ambulation and because of this, bladder emptying is almost never a problem. A further major advantage of local anaesthesia is the safety in repairing hernias in the elderly (see Table 1) and those with histories of serious cardiovascular and cerebrovascular disease. Many series exclude patients over 80 or those with accompanying serious disease and thus are highly selective. Local anaesthesia permits over 99% of such patients to have successful repairs.

The risk of serious morbidity is ever present in laparoscopic repairs. Few series have escaped the complications of visceral or vessel damage. These are exceedingly rare with the open approach.

Postoperative pain is markedly reduced by tension-free mesh repair compared to other suture techniques. Laparoscopic repair shows a definite advantage in the degree of pain in the first postoperative week. The time taken for return to work and normal activities is an important feature in assessing the choice of a hernia repair. There is now overwhelming evidence that tension-free open mesh repairs permit a return to normal activities in 1–2 weeks. Laparoscopic methods have not been shown to improve on this.[22,23,24]

The cost of repair under local anaesthesia as a day case is significantly less than repairs under general anaesthesia, and much below that of laparoscopic repair where, in addition, complex equipment and instrumentation are necessary and operating time is increased.

Not all hernias are the same. Direct hernias due to posterior wall weakness differ from indirect ones as in younger patients the sac is often preformed and may emerge through a firm internal ring with no posterior wall weakness. These in turn differ from large sliding hernias in older men and from large inguino-scrotal sacs with complete destruction of the wall of the canal. With the exception of the congenital indirect sac through a tight ring (Type I Gilbert or Nyhus) all other types benefit from a posterior wall replacement. Shulman argued that even in the Type I hernia it is justifiable to reinforce the wall by mesh as a routine. There is no proof that this is necessary in cases where the posterior wall is intact but we, like the Lichtenstein Clinic, have used it routinely in all cases largely because on many occasions it is difficult to tell whether the posterior wall is strong and intact. We believe it is safer to err on the side of caution even though a small number of patients may well have had a more extensive replacement than necessary. It is probably a less damaging procedure in this group than the deliberate division of a strong transversalis with resuture as in the Shouldice repair.

CONCLUSIONS

Non-tension mesh repair using local anaesthesia offers an exceedingly safe day-case operation for adults of all ages under local anaesthesia. It has almost no risk of serious morbidity and offers a return to work in 1–2 weeks. It is an inexpensive procedure requiring no complex instrumentation. Consistently good longer term results may be achieved in dedicated hernia units. The economic benefits to society are enhanced by the low complication and recurrence rates.

REFERENCES

1   Bassini E. Nuovo metodo operativo per la cura dell'ernia inguinale. *R. Stabilimento Prospevini, Padova,* 1889.

2   McGavin L. The double filigree operation in the radical cure of inguinal hernia. *BMJ* 1909; **2**:257–63.

3   Ball L. Repair of inguinal hernia and the use of filigrees. *Med J Austr* 1956; **1**:829.

4   Thomson W. Radical cure of inguinal hernia with a plastic insert. *Lancet* 1948; **2**:182–3.

5   Glassow F. Inguinal hernia repair using local anaesthesia. *Ann R Coll Surg Engl* 1984; **66**:382–7.

6   Usher F, Hill J, Ochsner J. Hernia repair with Marlex mesh. *Surgery* 1959; **46**:718–24.

7   Lichtenstein IL. Direct and indirect inguinal hernia repair including a new concept and introducing a tension-free repair. In Lichtenstein IL, ed. *Hernia repair without disability,* 2nd edn. St Louis: Ishyaku Euroamerica 1986: 65–118.

8   Shulman AG, Amid PK, Lichtenstein IL. The safety of mesh repair for primary inguinal hernias. *Ann Surg* 1992; **58**:255–7.

9   Stoppa R, Petit J, Henry X. Unsutured Dacron prosthesis in groin hernias. *Int Surg* 1975; **60**:411–12.

10 Rives J, Lardennois X, Flament JB et al. La piece en tulle de Dacron, traitement de choix des hernies de l'âiné de l'adulte. *Acta Chir Belg* 1971; **70**:284–6.

11 Gilbert AI. Sutureless repair of inguinal hernia. *Am J Surg* 1992; **163**:331–5.

12 Wantz GE. *Atlas of hernia surgery.* New York: Raven Press 1991:55.

13 Kark AE, Kurzer M, Waters KJ. Tension-free mesh hernia repair: review of 1098 cases using local anaesthesia in a day-unit. *Ann R Coll Surg Engl* 1995; **77**:299–304.

14 Medina M, Sillero M, Martinez-Gallego G et al. Risk factors of surgical wound infection in patients undergoing herniorrhaphy. *Eur J Surg* 1997; **163**:191–8.

15 Reid I, Devlin HB. Testicular atrophy as a consequence of inguinal hernia repair. *Br J Surg* 1994; **81**:91–3.

16 Wantz GE. Testicular atrophy as a sequel of inguinal hernioplasty. *Int Surg* 1986; **71**:159–63.

17 Rider MA, Baker DM, Locker A et al. Return to work after surgical hernia repair. *Br J Surg* 1993; **80**:1354–5.

18 Robertson GSM, Burton PR, Haynes IG. How long do patients convalesce after inguinal herniorrhaphy? Current principles and practice. *Ann R Coll Surg Engl* 1993; **75**:30–3.

19 Stock SE. Return to work after inguinal hernia repair. *Br J Surg* 1993; **80**:1489.

20 Amid PK, Shulman AG, Lichtenstein IL. Open 'tension-free' repair of inguinal hernias; the Lichtenstein technique. *Eur J Surg* 1996; **162**:447–53.

21 Salcedo-Wasicke CM, Thirlby RC. Post-operative course after inguinal herniorrhaphy: a case controlled comparison of patients receiving workers compensation vs. patients with commercial insurance. *Arch Surg* 1995; **130**:29–32.

22 Lawrence K, McWhinnie D. Randomised controlled trial of laparoscopic versus open repair of inguinal hernia: early results. *BMJ* 1995; **311**:981–5.

23 Brough W, Royston C. TAPP repair: the Hull and Stockport experience in laparoscopic inguinal hernia repair. In Darzi A, Monson JRT, eds. *Laparoscopic inguinal hernia repair.* Oxford: Isis Med Media 1994:56–7.

24 Kald A, Smed K, Anderberg B. Laparoscopic groin hernia repairs: results of 200 consecutive herniorrhaphies. *Br J Surg* 1995; **82**:618–20.

25 Rutkow IM, Robbins AW. 1669 mesh plug hernioplasties. *Contemp Surg* 1993; **43**:141–7.

26 Halverson K, McVay CB. Inguinal and femoral hernioplasty: a 22 year study of the authors' methods. *Arch Surg* 1970; **101**:127–35.

27 Moloney GE. Darning surgical hernias. *Arch Surg* 1972; **104**:129–30.

28 Kingsnorth AN, Gray MR, Nott DM. Prospective randomized trial comparing the Shouldice technique and plication darn for inguinal hernia. *Br J Surg* 1992; **79**:1068–70.

10 LICHTENSTEIN OPEN TENSION-FREE HERNIOPLASTY

Parviz Amid

For more than a century hernia repair success has been measured by its recurrence rate. In 1966, for the first time, the importance of the postoperative disability period of hernia repair was brought to the attention of surgeons by Lichtenstein.[1] With the goals of decreasing postoperative pain, recovery period and recurrence rate, the tension-free hernioplasty project was started at the Lichtenstein Hernia Institute in June 1984. The concept is based on:

- the degenerative origin of inguinal hernia, which results in destruction of the inguinal floor[2]
- the fact that the traditional tissue repair is associated with undue tension at the suture line.

TECHNIQUE OF ANESTHESIA

The procedure is performed under local anesthesia, which is our preferred choice for all reducible adult inguinal hernias.[3] The procedure is safe, simple, effective and economical, and has no side effects or risk of urinary retention. Furthermore, local anesthesia administered before incision produces a prolonged analgesic effect by inhibition of the build-up of local nociceptive molecules.[4-6] Several safe and effective anesthetic agents are currently available. Our choice, however, is a 50:50 mixture of 1% lidocaine (Xylocaine) and 0.5% bupivacaine (Marcaine), with 1/200 000 factory-added epinephrine.

An average of 45 ml of this mixture is usually sufficient for a unilateral hernia repair and is administered in the following fashion:

1 Subdermal infiltration (Fig. 1). About 5 ml of the mixture is infiltrated along the line of the incision with a 2-inch long 25 gauge needle inserted into the subdermal tissue parallel with the surface of the skin. Infiltration continues as the needle is advanced. Movement of the needle reduces the likelihood of intravascular infusion of the drugs because even if the needle penetrates a blood vessel, the tip will not

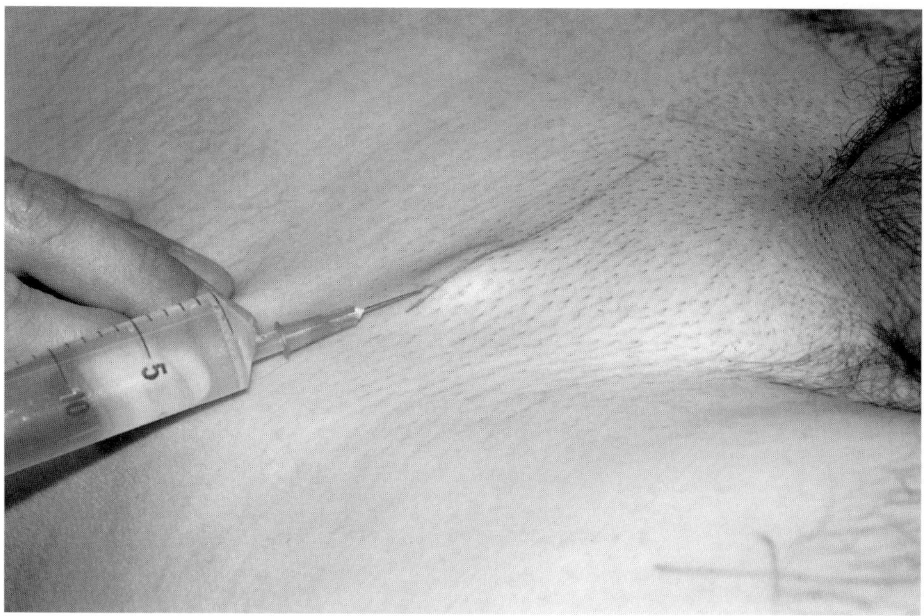

Figure 1. Subdermal infiltration. Local anaesthetic is infiltrated along the line of the incision with the needle inserted into the subdermal tissue parallel with the surface of the skin. Infiltration continues as the needle is advanced

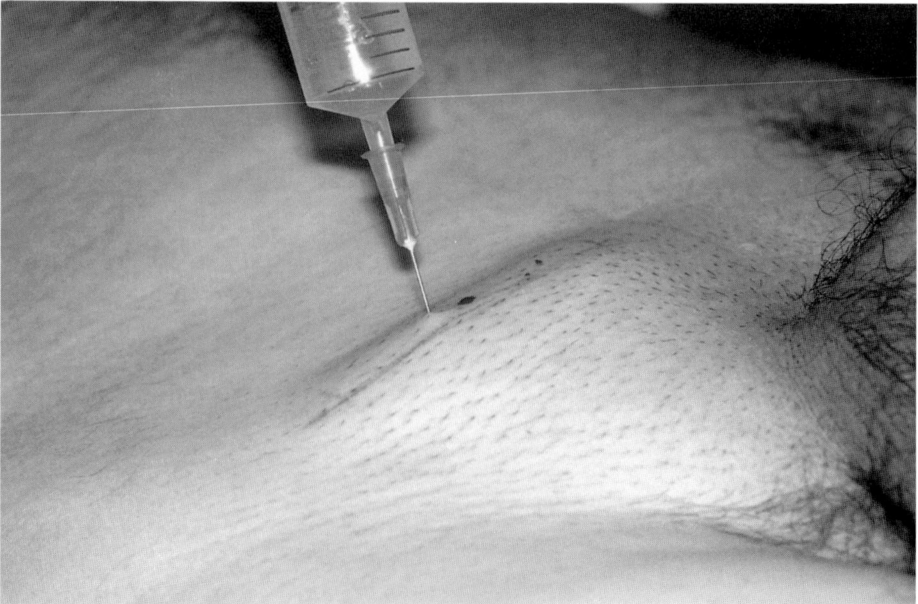

Figure 2. Deep subcutaneous injection. A total of 10 ml of the mixture is injected deep into the subcutaneous adipose tissue through vertical insertions of the needle (perpendicular to the skin surface) 2 cm apart

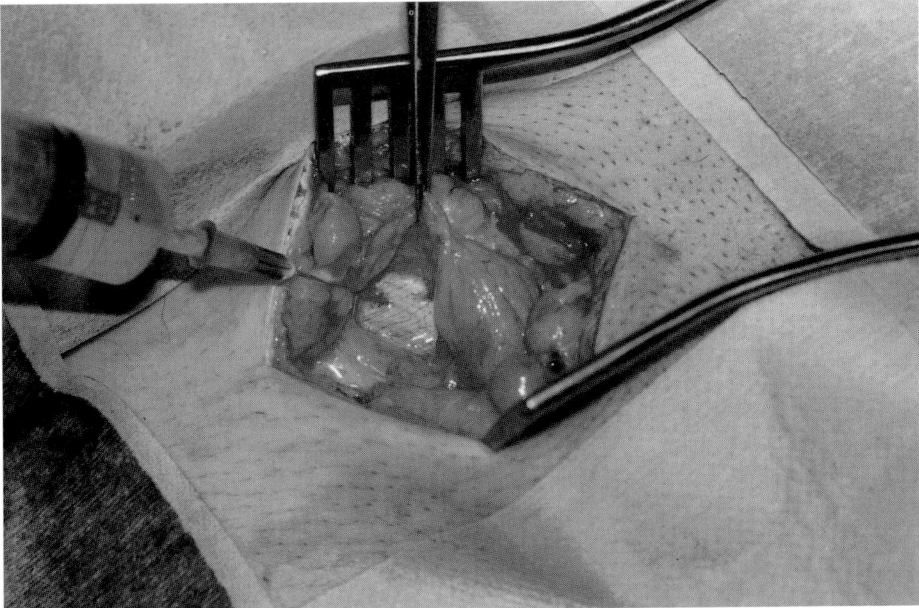

Figure 3. Right inguinal hernia viewed from the foot of the table. About 10 ml of the anaesthetic mixture is injected immediately underneath the aponeurosis of the external oblique muscle through a window created in the subcutaneous fat at the lateral corner of the incision

remain in the vessel long enough to deliver a substantial amount of the anesthetic agent intravenously. This step blocks the subdermal nerve endings and reduces the discomfort of the intradermal infiltration which is the most uncomfortable stage of local anesthesia.

2 Intradermal injection (making of the skin wheal). The needle in the subdermal plane is withdrawn slowly until the tip of the needle reaches the intradermic level. Without extracting the needle completely, the dermis is infiltrated by slow injection of about 3 ml of the mixture along the line of the incision.

3 Deep subcutaneous injection (Fig. 2). A total of 10 ml of the mixture is injected deep into the subcutaneous adipose tissue through vertical insertions of the needle (perpendicular to the skin surface) about 2 cm apart. Again, injections are continued as the needle is kept moving to reduce the risk of intravascular infusion.

4 Subaponeurotic injection (Fig. 3). About 10 ml of the anaesthetic mixture is injected immediately underneath the aponeurosis of the external oblique muscle through a window created in the subcutaneous fat at the lateral corner of the incision. This injection floods the enclosed inguinal canal and anesthetizes all three major nerves in the region while the remaining subcutaneous fat is incised. It also separates the

external oblique aponeurosis from the underlying ilioinguinal nerve, reducing the likelihood of injuring the nerve when the external oblique aponeurosis is incised. Occasionally it is necessary to infiltrate a few millilitres of the mixture at the level of the pubic tubercle, around the neck and inside the indirect hernia sac, to achieve complete local anesthesia. The local anesthesia can be further prolonged by splashing 10 ml of the mixture into the inguinal canal before closure of the external oblique aponeurosis and in the subcutaneous space before skin closure.

5 Epidural anesthesia. Epidural anesthesia is preferred for repair of nonreducible or bilateral inguinal hernias in obese patients. Sedative drugs given by the surgeon, or preferably by an anesthetist as 'conscious sedation' via infusion of rapid short-acting, amnesic and anxiolytic agents such as propofol, reduce the patient's anxiety. This also reduces the amount of local anesthetic agents required particularly for bilateral inguinal hernia repair.

TECHNIQUE OF OPERATION

A 5 cm skin incision, which starts from the pubic tubercle and extends laterally within the Langer's line, gives an excellent exposure of the pubic tubercle and the internal ring.

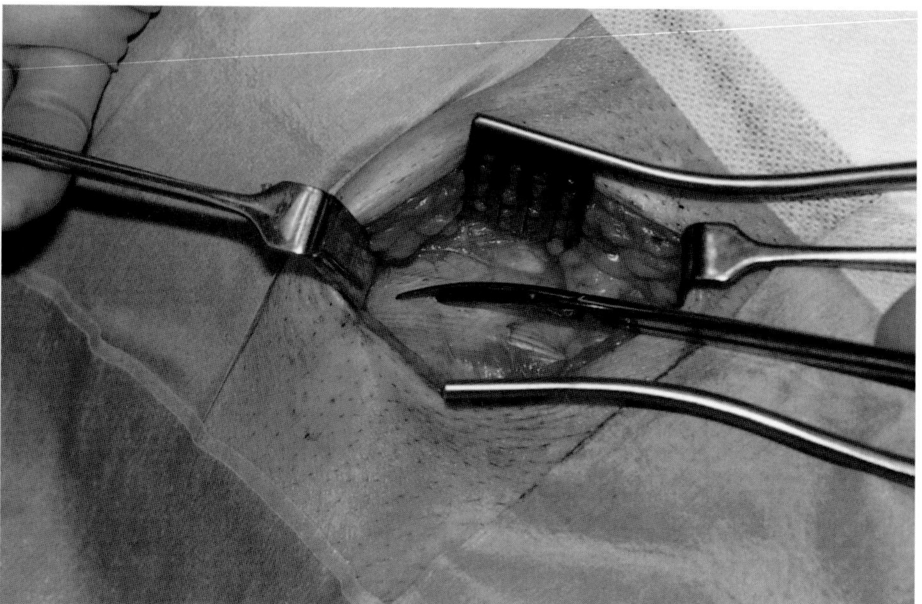

Figure 4. Opening the external oblique

After skin incision, the external oblique aponeurosis is opened (Fig. 4) and its lower leaf freed from the spermatic cord. The upper leaf of the external oblique is then freed from the underlying internal oblique muscle and aponeurosis for 3 cm above the inguinal floor (Fig. 5). The anatomical cleavage between these two layers is avascular, and the dissection can be done rapidly and nontraumatically. High separation of these layers has a dual benefit, as it visualizes the iliohypogastric nerve and creates ample space for insertion of a sufficiently wide sheet of mesh that can overlap the internal oblique by at least 3 cm above the upper margin of the inguinal floor. The cord with its cremaster covering is separated from the floor of the inguinal canal and the pubic bone for a distance of about 2 cm beyond the pubic tubercle (Fig. 6). The anatomic plane between the cremasteric sheath and the aponeurotic tissue attached to the pubic bone is avascular, so there is no risk of damaging the testicular blood flow. When lifting the cord, care should be taken to include the external spermatic vessels and the genital nerve with the cord. This assures that the genital nerve, which is always in juxtaposition to the external spermatic vessels, is preserved (Fig. 7).

Cutting or ligating the genital nerve can cause long-term incapacitating neuralgia.[7] The ilioinguinal and iliohypogastric nerves should also be preserved.

To explore the internal ring, for indirect hernia sacs, the cremasteric sheath is incised transversely (if thick) or longitudinally at the level of the deep ring (Fig. 8). The latter prevents disturbance of the retractibility of the testes. Complete stripping and excision

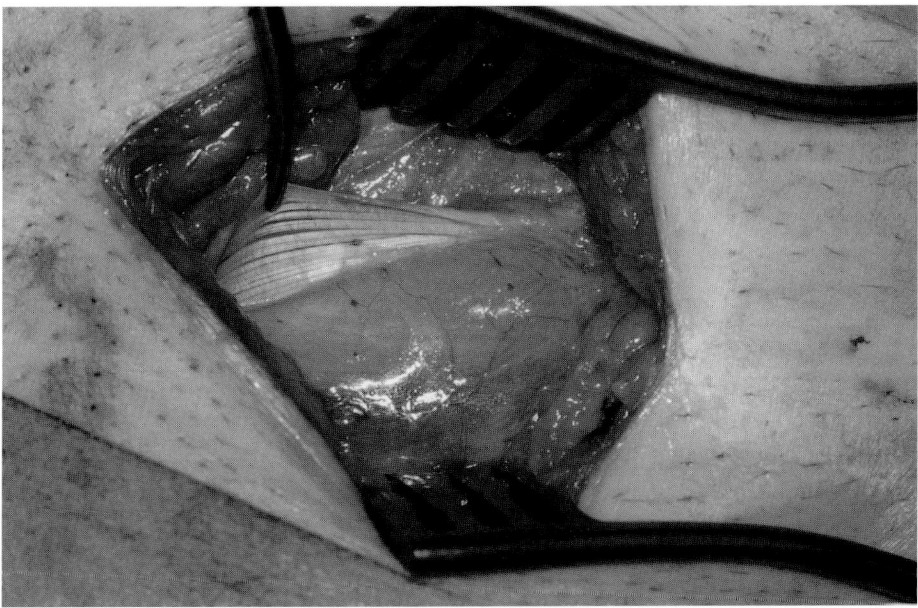

Figure 5.   The upper leaf of the external oblique is lifted

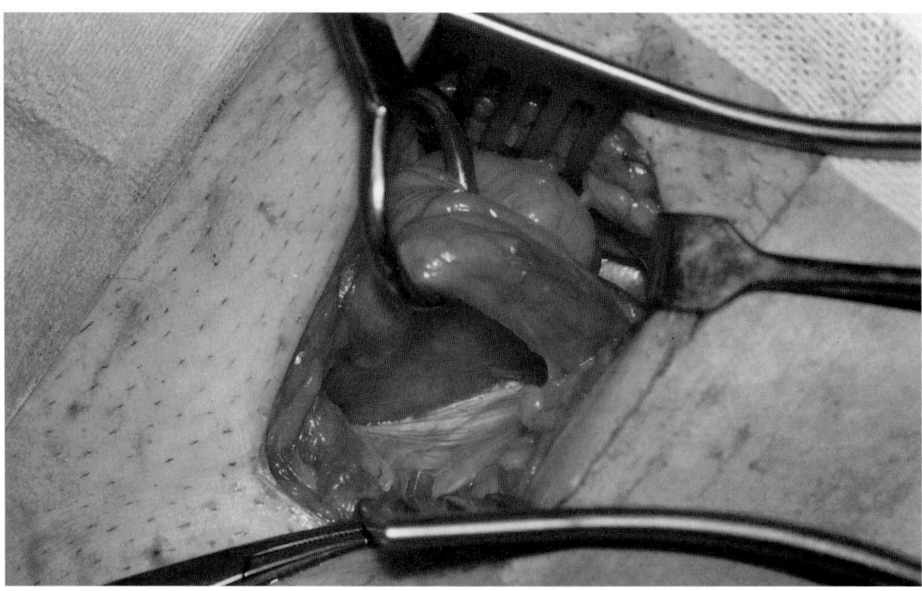

Figure 6. The spermatic cord with all its coverings is retracted superiorly exposing Poupart's ligament and the floor of the inguinal canal. In this case a direct sac is visible above the cord

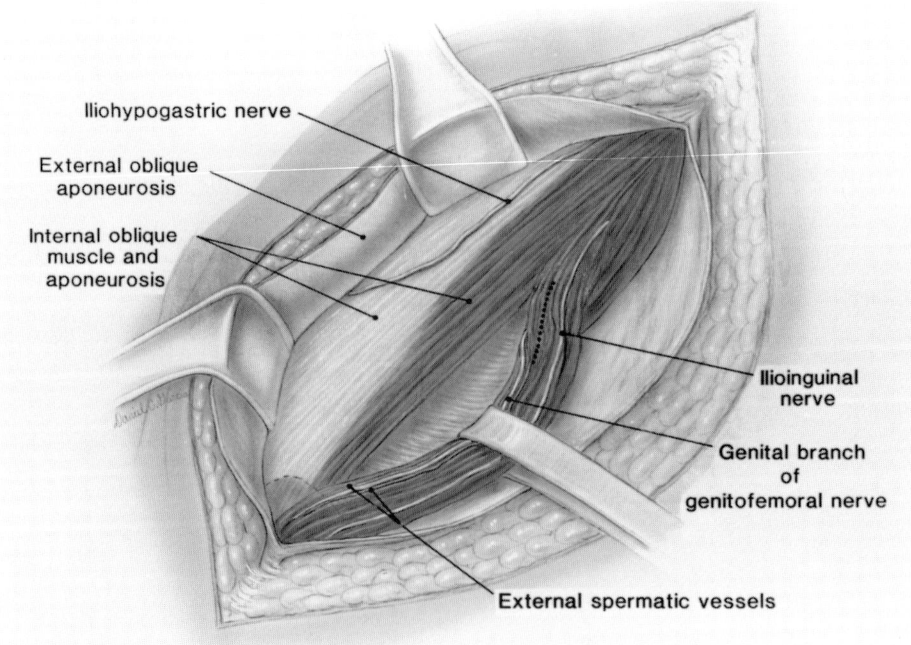

Figure 7. Spermatic cord together with its cremasteric covering, ilioinguinal nerve, external spermatic vessels and genital nerve is raised and the cremasteric fibers are cut transversely or longitudinally at the level of the internal ring

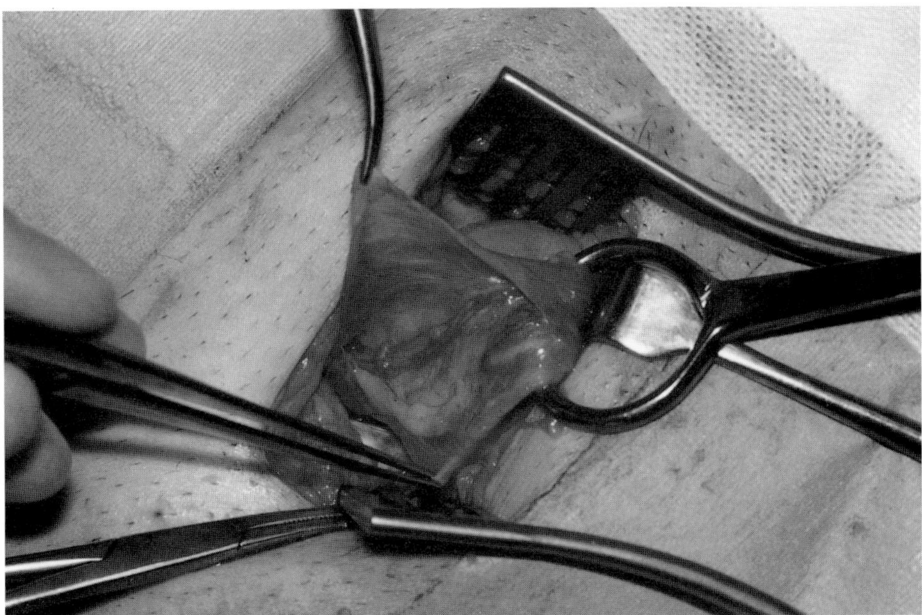

Figure 8. Cremaster incised longitudinally: this is atraumatic and results in minimal bleeding. A small lipoma of the cord and the vas deferens are visible

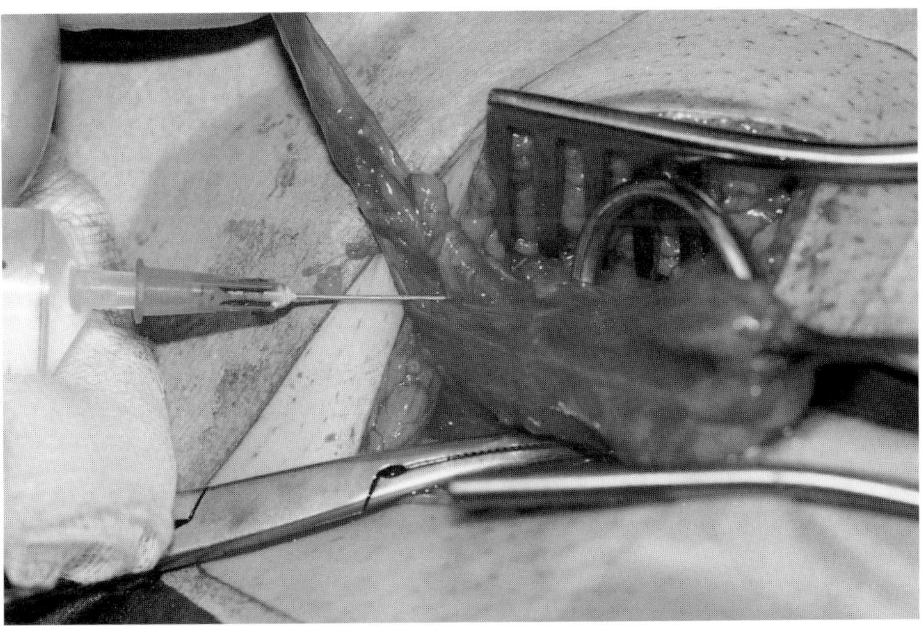

Figure 9. Indirect right inguinal hernia. In this case an indirect sac has been freed from the cord and local anaesthetic is being injected at the neck of the sac

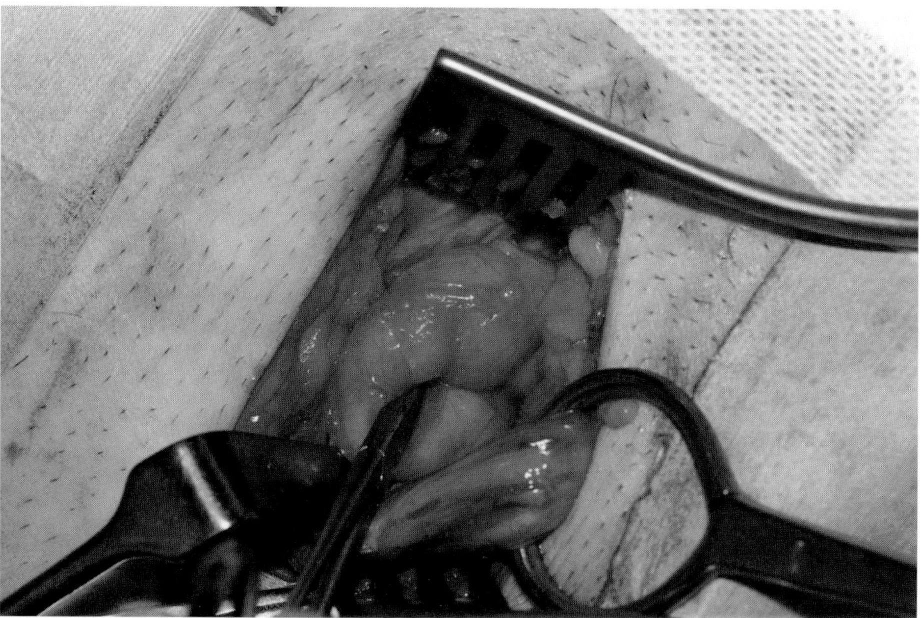

Figure 10. Direct left inguinal hernia. The spermatic cord is retracted inferiorly

of the cremasteric fibers is unnecessary, and can result in injury to the nerves, small blood vessels, and vas deferens.

Indirect hernial sacs are freed from the cord to a point beyond the neck of the sac (Fig. 9) and inverted into the abdomen without ligation. Due to mechanical pressure and ischemic changes, ligation of the highly enervated peritoneal sac is a major cause of postoperative pain.[8] It has been shown that nonligation of the indirect hernia sac does not increase the chance of recurrence.[9] To minimize the risk of postoperative ischemic orchitis, complete non-sliding scrotal hernia sacs are transacted at the midpoint of the canal, leaving the distal section in place. However, the anterior wall of the distal sac is incised to prevent postoperative hydrocele formation.

For large direct hernias, the direct sacs are inverted with an absorbable suture (Figs 10 and 11). A thorough exploration of the groin is necessary to rule out the coexisting intraparietal (interstitial) or femoral hernias. The femoral ring is routinely evaluated through the space of Bogros via a small opening in the canal floor.

An 8×16 cm sheet of mesh is used. We prefer monofilamented polypropylene meshes (such as Atrium, Marlex, Prolene and Trelex) because their surface texture promotes fibroplasia and their monofilamented structure does not promote or harbor infection.[10] The medial end of the mesh is rounded to the shape of the medial corner of the inguinal canal (Fig. 12).

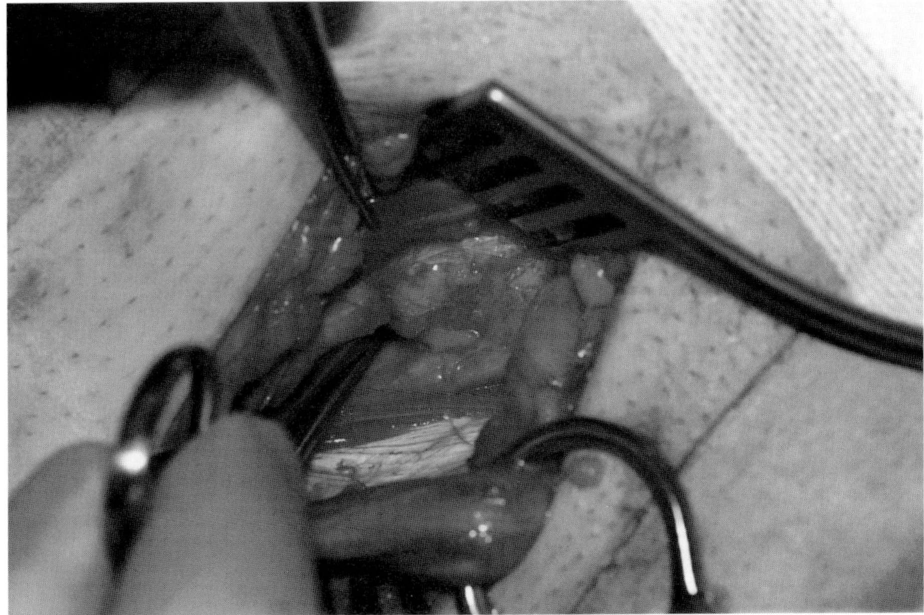

Figure 11. Direct left inguinal hernia. The direct sac is inverted prior to plication

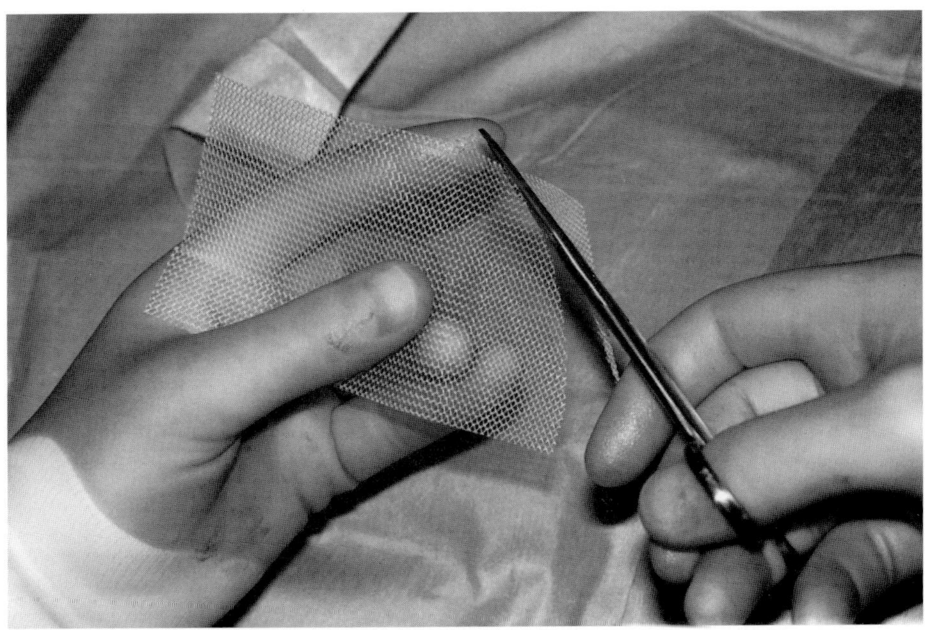

Figure 12. Cutting the mesh to size and shape

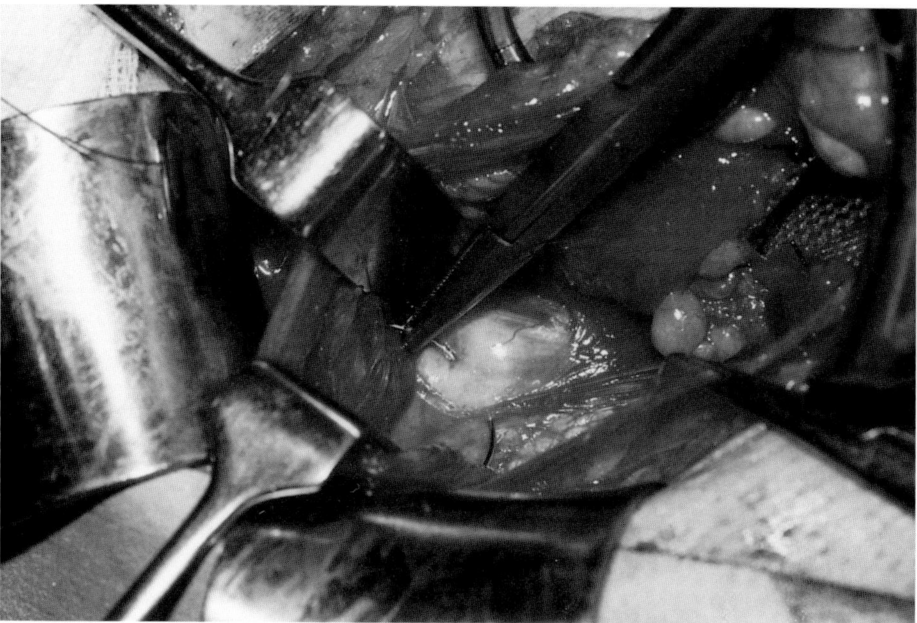

Figure 13. Left inguinal hernia viewed from the left and below. The needle takes in the aponeurotic tissue overlying the pubic tubercle but the periosteum of the bone is avoided

With the cord retracted upwards, the rounded corner is sutured, with a nonabsorbable monofilamented suture material, to the aponeurotic tissue over the pubic bone and overlapping the bone by 1–1.5 cm (Figs 13–16). This is a crucial step in the repair because failure to cover this bone with the mesh can result in recurrence; the periosteum of the bone is avoided. This suture is continued (as a running suture with up to five passages) to attach the lower edge of the patch to Poupart's ligament up to a point just lateral to the internal ring. Suturing the mesh beyond this point is unnecessary and could injure the femoral nerve. If there is a concurrent femoral hernia, the mesh is also sutured to Cooper's ligament 1–2 cm below its suture line with the inguinal ligament to close the femoral ring.

A slit is made at the lateral end of the mesh creating two tails, a wide one (two-thirds) above and a narrower one (one-third) below (Fig. 17). The upper wide tail is grasped with a hemostat and passed towards the head of the patient from underneath the spermatic cord (Fig. 18); this positions the cord between the two tails of the mesh (Figs 19–21). The wider upper tail is crossed and placed over the narrower one and held with a hemostat (Fig. 22). With the cord retracted downwards and the upper leaf of the external oblique aponeurosis retracted upwards, the upper edge of the patch is sutured in place with two interrupted absorbable sutures, one to the rectus sheath and the other to the internal oblique aponeurosis, just lateral to the internal ring. Sharp retraction of the

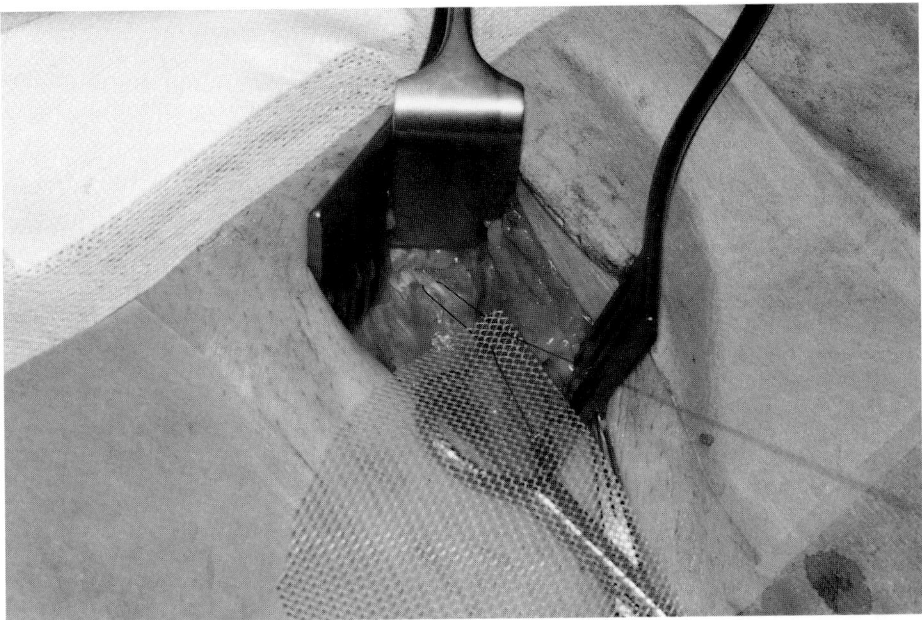

Figure 14. Right inguinal hernia viewed from the right and above. The inferomedial corner of the mesh is attached to the aponeurotic tissue overlying the pubic tubercle using a nonabsorbable suture

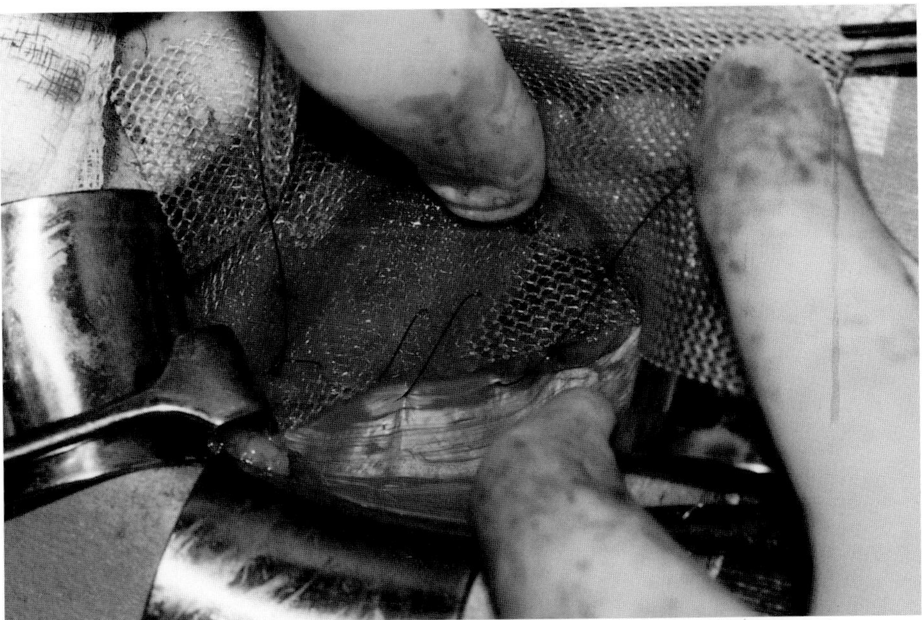

Figure 15. Loft inguinal hernia viewed from below. The inferomedial corner of the mesh has been attached to the aponeurotic tissue overlying the pubic tubercle and the suture is continued along the inferior border of the mesh attaching it to Poupart's ligament

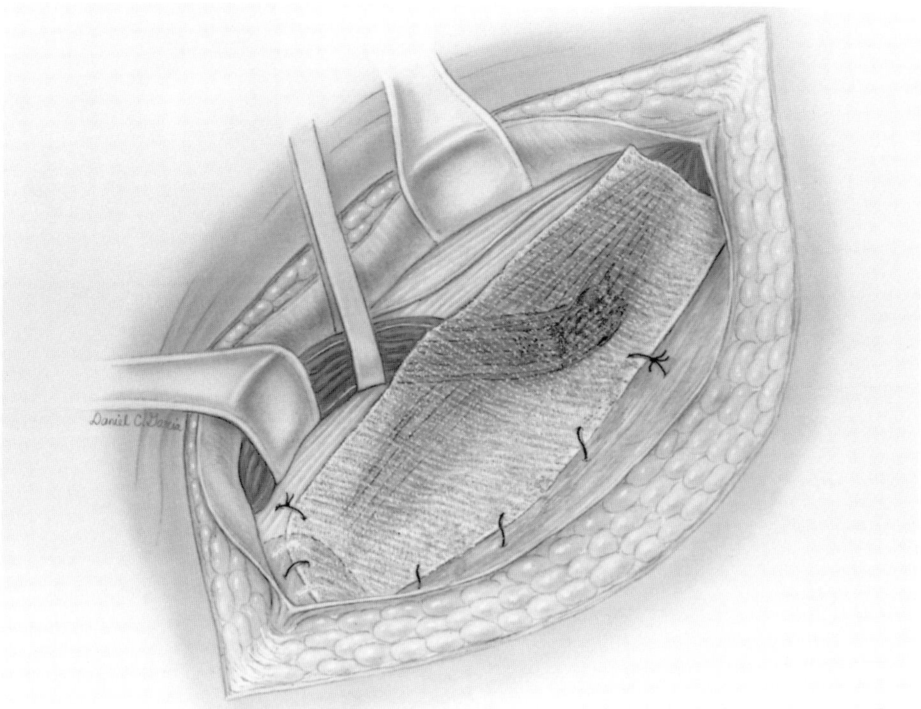

Figure 16. Medial corner of the patch overlaps the pubic bone by 1–1.5 cm

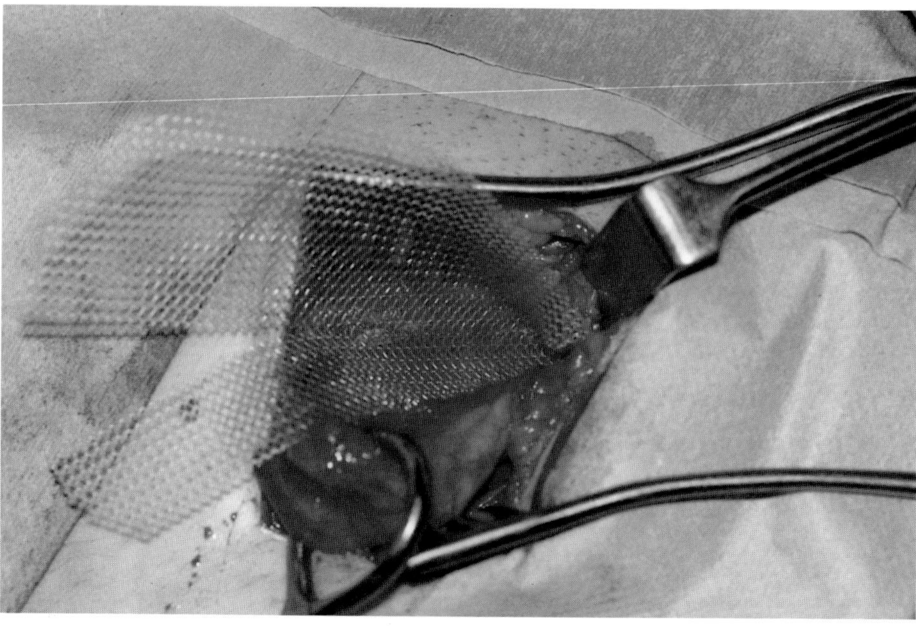

Figure 17. A slit is made at the lateral end of the mesh creating two tails, a wide one (two-thirds) above and a narrower (one-third) below

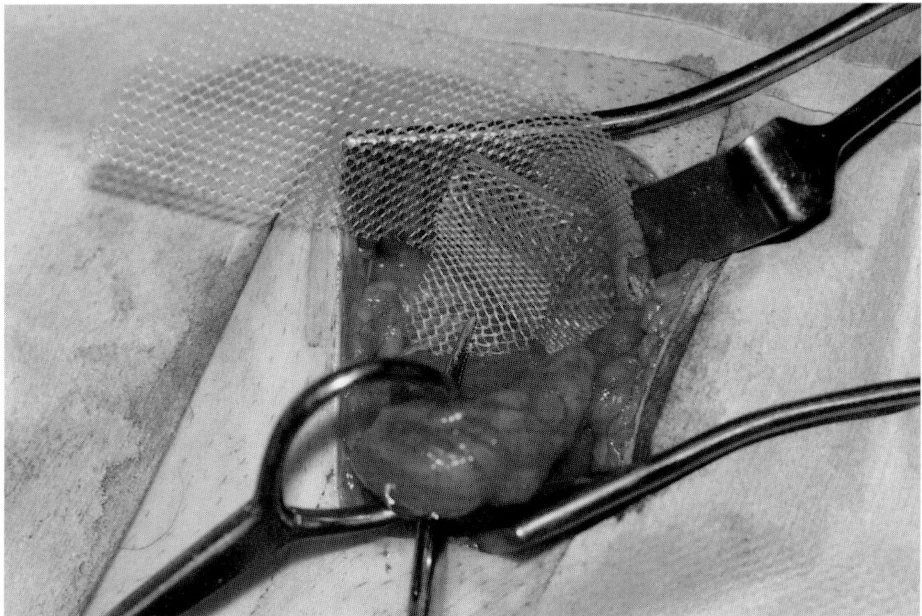

Figure 18. The upper wide tail is grasped with a haemostat and passed underneath the spermatic cord

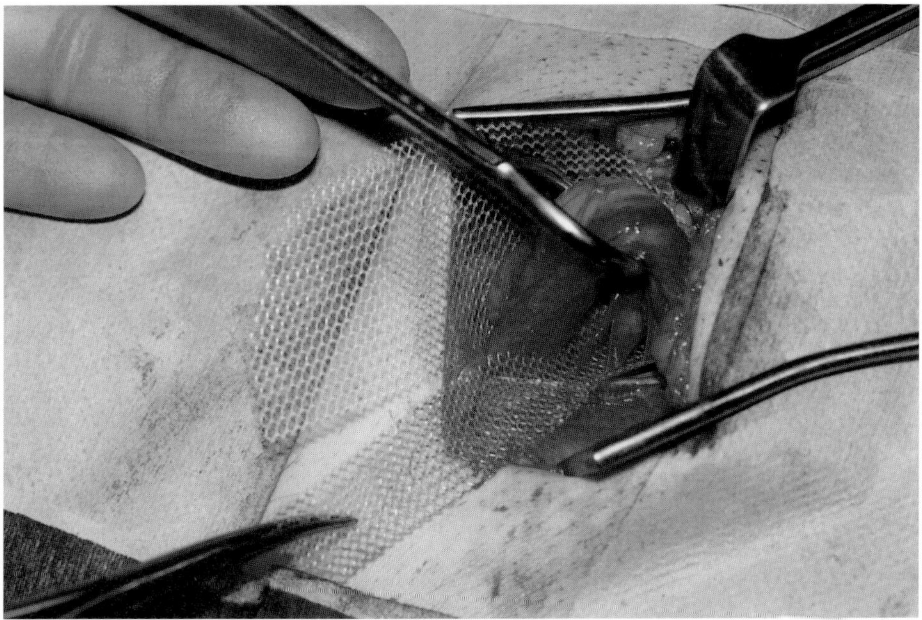

Figure 19. This positions the cord between the two tails of the mesh

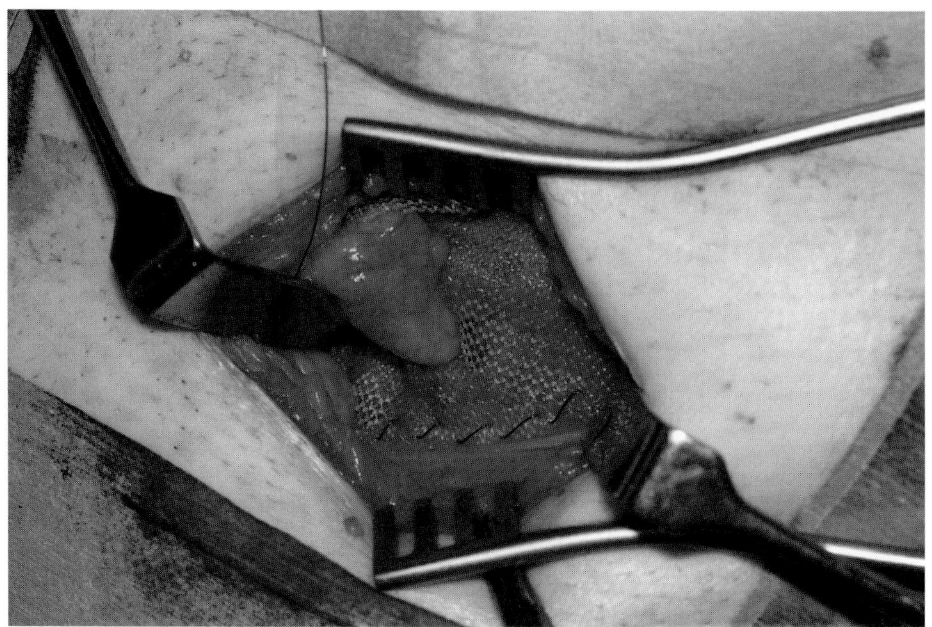

Figure 20.   Completed attachment of the inferior border of the mesh to Poupart's ligament

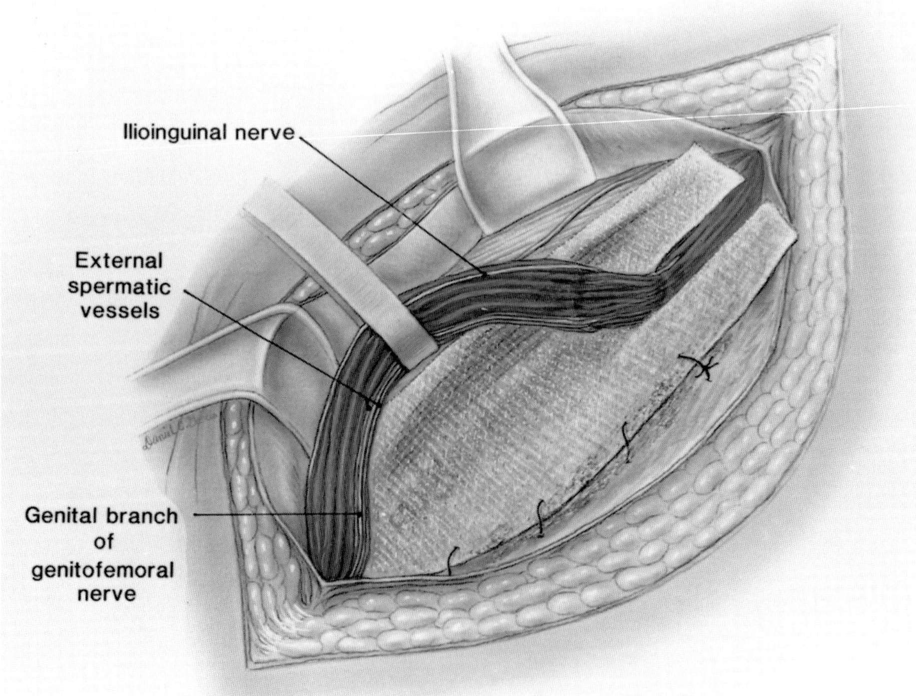

Figure 21.   Spermatic cord is placed in between the two tails of the mesh

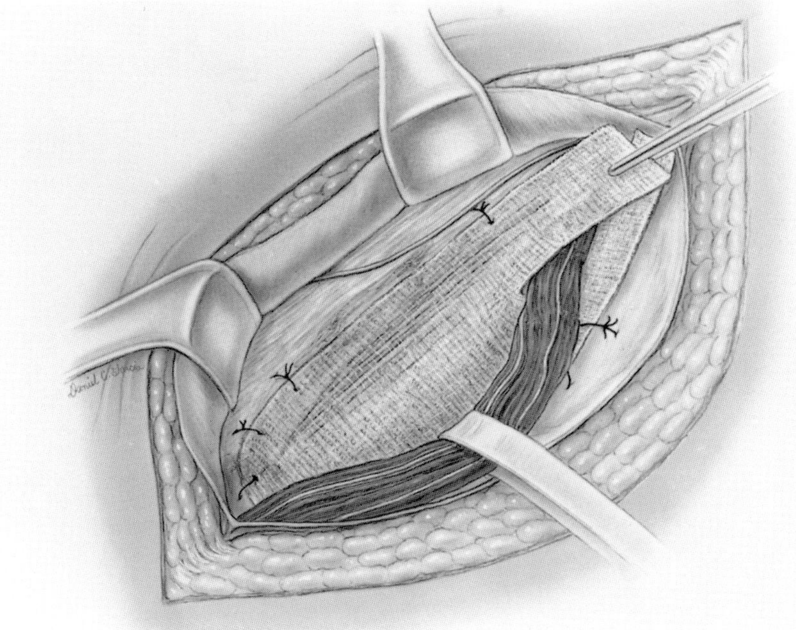

Figure 22.   Crossing of the two tails

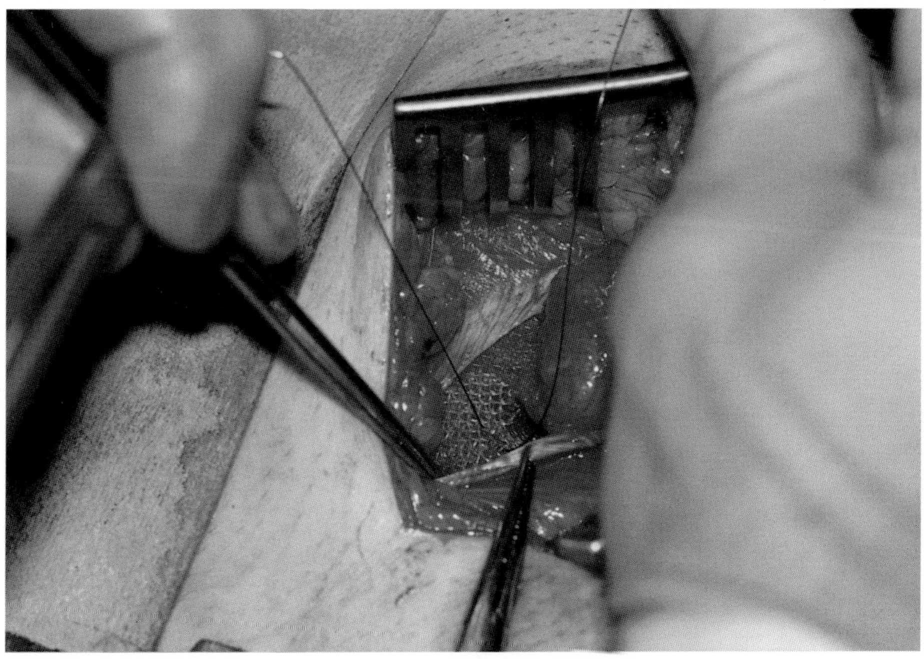

Figure 23.   Left inguinal hernia viewed from below. Using a single nonabsorbable monofilamented suture, the lower edge of each of the two tails is fixed to Poupart's ligament

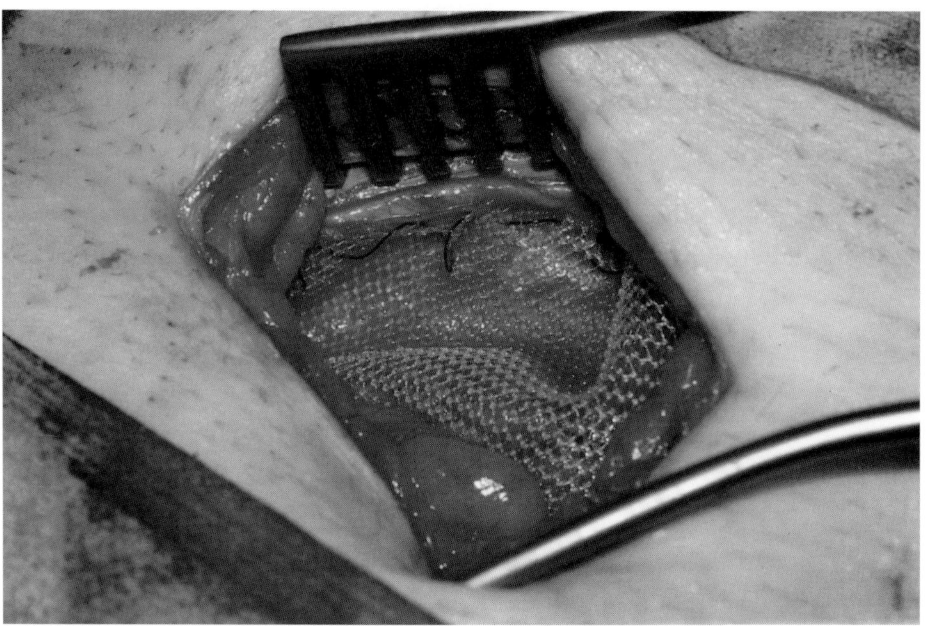

Figure 24. Left inguinal hernia viewed from the left and the foot of the table. The upper border of the mesh has been attached, in this case with a continuous suture. The slight laxity of the mesh ensures a 'tension-free' repair

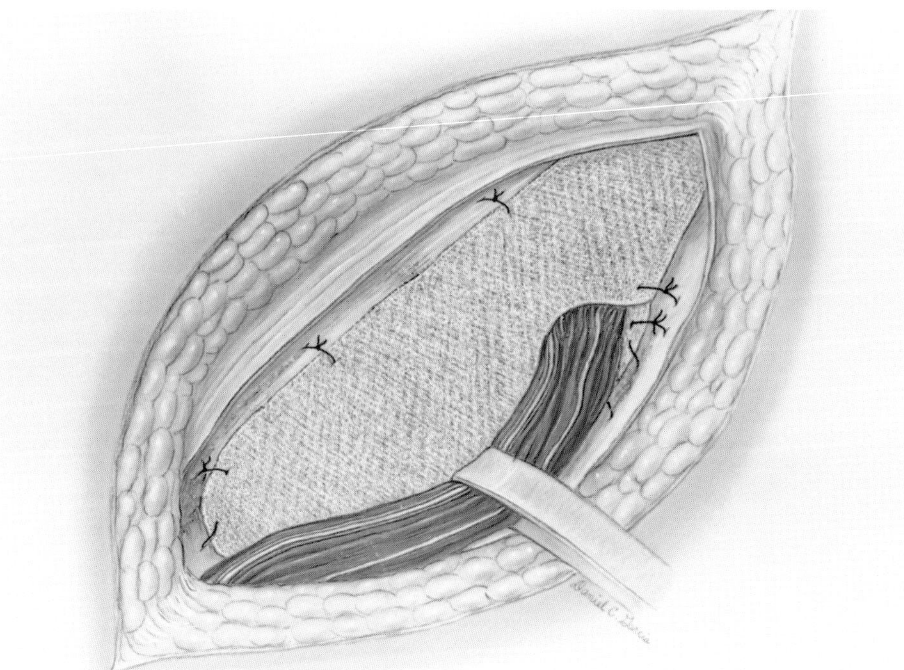

Figure 25. The lower edges of the two tails are sutured to the shelving margin for creation of a new internal ring made of mesh

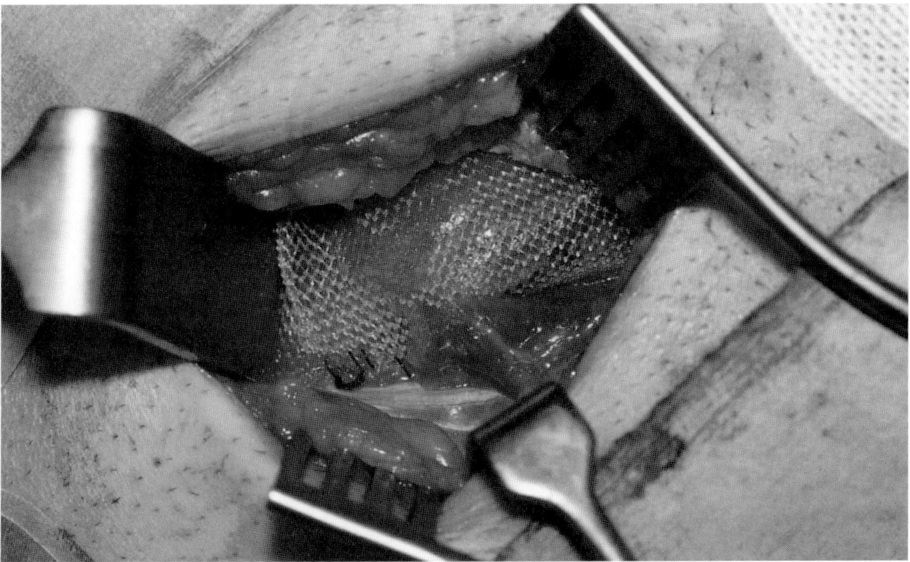

Figure 26. Right inguinal hernia viewed from the right and below. The lower edges of each of the two tails of the mesh have been attached to Poupart's ligament lateral to the emergence of the spermatic cord through the 'new' deep ring. Note the preserved ilioinguinal nerve lying on cremaster

upper leaf of the external oblique during this phase of the repair is important because it achieves the appropriate amount of subsequent laxity for the patch.[8] When the retraction is released, the mesh buckles slightly, and this laxity assures a true tension-free repair and is taken up when the patient strains on command during the operation or resumes an upright position.

Using a single nonabsorbable monofilamented suture, the lower edges of each of the two tails are fixed to Poupart's ligament just lateral to the completion knot of the lower running suture (Fig. 23). This creates a new internal ring made of mesh (Figs 24, 25). The crossing of the two tails produces a configuration similar to that of the normal transversalis fascia sling, which is assumed to be largely responsible for the normal integrity of the internal ring.

The excess patch on the lateral side is trimmed, leaving at least 5 cm of mesh beyond the internal ring. This is tucked underneath the external oblique aponeurosis (Fig. 26), which is then closed over the cord with an absorbable suture.

RESULTS

A total of 5000 primary inguinal hernias in 4000 adult male patients were performed under local anesthesia at the Institute from 1984 to 1995. The series included 1000 bilateral inguinal hernias, which were repaired simultaneously under local anesthesia.[11] The patients were age 19 to 86 years; 44% had indirect, 43.1% had direct, and 12.5% had a combination of indirect and direct inguinal hernias; 78% were of normal weight or up to 20 pounds overweight whereas 20% were 20–50 pounds overweight, and 2% were more than 50 pounds overweight; 27% had bilateral inguinal hernias and 11.4% had sliding hernias; and 60.2% had sedentary jobs, and 38.8% performed hard manual labor duties. The operative time, including the administration of local anesthesia was 20–45 min depending on the complexity of the hernia.

Outpatient surgery was performed on 99% of the patients, who had a 2–3 h hospital stay after the operation. One per cent of patients were admitted to the hospital because of unrelated medical or personal reasons. Analgesic requirement for postoperative pain was 0–20 (mean, 8) tablets of Vicodin (hydrocodone bitartrate 5 mg and acetaminophen 500 mg) for 1–4 days. Postoperative unrestricted activity was encouraged. Patients returned to their usual work activities with no restrictions between 2 and 14 days. There was one chronic postoperative neuralgia, and no patient developed a seroma requiring aspiration.

Recurrences

Early in the evolution of this technique, four patients developed recurrences as a result of technical errors. Three hernias recurred at the pubic tubercle because of failure to overlap the bone with the mesh. One recurrence resulted from total disruption of the mesh from the inguinal ligament because the mesh was too narrow. There has been only one recurrence in those patients operated on within the last 6 years.

Importance of follow-up

Reported recurrence rates by individuals or institutions are scientifically meaningless unless the method of follow-up is known and the length of observation is sufficient. The only reliable method of follow-up is by physician examination. Written questionnaires and telephone inquiries are notoriously unreliable and associated with 50% inaccuracy.[12,13] Short-term follow-up, particularly after mesh repair, solely reveals the therapeutic value of the repair.[8] A long-term follow-up of 10 years or more is required to evaluate the therapeutic value of the repair as well as its prophylactic effectiveness.[8]

Technical considerations

The use of a wide piece of mesh to overlap with tissues beyond the boundary of the Hesselbach's triangle for 3–4 cm is important to reduce the chance of recurrence. After incorporation is complete, this overlap results in uniform distribution of intra-abdominal pressure over the much wider surface of the overlapped area rather than just the line where the mesh is joined to the tissue.

Because the mesh is placed behind the external oblique aponeurosis, the intra-abdominal pressure works in favor of the repair. The external oblique aponeurosis keeps the mesh tightly in place by acting as an external support when intra-abdominal pressure rises.[8,14] Placement of the mesh underneath the transversalis fascia (such as the Rives procedure),[15] although a sound concept, requires unnecessary dissection and leads to excessive surgical trauma.

Proper fixation of the margins of the mesh to the groin tissue is another important step in the prevention of recurrence. In mobile areas such as the groins, there is a tendency for the prosthesis to fold, wrinkle, or curl around the cord. More importantly, *in vivo*, mesh prostheses lose approximately 20% of their size due to shrinkage.[10] The slightest movement of the mesh from the pubic tubercle, the inguinal ligament and the area of the internal ring, due to the above factors, is a leading cause of failure of mesh repair of inguinal hernias. Adequate laxity of the mesh must be allowed during fixation to totally eliminate tension and compensate for the increased intra-abdominal pressure that results when the patient stands or strains. A completely flat mesh with no ripple, in a patient under sedation and in a recumbent position, will be subject to tension in the standing position and with straining.[8]

Use of a plug

Creation of a new internal ring by crossing the tails of the mesh is a critically important part of the mesh hernioplasty. Insertion of a plug into the ring to secure the ring and to safeguard the repair by placement of the prosthesis in the preperitoneal space is not as effective as crossing the tails of the mesh.

The idea of using a plug, made of mesh, in hernia surgery was described by Irving Lichtenstein more than two decades ago for the purpose of repairing femoral hernias and selected cases of recurrent inguinal hernias. Recently, the plug repair method has been much commercialized and widely advertised as an appropriate alternative for the repair of inguinal hernias. Although completely sound for the repair of femoral hernias, the plug is not suitable for the repair of most inguinal hernias for the following reasons:

- Contrary to femoral hernias that occur through the femoral canal, which is a three-dimensional canal, inguinal hernias occur through a two-dimensional defect in the flat surface of the transversalis fascia. Therefore, the repair is not as effective because the contact surface of the plug is only the surface ring of the defect.
- Similar to the loose handmade plugs that after implantation lose up to 75% of their diameter,[16] the commercially available plugs, due to their looseness, can shrink and this result in recurrence of the hernia. More importantly, the shrunken plug can erode into the bladder or intestines.[10]

Therefore, besides being costly, these plugs are not an effective mean of securing the deep ring. An effective plug must be firm, because a soft plug that can be collapsed by pinching it between two fingers (the pinch test) would shrink as a result of the patient's own scarring process.[16] Even a firm plug, after its implantation, loses 5–10% of its diameter and fails to safeguard the internal ring as securely as crossing the tails of the mesh. Furthermore, plugs cannot act as an adequate preperitoneal prosthesis because they are far smaller than 10×15 cm, which is the minimum requirement of an adequate preperitoneal prosthesis.[15,17]

CONCLUSION

Use of the tension-free technique in conjunction with local anesthesia has drastically reduced the hospital stay, postoperative discomfort, recovery period, recurrence rate and cost of hernia surgery. Since its introduction, open tension-free hernioplasty has been employed by many surgeons worldwide with outcome measures identical to ours. A survey of 70 surgeons with no special interest in hernia surgery, who had done 22 300 Lichtenstein open tension-free hernioplasties, gave similar results.[18]

It is a testimony to the simplicity, safety, and effectiveness of open tension-free hernioplasty that the results from surgeons with no special interest or expertise in hernia repair are identical to those with a special interest in this subject.

The procedure is simple and safe and achieves all the goals of modern surgery, such as a more comfortable postoperative course and a rapid return to unrestricted activity, with a recurrence rate of virtually zero (0.1% from early operations). It also avoids the need for general anesthesia and invasion of the peritoneal or preperitoneal spaces and their associated complications.

REFERENCES

1 Lichtenstein IL. Immediate ambulation and return to work following herniorrhaphy. *Indust Med Surg* 1966; **35**:754–9.
2 Read RC. A review: the role of protease–antiprotease imbalance in the pathogenesis of herniation and abdominal aortic aneurism in certain smokers. *Postgrad Gen Surg* 1992; **4**:161–5.
3 Amid PK, Shulman AG, Lichtenstein IL. Local anesthesia for inguinal hernia repair step-by-step procedure. *Ann Surg* 1994; **220**(6):735–7.
4 Woolf CJ. Recent advances in the pathophysiology of acute pain. *Br J Anaesth* 1989; **63**:139–46.
5 Wall PD. The prevention of postoperative pain (editorial). *Pain* 1988; **33**:289–90.
6 Dubner R. Neuronal plasticity and pain following peripheral tissue inflammation of nerve injury. In Bond MR, Charlton JE, Woolf CJ, eds. *Proceedings of the VIth World Congress of Pain*. Amsterdam: Elsevier 1991; 263–76.
7 Lichtenstein IL, Shulman AG, Amid PK, Montllor M. cause and prevention of postherniorrhaphy neuralgia: a proposed protocol for treatment. *Am J Surg* 1988; **155**:786–90.
8 Amid PK, Shulman AG, Lichtenstein IL, Hakakha M. The goals of modern hernia surgery. How to achieve them: open or laparoscopic repair? *Probl Gen Surg* 1995; **12**:165–71.

9 Smedberg SGG, Broome AEA, Gullmo A. Ligation of the hernia sac? *Surg Clin North Am* 1984; **64**:299.

10 Amid PK. Classification of biomaterials and their related complications in abdominal wall hernia surgery. *Hernia* 1997; **1**:15–21.

11 Amid PK, Shulman AG, Lichtenstein IL. Simultaneous repair of bilateral inguinal hernias under local anesthesia. *Ann Surg* 1996; **223**:249–52.

12 Abramson JH, Gafin J, Hopp C, *et al.* The epidemiology of inguinal hernia: a survey in western Jerusalem. *J Epid Commun Health* 1978; **32**:59.

13 Panos RG, Beck DE, Maresh JE, Harford FJ. Preliminary results of a prospective randomized study of Cooper's ligament versus Shouldice herniorrhaphy technique. *Surg Gynecol Obstet* 1992; **175**:315–18.

14 Shulman AG, Amid PK, Lichtenstein IL. Mesh between the oblique muscles is simple and effective in open hernioplasty. *Ann Surg* 1995; **4**:326–7.

15 Stoppa RE, Rives JL, Warlaumont CR, *et al.* The use of Dacron in the repair of hernias of the groin. *Surg Clin North Am* 1984; **64**:269–86.

16 Amid PK, Shulman AG, Lichtenstein IL. Hernioplasty. In Bendavid R, ed. *Prostheses and Abdominal Wall Hernias.* Austin, Texas: RG Landes Co 1995; 389–94.

17 Wegener ME, Arregui ME. Laparoscopic totally extraperitoneal herniorrhaphy. *Probl Gen Surg* 1995; **12**:185–9.

18 Shulman AG, Amid PK, Lichtenstein IL. A survey of non-expert surgeons using the open tension-free mesh repair for primary inguinal hernias. *Int Surg* 1995; **80**:35–6.

11 THE MARLEX MESH PERFIX PLUG GROIN HERNIA REPAIR

Ira M Rutkow and Alan W Robbins

Since the early 1990s, surgical techniques used to repair groin hernias have undergone a profound transformation. In 1998 these changes are highlighted by the fact that a mesh prosthesis will be used in almost 75% of all inguinal herniorrhaphies done in the United States. American surgeons are increasingly interested in a 'tension-free' hernia repair in which a prosthetic mesh *is not* used to buttress or support a primarily sutured herniorrhaphy but *is* the actual repair. Of the newer mesh-based hernioplasties, the Marlex mesh PerFix plug (manufactured by CR Bard Inc.) repair has garnered the support of a growing number of surgeons. Because it is so simple the PerFix repair can be used for essentially all primary and recurrent inguinal and femoral hernias.[1-8] The 15–20 min surgical operation is done on an ambulatory basis and patients are discharged less than 2 h after completion of the procedure.

PREOPERATIVE ROUTINE

Epidural anaesthesia is used routinely, except in instances where back and spinal surgery contraindicates its application. Such regional anaesthesia allows the patient to cough or strain on command and assist in testing the integrity of the plug repair. The epidural agent (a 20 cm³ ampule of 3% chloroprocaine [Nesacaine] to which is added a 2 cm³ ampule of sublimaze [Fentanyl]) in addition to midazolam (Versed), preserves most motor function, which permits patients to move their lower extremities while under a profound sensory block with little peritoneal sensation. Because chloroprocaine has rapid onset and short duration, patients are able to walk within 60 min of the end of the procedure (Fig. 1).

The operative site (only the skin where the incision is to be made) is shaved just prior to the procedure. The skin is prepared with povidone/iodine and alcohol and a self-adhesive clear plastic drape is placed on the operative site, followed by customary draping. Antibiotics are not given, nor is the PerFix plug (Fig. 2) soaked in an antibiotic solution.

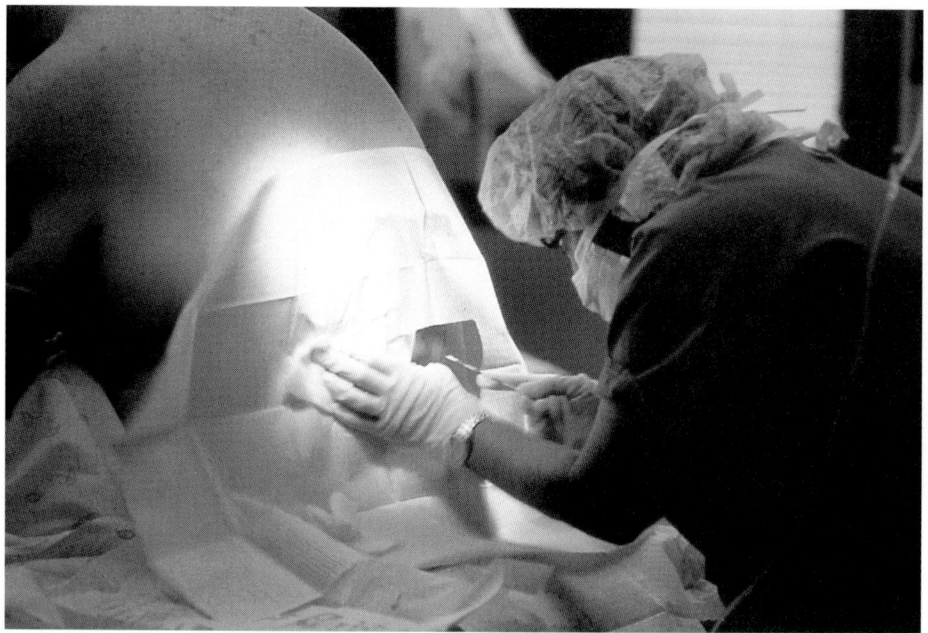

Figure 1. Administration of epidural anesthesia

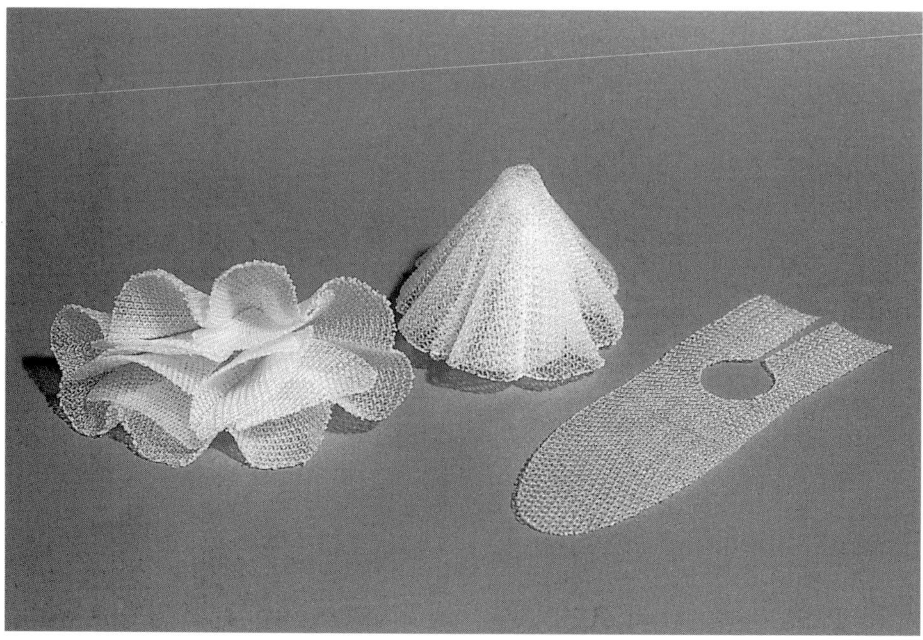

Figure 2. Marlex mesh PerFix hernia plug and onlay patch

REPAIR TECHNIQUE

An oblique, 4–6 cm incision of the epidermis, overlying the internal ring, is made with a scalpel (Fig. 3). All subsequent tissue dissection, including that of the hernial sac off the spermatic cord structures, is done with electrocautery. This instrument provides excellent haemostasis and helps reduce postoperative haematoma and seroma formation. The usual blood loss during a routine PerFix plug hernia repair is less than 5 ml.

The external oblique aponeurosis is opened and a self-retaining blunt-tipped Beckmann retractor together with a hand-held double-sided retractor provide excellent exposure. If the ilioinguinal and genitofemoral nerves are found they are preserved otherwise they receive no special attention. The spermatic cord is mobilized at the level of the pubic tubercle and a rubber drain is placed around the cord structures.

For indirect hernias, including large scrotal ones, the sac is approached initially by separating the cremasteric fibers longitudinally along the spermatic cord, so as not to destroy the cremasteric reflex. In completing an indirect herniorrhaphy, the most important element is a high dissection of the sac, not a high ligation. As the peritoneum is a sensitive structure, the long-held belief that ligating a sac is an

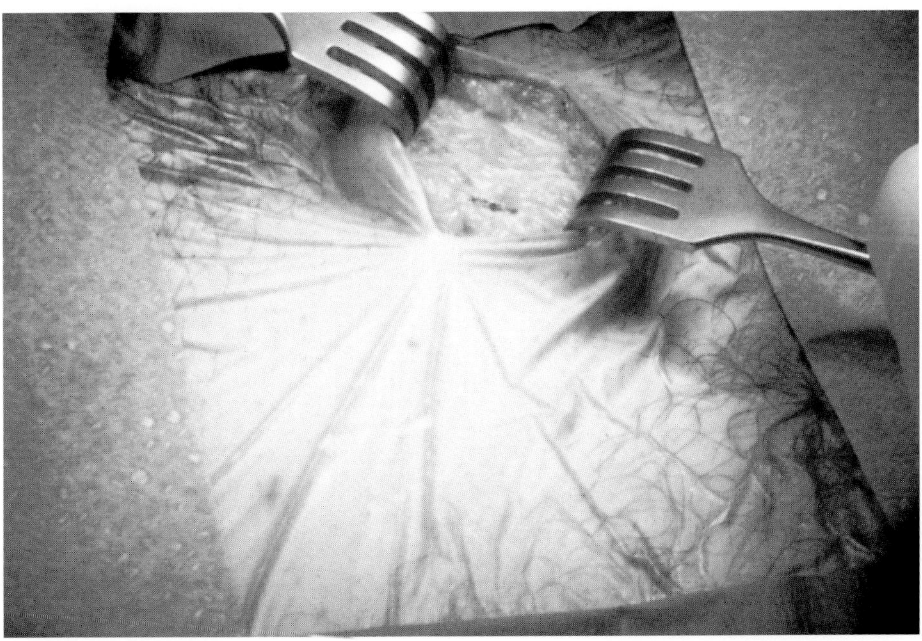

Figure 3. An oblique, 4–6 cm incision of the epidermis. All dissection, including that of the hernial sac off the spermatic cord structures, is completed with electrocautery

important part of any groin hernia operation does nothing more than lead to a 'miniature peritonitis' at the ligation site, causing increased postoperative discomfort. A high dissection is considered to be complete once the preperitoneal fat pad at the base of the indirect sac is visualized. The freely dissected unopened sac and any adjacent lipomata are then simply placed back through the internal ring into the abdominal cavity. A 'large' PerFix plug is inserted, tapered end first, through the internal ring and placed into position just beneath the crura (Fig. 4a–c). In small indirect hernias, the plug is kept in place by putting one or two interrupted sutures (3-0 polyglactin 910 [Vicryl]) through the outside fluted portion of the prosthesis and the crura. These are not meant to be strength stitches and any crural tissue, regardless of how flimsy it may appear, usually suffices. In larger indirect and scrotal hernias, the plug should always be secured to the margins of the patulous internal ring with multiple interrupted sutures. In any PerFix repair, if the plug's bulk is considered excessive, then some of the inside mesh 'petals' can be removed.

In both fusiform and saccular direct hernias, the attenuated transversalis tissue is raised with a clamp and the sac is circumscribed at its midportion so as to expose

(a)

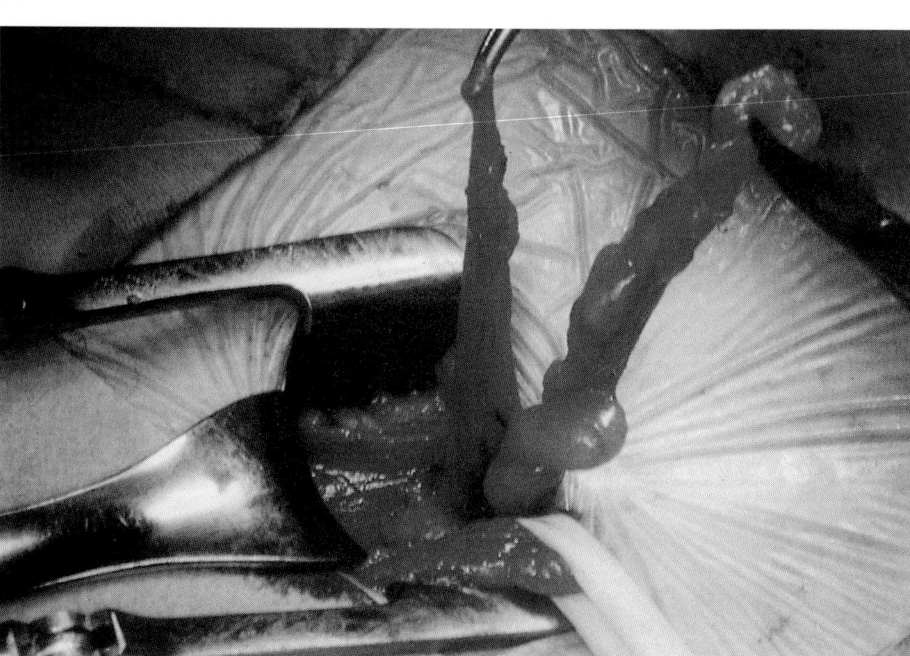

Figure 4. (a) An indirect hernia sac and its accompanying lipoma are dissected off the spermatic cord structures

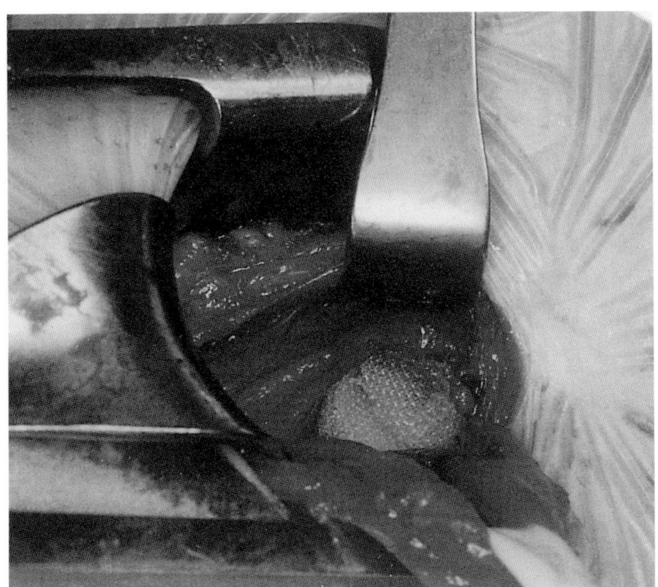

(b) Marlex mesh PerFix plug is placed into the internal ring and secured in position with interrupted sutures

(b)

(c)

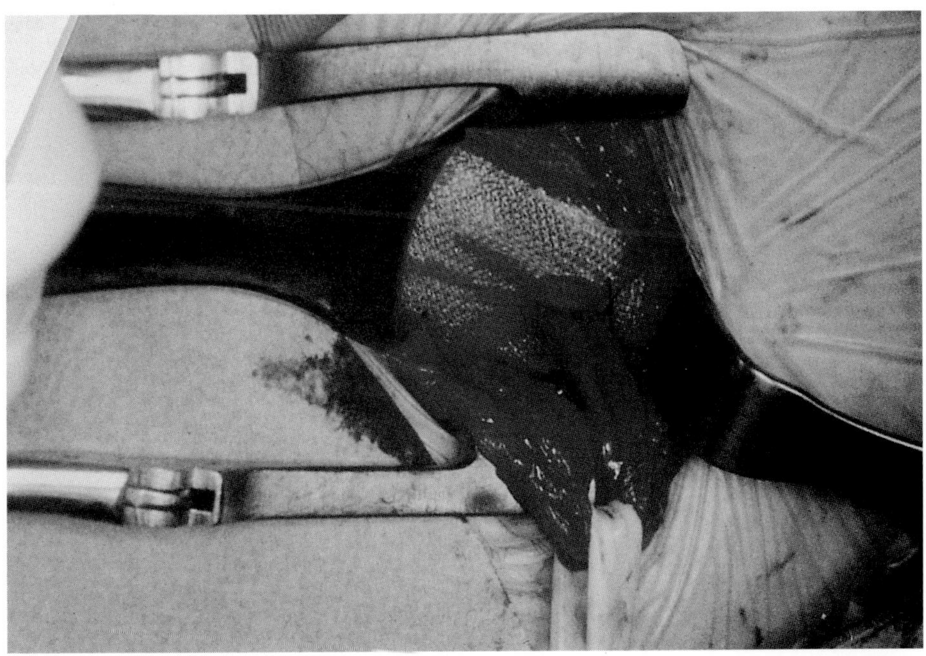

(c) An onlay patch encircles the spermatic cord while helping to strengthen the undisturbed direct space

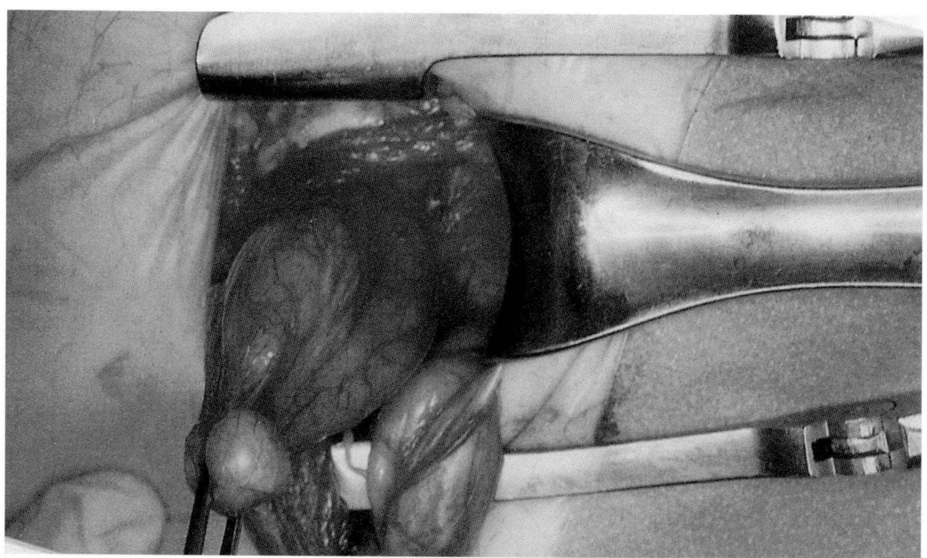

Figure 5. (a) A direct hernia sac is raised

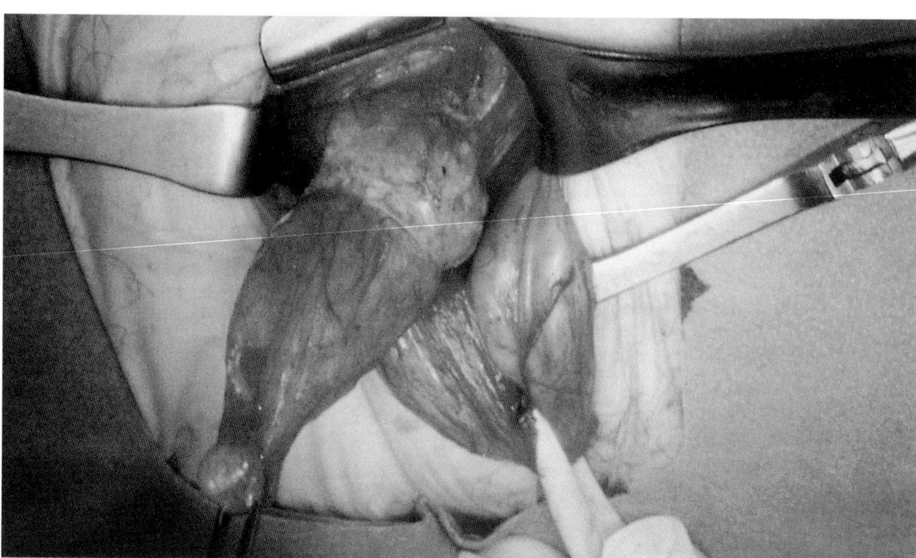

(b) Attenuated transversalis fascia of the raised defect is circumscribed so as to expose preperitoneal fat

preperitoneal fat (Fig. 5a–d). This creates an opening into the preperitoneal plane, where the PerFix plug must ultimately lie. The freed sac and overlying attenuated transversalis fascia/transversus abdominis aponeurosis layer are invaginated. As in an indirect repair, a plug is inserted narrow end first through the newly created defect in

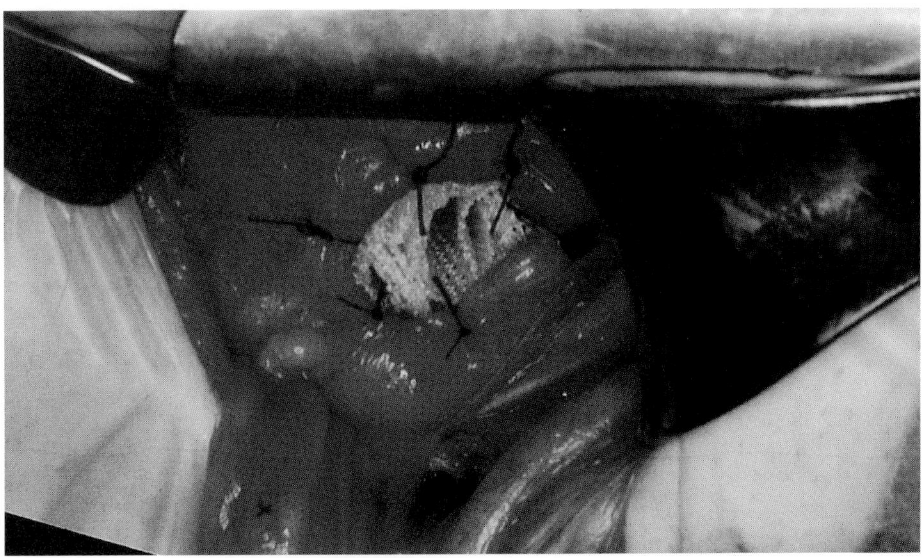

(c) Marlex mesh PerFix plug is placed through the direct defect and secured in a preperitoneal position with interrupted sutures

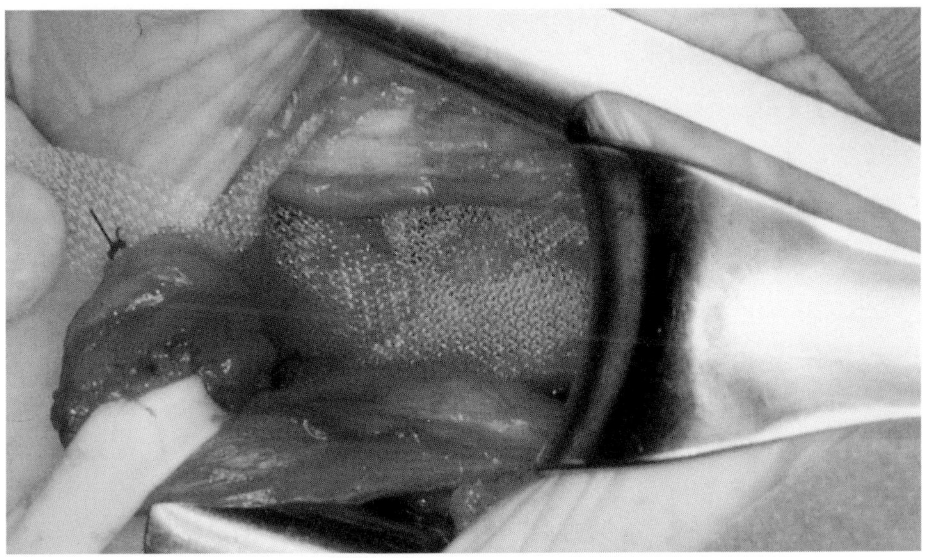

(d) An onlay patch encircles the spermatic cord to help strengthen the area of the internal ring, while lying on top of the previously placed PerFix plug

the floor (thereby serving as a toggle-like device) and secured with multiple interrupted sutures to surrounding intact tissue. Because Marlex mesh has a well-documented 'Velcro-like' reaction to tissue, any surface usually suffices to help hold the plug in position. For large direct or pantaloon hernias, the placement of two or even more

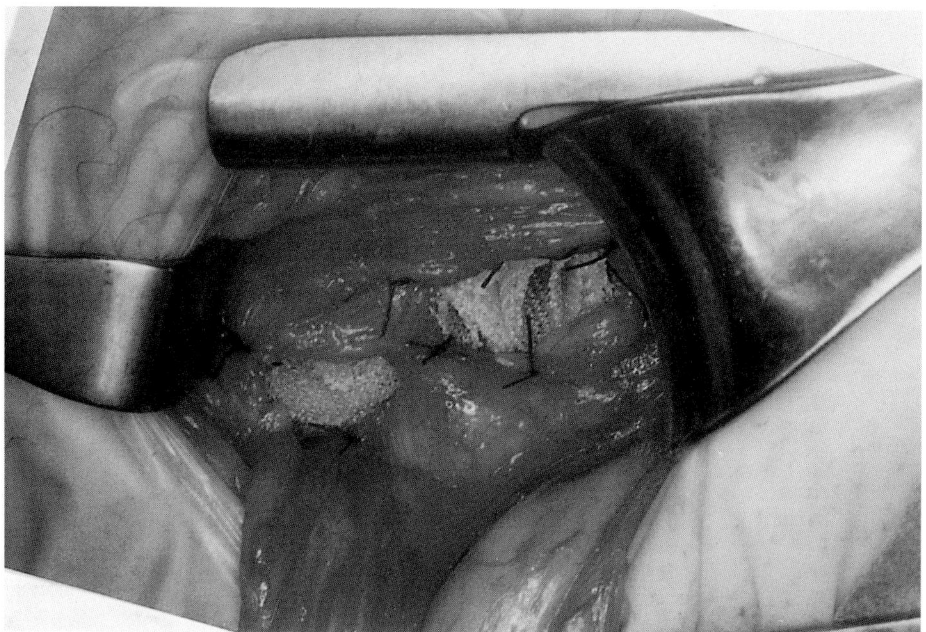

Figure 6. In a pantaloon hernia, two plugs are easily used

plugs has been successful (Fig. 6). Where such plugs abut they should be joined together with sutures.

All indirect and direct primary hernioplasties are reinforced with a second piece of flat Marlex mesh. This onlay patch is placed using a sutureless technique on the anterior surface of the posterior wall of the inguinal canal from the pubic tubercle to above the internal ring. The lateral portion of the pre-shaped onlay patch includes an aperture for the spermatic cord. This split section is sutured back to itself to provide an opening for the cord while functioning as a pseudo-internal ring. It is important to understand that the onlay patch is intended solely to strengthen the direct space in an indirect repair and the area of the internal ring in a direct repair. The onlay piece of mesh is not an integral part of the current repair, but is meant to serve as a form of further prophylaxis against future herniation.

Cord structures are placed on the anterior surface of the onlay patch. The external oblique aponeurosis is reapproximated over the cord structures with a continuous absorbable suture. Scarpa's fascia and subcutaneous tissues are brought together and the skin edges are coapted with a running subcuticular stitch of the same material. A transparent self-adhesive dressing is placed over the incision.

The PerFix plug repair is applicable for femoral hernioplasty. Using an infrainguinal approach, the mushroom-like appearance of a femoral hernia can be seen extending from the femoral canal. Adhesions between the hernial sac and surrounding tissues are freed. If the femoral opening is too small and the sac too bulky to be reduced adequately, the sac is divided and ligated. It should then be possible to reduce the remaining proximal portion of the sac. The sac is reduced from outside in through the femoral canal. Using a 'medium-sized' PerFix hernia plug, all inside 'petals' are removed and only the outside fluted layer of mesh is placed through the opening of the femoral canal. After proper positioning, the plug is secured with interrupted sutures to the surrounding fascia or other tissues which compromise the opening of the femoral canal. An onlay patch is not required.

The PerFix plug technique is suitable for virtually all recurrent groin hernias (Fig. 7a–c). In operating on such defects, the rule is to dissect as little as possible. Therefore, no routine attempts to identify fused anatomic layers are made. Unlike primary repairs, with a recurrent hernia the spermatic cord is not mobilized routinely as attempts at such mobilization can cause damage to an already compromised cord. The recurrent direct sac, be it fusiform or saccular, is simply dissected down to its base on the inguinal floor. Although disparate elements of the spermatic cord may be intimately attached to the sac, all that is necessary is a gentle dissection to peel such structures off the wall of

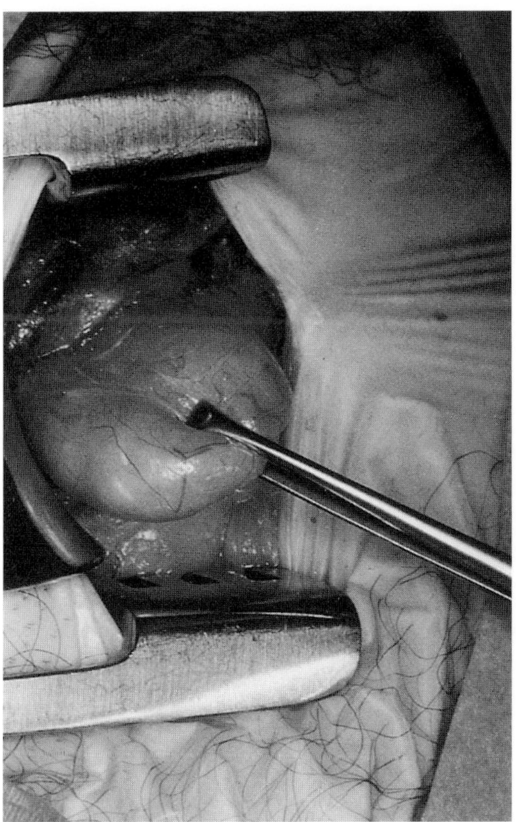

Figure 7. (a) A recurrent hernia sac is raised. Note the undisturbed spermatic cord vessels lying above the sac

147

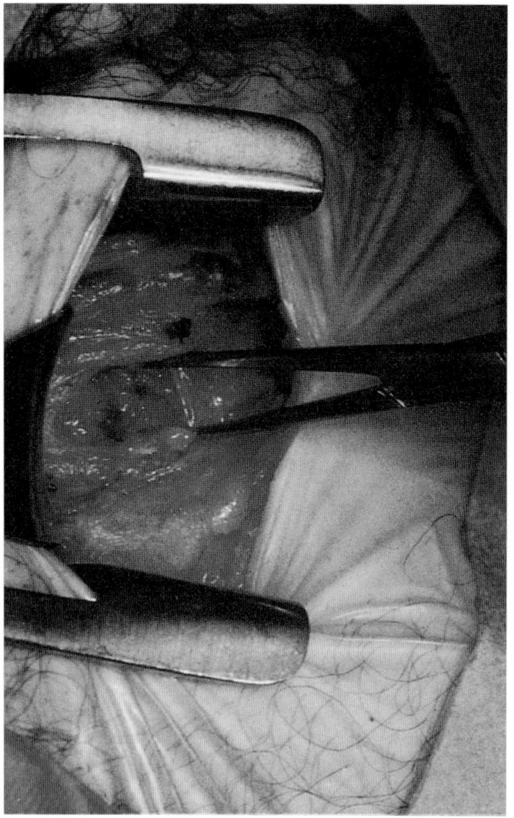

(b) Attenuated transversalis fascia is circumscribed, and the sac reduced into its preperitoneal position revealing a 1.5 cm direct defect

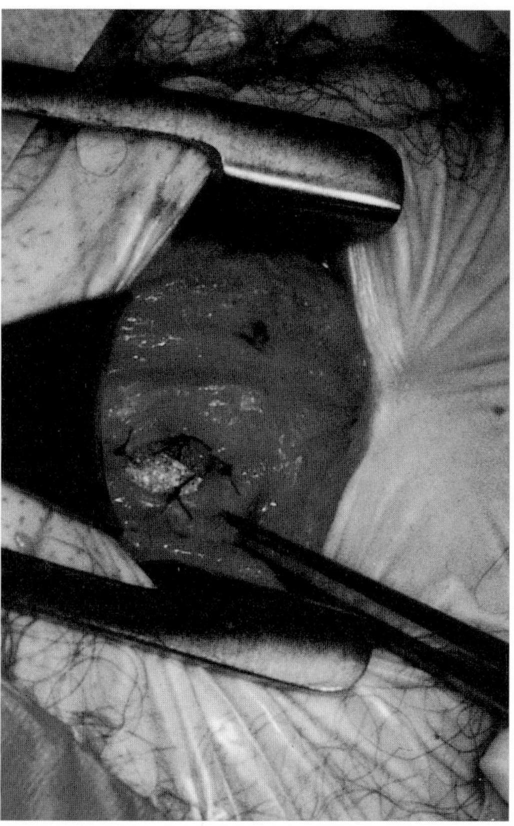

(c) Marlex mesh PerFix plug is placed through the recurrent defect and secured in a preperitoneal position with interrupted sutures

the sac. The base is circumscribed to help release the sac completely from adjacent scarred areas. The recurrent indirect sac is similarly freed, albeit to the level of the internal ring. The sac is reduced without ligation or excision. The plug is inserted into the defect and always secured with several anchoring sutures between it and the scarred margins of the rigid defect in the inguinal floor or the scarred internal ring. An onlay patch may be used if there is sufficient room (i.e. in the course of the dissection the spermatic cord was mobilized off the inguinal wall) to place it in position.

POSTOPERATIVE ROUTINE

Patients are discharged within 2 h of the end of the operation. The only analgesic used postoperatively is a single intramuscular injection of ketorolac tromethamine (Toradol) given in the recovery room. On discharge, patients are provided a prescription for propoxyphene napsylate and acetaminophen tablets (Darvocet N-100). All patients are encouraged to remain active, but are requested not to shower or drive a car for 24 h. They are instructed to begin lifting weights of up to 5 kg, whenever they like. All patients, assuming that they will feel all right, are told to resume normal daily activities (e.g. dinner engagements, gardening, light exercise, walking, and so on), including return to work, at their own discretion. Manual labour may be resumed in 2 weeks and other intensive activities (such as bicycling, jogging, and tennis) in a proportionally shorter time. All reasonable activities may be resumed by the end of the second to third postoperative weeks. They have their postoperative checkup during the first or second week, when the self-adhesive dressing is removed.

DISCUSSION

Nine years' experience (1989–1997) of over 3100 patients shows that the Marlex mesh PerFix plug groin hernioplasty is a simple surgical operation, and in a standardized form can be used to repair virtually any primary or recurrent inguinal or femoral hernia. Recurrence rates remain acceptably low (1% in primary and 3% in recurrent repairs), and most importantly, operative morbidity and short- and long-term complications are essentially eliminated. People are able to resume their normal daily activities promptly and return to work expeditiously.

REFERENCES

1   Robbins AW, Rutkow IM. The mesh-plug hernioplasty. *Surg Clin North Am* 1993; 73:501–12.
2   Rutkow IM, Robbins AW. 'Tension-free' inguinal herniorrhaphy: a preliminary report on the 'mesh plug' technique. *Surgery* 1993; **114**:3–8.
3   Rutkow IM, Robbins AW. 1669 mesh-plug hernioplasties. *Contemp Surg* 1993; **43**:141–7.
4   Rutkow IM, Robbins AW. Mesh plug hernia repair: a follow-up report. *Surgery* 1995; 117:597–8.
5   Rutkow IM, Robbins AW. Open mesh plug hernioplasty. *Prob Gen Surg* 1995; **12**:121–7.
6   Rutkow IM, Robbins AW. Groin hernia surgery in an office-based surgical suite. In Nyhus L, Condon R, eds. *Hernia*, 4th edn. Philadelphia: Lippincott 1995: 250–2.
7   Rutkow IM, Robbins AW. The management of groin hernia. In Cameron J, ed. *Current surgical therapy*, 5th edn. St Louis: Mosby 1995: 481–6.
8   Rutkow IM, Robbins AW. Hernia repair: the mesh plug hernia repair. In Carter DC, Russell RCG, Pitt HA, eds. *Atlas of general surgery*, 3rd edn. London: Chapman & Hall 1996: 59–67.

12 GROIN DISRUPTION IN SPORTSMEN

O Jeremy A Gilmore

INTRODUCTION

Injuries to the groin affect 5% of patients referred to sports medicine clinics[1] but account for a far greater loss of time from sport. Groin injuries may be acute but more often are chronic. In many patients, this chronic groin pain presents a complex management problem. It may be related to injury of the soft tissues, bones or joints and it may be neurological, orthopaedic, urological, gynaecological or general surgical in origin (Table 1).

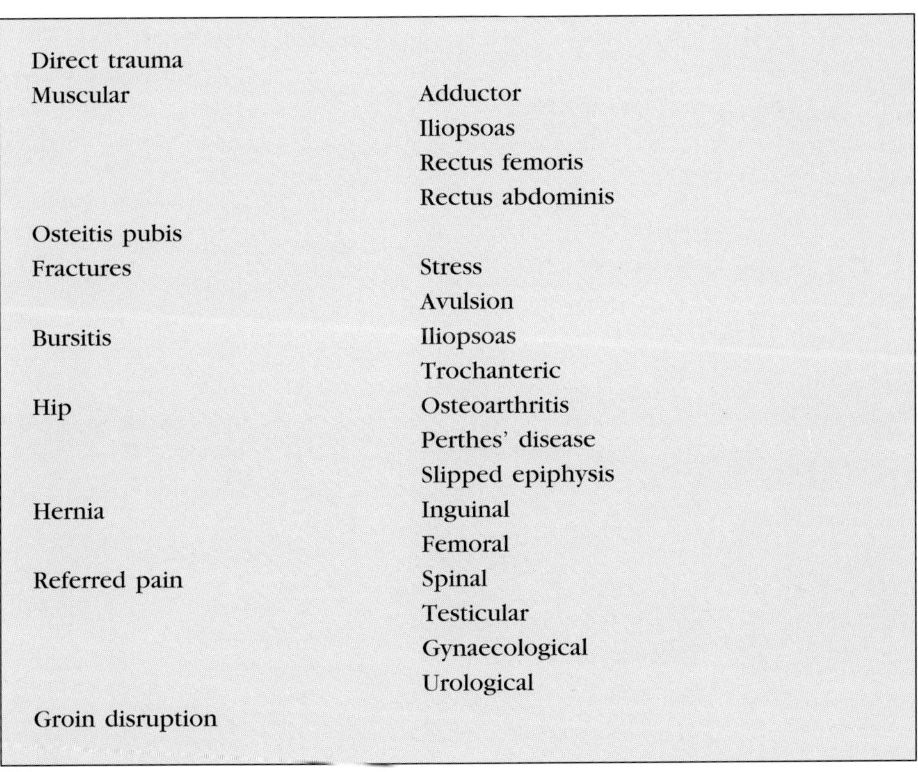

Direct trauma	
Muscular	Adductor
	Iliopsoas
	Rectus femoris
	Rectus abdominis
Osteitis pubis	
Fractures	Stress
	Avulsion
Bursitis	Iliopsoas
	Trochanteric
Hip	Osteoarthritis
	Perthes' disease
	Slipped epiphysis
Hernia	Inguinal
	Femoral
Referred pain	Spinal
	Testicular
	Gynaecological
	Urological
Groin disruption	

Table 1. Causes of groin pain

Sport	Total referred	Operation	Percentage
Association football	1598	1097	69
Rugby union	204	101	50
Rugby league	50	40	80
Athletes	61	25	41
Racquet games	74	20	27
Cricket	49	31	63
Hockey	29	14	48
Other sports/general fitness	241	72	30
Total	2306	1400	61

Table 2. Incidence of operation related to sport from 1980 to 1995

Groin disruption is *not* a hernia; there is no protrusion of a viscus beyond its normal confines. Groin disruption is a severe musculotendinous injury of the groin which can be successfully treated by the surgical restoration of normal anatomy.[2,3,4]

The syndrome was first recognized in 1980 following the successful treatment of three professional footballers from the Premier Division who had been unable to play for many months because of undiagnosed injuries of the groin. Since 1980, 2306 cases have been referred and 1400 have required operation. Of these, just over 100 had undergone previous exploration elsewhere. Of patients referred, 98% were male with the majority being soccer players.

Groin injury also occurred in other sports including rugby union, rugby league, athletics, racquet games, cricket, hockey and also in general fitness training and gym workouts. The incidence of surgery varied with each sport (Table 2) and according to the sportsmens' commitment. In football players, the incidence was 82% in professionals, 58% in the semi-professional and 54% in amateurs.

In amateurs, an operation is indicated if everyday life is affected or the loss of sport reduces their quality of life. In professionals, an operation is required if they are unable to play, or their game is deteriorating and conservative treatment has failed.

AETIOLOGY

The studies we have undertaken on soccer players show the underlying problems in groin disruption are muscle imbalance and overuse (Fig. 1). The strong hip flexors that are used to kick the ball tilt the pelvis forward; the forward tilted pelvis stretches the abdominal muscles, which become weak and fail to stabilize the pelvis; and excessive

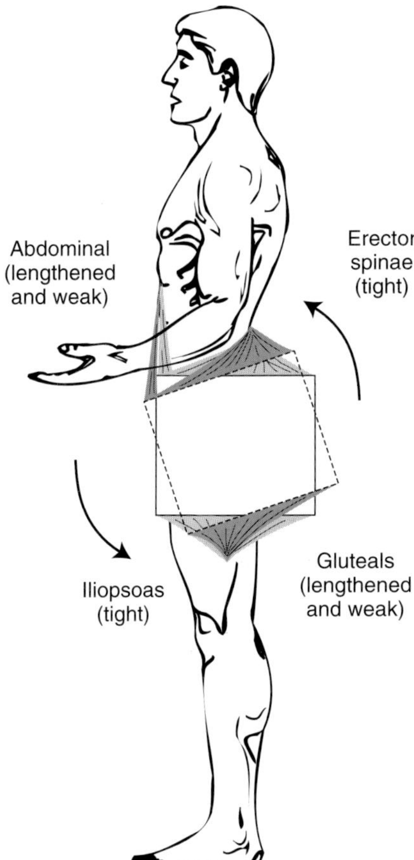

Figure 1. The pelvic crossed syndrome

physical activity results in tears of the groin and groin disruption. These patients also often have hamstring problems (recurrent tears) and back problems, often lordosis.

PATHOLOGY

The severity of pathology found at operation varies. However, the main features include:

- torn external oblique aponeurosis
- torn conjoined tendon
- conjoined tendon torn from the pubic tubercle
- dehiscence between conjoined tendon and inguinal ligament
- *no inguinal hernia is present,* either direct or indirect

Oedema and occasionally evidence of haemorrhage are present in acute cases. The severity of the tears usually correlates with the patient's symptoms.

153

SYMPTOMS

Symptoms from the largest single group, professional footballers, have been analysed: 814 cases have been referred and 664 required operation. Patients were from 77 of the 92 English football league clubs, while others came from Scotland, Ireland, Europe and the Middle East.

All patients presented with pain in the groin, mostly unilateral in the inguinal region. The site of the pain was not related to the patients' dominant side (right 47%, left 38%). In 15% of patients, symptoms were bilateral; 60% also had adductor pain and 6% had pain in the perineum.

The onset of symptoms was insidious in 70% of patients and there was a record of a specific injury in only 30%. The specific injuries included overstretching, excessive or mis-kicking, and abduction and eversion injuries.

The duration of symptoms varied from 2 days to 5 years, while the time since the last game, a most important consideration in a professional sportsman, varied from 1 to 57 weeks. During the first 3 years of the study, the average delay before referral was 15 weeks. During the next 4 years the average delay was 6 weeks, while more recently most players were referred within 3 weeks.

Players' symptoms vary with their team position: goalkeepers complain of pain with dead ball kicking; fullbacks and central defenders complain of pain with long ball kicking and turning; midfield players, who are often smaller and faster, find their game inhibited and their high work rate slowed; strikers and wingers lose acceleration and speed. Patients with adductor tears complain of pain with instep kicking.

Pain in the groin increases throughout a game, particularly during the last 20 min and is exacerbated by specific movements (Table 3). The day after a game, turning or getting out of bed or a car often causes pain, as does vigorous sexual intercourse.

During sport	After sport	
Sudden movement	Coughing	
Sprinting	Sneezing	
Striding	Sit-ups	
Accelerating		
Twisting and turning	Turning in bed	
Side stepping	Getting out of bed	Especially day
Dead ball kicking	Getting out of car	after game
Long ball kicking	Sexual intercourse	

Table 3. Causes of increased pain in groin disruption

PHYSICAL SIGNS

There are no visible physical signs, there is *no* hernia or swelling, and rarely any bruising except in acute cases. The physical signs, however, are palpable. The diagnosis is made by inverting the scrotum and placing the examining little finger in each superficial inguinal ring in turn. On the affected side the ring is usually dilated, there is a cough impulse and, most importantly, there is tenderness. Sometimes the tenderness is exquisite, but in patients who have been resting it may be minimal. In these patients, resumption of training is advised with a review at 10 days.

Adductor weakness is present in 60% of patients, and presents a particular problem. From experience, the solution to this problem is to repair the groin disruption, undertaking intensive adductor exercises both before and after surgery.

INVESTIGATIONS

Groin disruption is a clinical diagnosis based on history and examination. Pelvic instability must be excluded. Stork or flamingo views of the pelvis are taken and movement of the symphysis should be less than 3 mm. A herniogram is not diagnostic in groin disruption, since it is not a hernia, and this investigation usually fails to demonstrate musculotendinous tears.

An isotope bone scan is useful to exclude osteitis pubis, or hip, pelvic and spinal pathology. An MRI (magnetic resonance imaging) scan may show acute tears, but it is not reliable in chronic cases.

TREATMENT

Surgery is indicated in patients who fail to respond to a standard rehabilitation programme (Table 4). Successful treatment depends on an accurate diagnosis, meticulous surgery repairing each element of the disruption and vigorous rehabilitation.

Week	Activity
1	Walk four times a day plus stretching
2	Jog in straight lines, start adductor exercises and limited sit ups
3	Run in straight lines, increase adductor exercises
4	Sprint, start kicking, may play after one week of sprinting

Table 4. Groin disruption rehabilitation programme

Patients are admitted on the day of operation and return home following postoperative physiotherapy, usually within 24 hours.

Operation consists of diagnostic exploration of the groin and surgical repair of each element using a six-layered suture technique. Exploration is carried out through a 5–6 cm incision and each element of the disruption is identified. The external oblique, conjoined tendon, rectus abdominis, transversalis fascia, inguinal ligament, pubic tubercle, lacunar ligament and the adductor insertion are all examined and checked for contusions, tears and dehiscence. Normal anatomy is restored by repairing each element: the conjoined tendon and transversalis fascia are repaired, and also the rectus abdominis when torn; the repaired conjoined tendon is re-attached to the pubic tubercle and approximated to the inguinal ligament at a constant tension, repairing the inguinal ligament at the same time if necessary. The torn external oblique aponeurosis is repaired before Scarpa's fascia is closed, and the skin is closed using a subcuticular suture. Very rarely an adductor tenotomy is indicated.

RESULTS

Surgery in professional soccer players was considered successful in 643 out of 664 cases as measured by a return to league football. During the first 8 years of the study, the average time of return was at 6 weeks (range, 4–10 weeks). During the next 8 years the average return was at 5 weeks (range, 20 days to 7 weeks).

During the course of the study, 10% of patients returned within 1–5 years with contralateral disruption, having recognized the symptoms themselves. Complications have been minimal, most patients being young, slim and fit. There has been one wound infection. Eight patients subsequently required removal of the anchor stitch through the pubic tubercle and 10 required re-exploration for recurrent disruption.

During 16 years, 114 international soccer players – mostly from England, Scotland, Wales and Ireland with 25 coming from outside the UK – have been successfully treated.

DISCUSSION

Although soccer players are the commonest patients with groin disruption, other sportsmen (Table 2) and a few sportswomen (12 operations in 16 years) are affected.

In rugby union, half of the 204 patients referred required surgery; the majority were wing forwards, scrum halves and centres, that is, those players most involved in the game. Surgery was successful in 96 out of 101 patients.

In rugby league, players from any position can have groin disruption (indicating the difference between rugby union and rugby league in terms of mobility and involvement), and 50 patients were referred. Surgery was successful in 38 out of the 40 that required an operation.

Most cricketers with groin disruption were fast bowlers who complained of pain in the groin of their landing leg. A history of specific injury was unusual, and the symptoms had usually been present for months: 49 cricketers were referred and 31, including nine English fast bowlers, required surgery, which had a successful outcome in 29.

In racquet games, groin disruption makes twisting and turning especially painful, and the player's game is slow and inhibited. In tennis, the patients complained of pain in the groin on their serving side. Track athletes presenting with groin disruption were almost invariably middle and long distance runners plus the occasional hurdler.

For hockey players, a history of specific injury was rare; most patients were midfield players, playing two or more games a week on artificial surfaces.

During 16 years of experience, 48 international sportsmen (not soccer players) have required surgery including those participating in rugby league (15), rugby union (7), cricket (10), hockey (4) and athletics (4).

SUMMARY

Groin disruption is a severe musculotendinous injury; it is *not* a hernia – if it were a hernia the diagnosis would have been established long ago. The incidence of groin disruption is increasing in all sports as more games are played and fewer players take breaks between seasons. The incidence of diagnosis is also increasing as more doctors and physiotherapists have become aware of the syndrome. Previously many patients were diagnosed as suffering from osteitis pubis and were subjected to long periods of rest; a few underwent unnecessary pubic symphysis fusion; and some professional sportsmen were forced to retire.

Careful rehabilitation is effective in some – especially younger – patients with less severe disruption. However, many do not recover, even with prolonged rest. In chronic cases, healing will not occur because the torn conjoined tendon is separated from the pubic tubercle and the inguinal ligament, and no amount of rest will result in the approximation of these structures.

The recognition and surgical treatment of the groin disruption has resulted in the rapid restoration of many sportsmens' careers.

REFERENCES

1   Renstrom P. Swedish research in sports traumatology. *Chir Orthop* 1994; **191**:144–58.
2   Gilmore OJA. Gilmore's groin: ten years experience of groin disruption – a previously unsolved problem in sportsmen. *Sports Med Soft Tissue Trauma* 1991; 3:12–14.
3   Gilmore OJA. Gilmore's groin: a previously unsolved problem in sportsmen. In MacLeod DAD, Maughan RJ, Williams C *et al*, eds. *Intermittent high intensity exercise – preparation, stresses and damage limitation.* London: E & FN Spon 1993; 477–86.
4   Gilmore, OJA. Gilmore's groin. Physiotherapy in sport. *J Ass Chartered Physiother Sport* 1995; **18**:14–15.

13 HERNIOGRAPHY

Terry Irwin, John Lawson and Nial Eames

INTRODUCTION

Although herniography has been available for many years, it has not proved popular, except in a few specialized units.[1–4] Many surgeons are simply unaware of the technique and the indications for it. Herniography in children has been abandoned.[5]

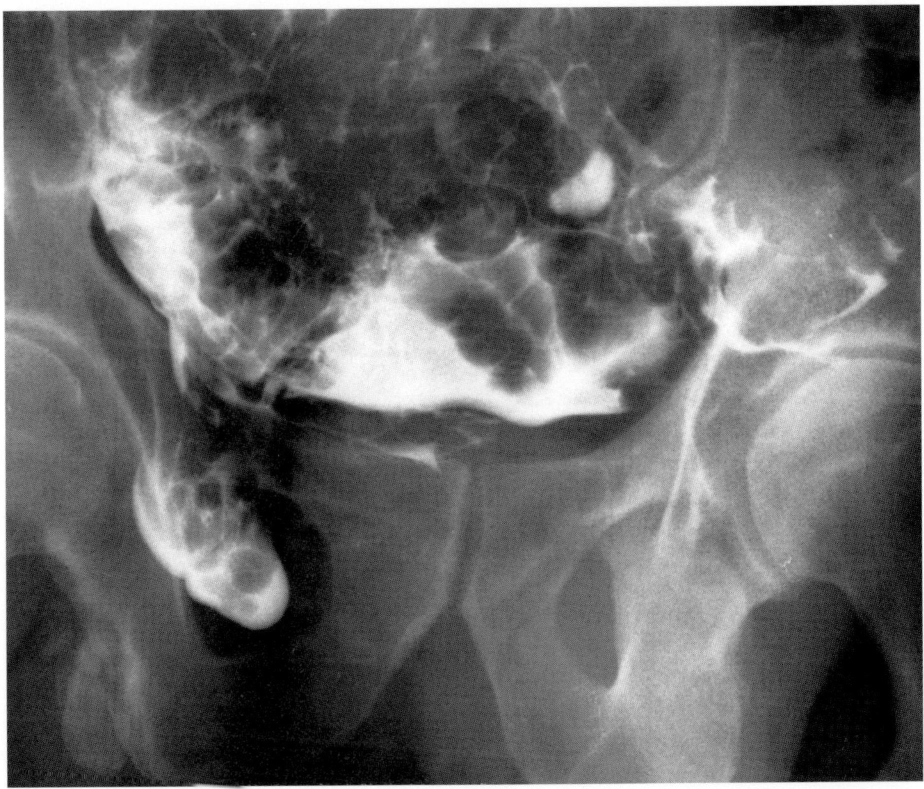

Figure 1. This young man with chronic groin pain had a positive herniogram, but his adductor periostitis was the cause of his pain

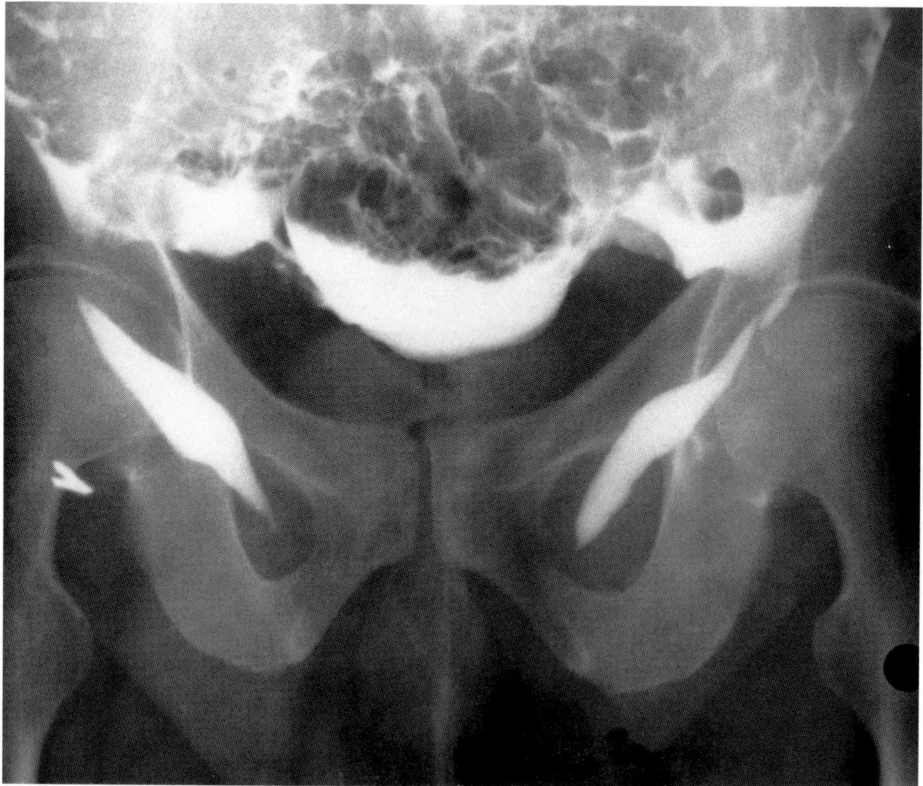

Figure 2.   Bilateral indirect inguinal hernia: only the right side was symptomatic

Herniography is not a panacea for all groin pain, and demonstrated hernias are not necessarily the cause of the groin pain (Fig. 1). Indeed, asymptomatic, contralateral hernias are frequently demonstrated[6] (Fig. 2). This raises the question, what should be done about herniographically demonstrated but clinically occult hernias, and long-term follow-up studies will be needed to provide rational answers.

Our own experience suggests that herniography yields returns only when careful selection criteria are applied. In our first 52 cases,[7] performed at a time when the technique was largely restricted to one consultant surgeon's practice, over one-third of herniograms were positive. With wider use of the technique by other practitioners, during the next 50 cases, only 9 of 88 investigations were positive.

INDICATIONS

The commonest indication for herniography is the presence of pain in the groin, located in or near to the inguinal canal or radiating into the scrotum.[1,2,7–11] In most cases this is the main presenting symptom and no swelling can be palpated.[7,12,13] Obviously, without saying that other causes of such pain must be excluded before embarking on herniography. Such causes will include direct trauma, acute groin strains, muscular injuries to the adductors, iliopsoas and rectus femoris, osteitis pubis, stress fractures, avulsion injuries, iliopsoas and trochanteric bursitis, osteoarthritis, avascular necrosis and Perthes' disease of the hip and referred pain from the lumbar spine.

We do not routinely use herniography in sportsmen with 'Gilmore's groin'[14] and the role of herniography is controversial in the assessment of such patients, with some authors advocating the technique[2,15–17] though Gilmore himself emphasizes that there is usually no hernia present (see Chapter 12). Rather, the pathology is disruption of the external oblique aponeurosis or conjoined tendon, or the conjoined tendon is torn off either the inguinal ligament or the pubic tubercle,[14] and herniography is negative.

Herniography is also useful in assessing patients with a history of groin swelling suggestive of a hernia, but where no hernia can be palpated in the outpatient clinic.[7] Most surgeons feel that a reliable history is sufficient evidence on which to proceed to repair. However, there may be an unreliable history, or – embarrassing as it might seem – uncertainty about whether the hernia is inguinal or femoral. If there is uncertainty, the usual practice is to review the patient after a few months. However, this is inconvenient for the patient and delays the establishment of an accurate diagnosis. Routine preoperative herniography cannot be justified in all cases of inguinal hernia,[18] though some authors would use it to define difficult anatomy.[19]

Occasionally patients who have had a previous inguinal hernia repair will present with groin pain after a symptom-free interval. It is important to exclude those patients who have had ilioinguinal nerve or genitofemoral nerve pain since the time of surgery. Herniography can accurately define the presence and site of recurrent hernia in some of these patients (Fig. 3).[7,8,20,21] However we do not feel that herniography is necessary in assessing recurrent hernias that are clinically obvious, though others have suggested that this is valuable.[19]

Smedberg *et al.*[22] have suggested that herniography be used for routine follow-up after hernia repair, in order accurately to gauge the recurrence rate, a policy that seems both extreme and unnecessary to us.

It is increasingly being accepted that ligation of the hernial sac is unnecessary at hernia repair. Although an inverted sac might be expected to show up on subsequent herniography, after dealing with the sac in this way the herniogram is usually normal.[22] Interestingly, Kahn and Hamlin[23] have demonstrated that herniography does not lead to false-positive results after mesh plug repairs.

It is well recognized that distinguishing direct from indirect inguinal hernia can be difficult.[24] Although this important observation has altered teaching and examination practice, it cannot be used to justify herniography, since modern hernia surgery is not usually affected by the type of hernia present. There are occasional patients whose body habitus makes distinguishing an inguinal from a femoral hernia challenging, much as this might embarrass the surgeon. While it is an attractive proposition that herniography might be useful here,[25] radiological differentiation of

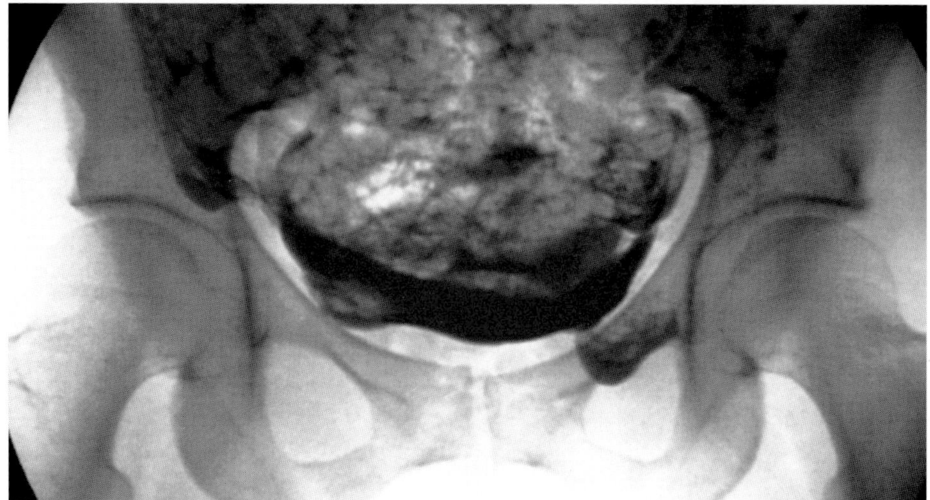

Figure 3. Recurrent inguinal hernia

a femoral from an indirect inguinal hernia is not always easy, though accuracy does improve with experience.[2,26]

Herniography has been used to diagnose rarer variants of hernia,[27,28] including obturator[29] and Spigelian hernias (Fig. 4).[30,31] Unfortunately the technique appears unreliable in this regard,[29] nor have we found it useful in lumbar or incisional hernia. Our normal practice is to assess Spigelian hernias using computerized tomography.

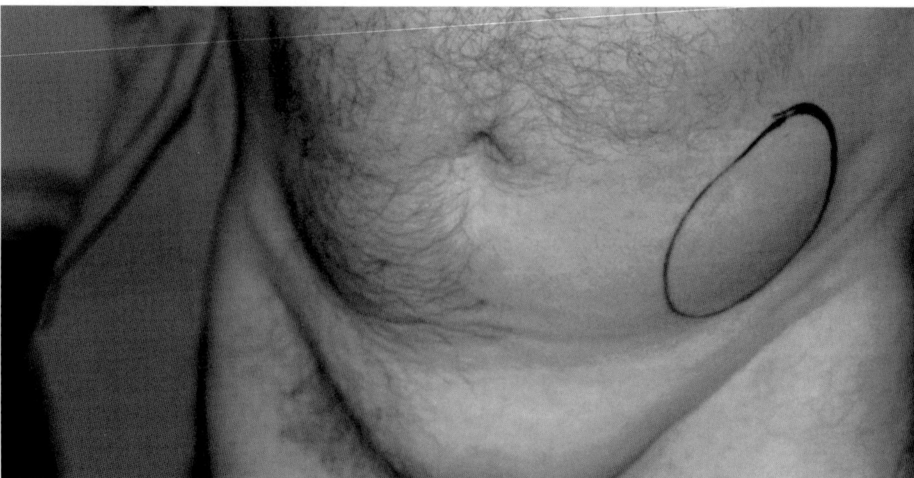

Figure 4. (a) An unusual position for a 'classical' inguinal hernia, higher and more lateral. Herniography may be useful in establishing or cofirming the diagnosis of a Spigelian hernia. (b) Large Spigelian hernia sac at aperation, emerging at the function of the transversus and internal oblique muscles with the rectus muscle. (c) Spigelian hernia sac reduced and held in position with artery forceps at the lateral border of the rectus muscle

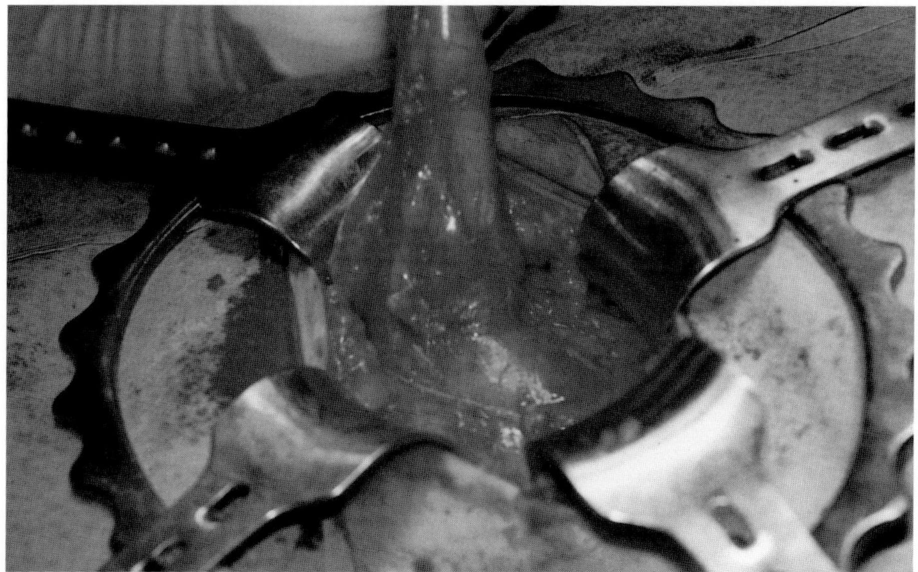

(b)

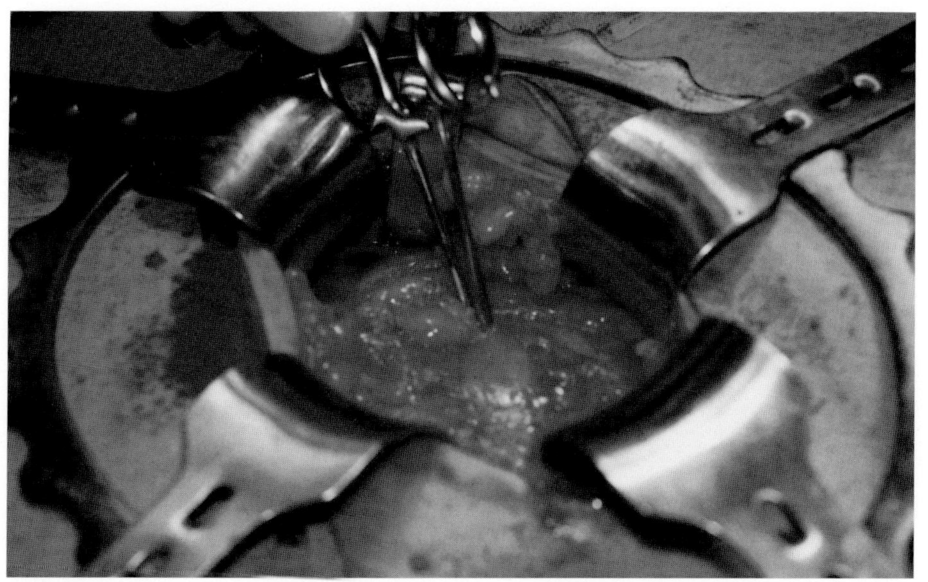

(c)

TECHNIQUE

The examination is performed as an outpatient procedure. Patients can eat normally until the evening before the examination and can have a light breakfast approximately 3 hours pre-examination. Patients are asked to empty their bladder immediately before the procedure which is performed on a tilting X-ray table under aseptic conditions. Our patients are sent an explanatory leaflet prior to the procedure and a consent form is completed in all cases.

A side marker (left or right) is taped to the nonsymptomatic side to enable orientation on all radiographs. The skin of the anterior abdominal wall is cleansed and draped, and the procedure is performed under local anaesthesia. Initially the puncture site chosen was in the left iliac fossa, but due to the risk of perforation of the sigmoid colon this has been changed to a subumbilical approach. A point is chosen 4–5 cm caudal to the umbilicus and is infiltrated with local anaesthetic (5 ml of lignocaine 2%, Astra Pharmaceuticals). A 20 gauge disposable lumbar puncture needle is then inserted and the stylet withdrawn. We currently inject 50 ml of nonionic water-soluble contrast (iopamidol 300 mg iodine per ml, E Merck Pharmaceuticals). It is important to screen the contrast injection, particularly at the beginning, to ensure free spread of contrast within the peritoneal cavity. If contrast is seen to loculate around the tip of the needle,

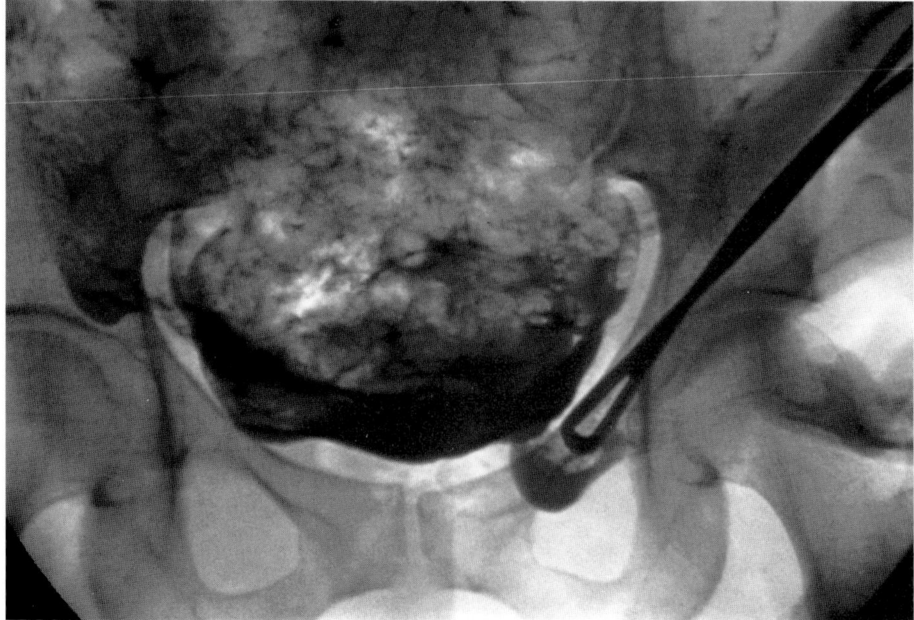

Figure 5. Excellent correlation between the site of pain and the site of herniation.

or lie within the bowel lumen, the needle is simply repositioned, usually by withdrawing slightly. Once the contrast has been injected the patient is asked to turn prone and the table is tilted to approximately 35–40° foot down. The X-ray tube is angled approximately 35° cranially. The images are taken with the patient lying prone and then angled approximately 40° to the left and to the right. The patient is also asked both to cough and to perform the Valsalva manoeuvre. Conventional or digital radiographs are taken in these positions. The table is tilted up so that the patient is standing vertically and the X-ray tube is brought horizontal; anteroposterior and lateral radiographs are performed and oblique and additional spot radiographs are taken if required.

The patient is also asked to indicate the site of symptoms with a pair of forceps and the relationship of this site to any hernia is recorded on film (Fig. 5). With positive examinations there is often an accurate correlation between the site indicated by the patient and the hernia. Following the examination, the patient is given refreshments and observed in the X-ray department for 20–30 min. They are advised to refrain from strenuous activity for the remainder of that day and to contact the department or their doctor should they develop significant abdominal pain.

Initially we performed herniography using an ionic water-soluble agent and several patients experienced abdominal pain.[7,32] Although some patients are aware of a sensation when the nonionic contrast is injected, significant pain is not a feature. Injections may be misplaced into the anterior abdominal wall or retroperitoneum, loculated within the mesentery, or injected into bowel or blood vessels. This is readily identified with screening, and we have not seen any significant complications related to misplaced injection.

We would not perform herniography in a patient sensitive to iodine containing contrast media. Extensive abdominal surgery is a relative contraindication, but we have performed many herniograms in this situation without complication.

INTERPRETATION

A positive herniogram is defined as an outpouching of the peritoneal cavity which can be outlined by contrast and may or may not contain a bowel loop. If obstructed, the hernial sac will not outline with contrast and will not be demonstrated by a herniogram. Any hernia which does not have a peritoneal sac will not be detected by a herniogram and this may include Gilmore's groin.

With the patient positioned as described, the contrast medium pools in the dependant part of the peritoneal cavity. By asking the patient to tilt from side to side and to perform the Valsalva manoeuvre and cough, contrast will outline a peritoneal sac and demonstrate a hernia.[1,3]

The appearance of the normal groin anatomy and the common types of hernia are demonstrated in Figures 6–9. There is considerable variation in the appearance of the normal herniogram, with the peritoneal folds and recesses being much more conspicuous in some patients than others, and there is often a degree of asymmetry between the

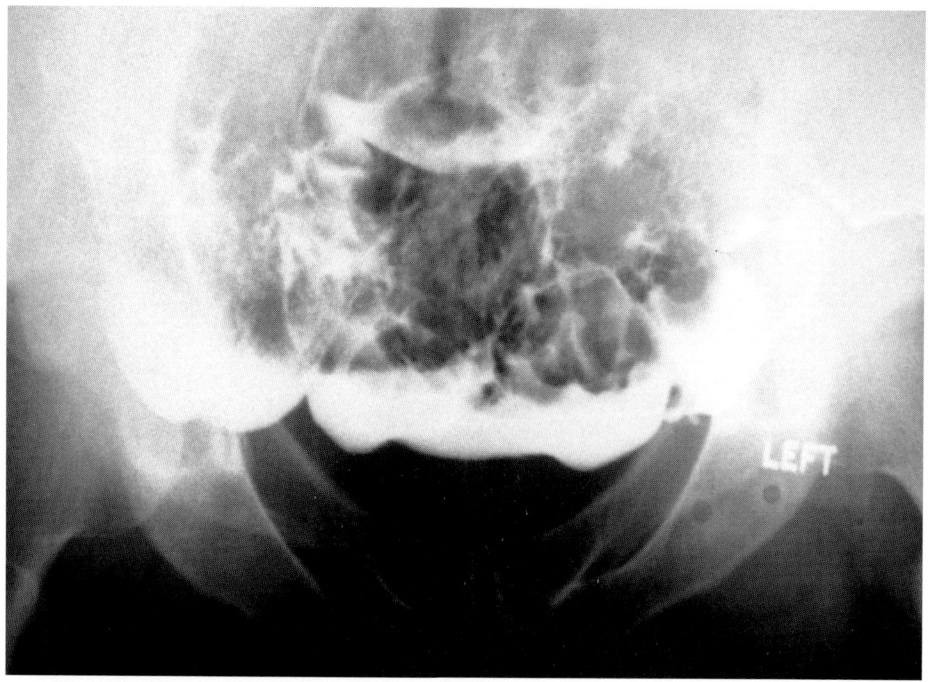

Figure 6. The important anatomical landmarks to be found on a normal herniogram. The median umbilical fold represents the obliterated urachus, the medial umbilical folds represent the obliterated umbilical vein and the lateral umbilical fold is the site of the inferior epigastric vessels

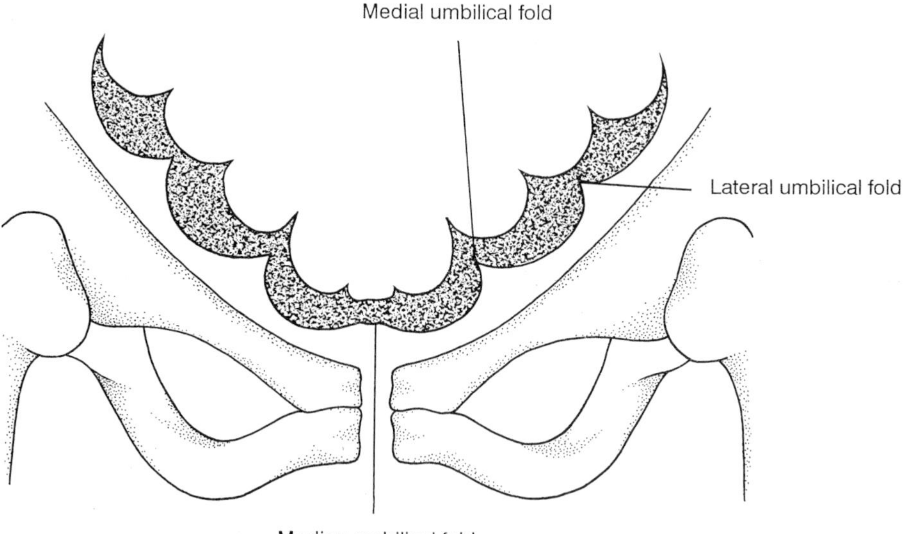

Figure 7. The normal anatomical landmarks in the groin are shown. The median umbilical fold represents the obliterated urachus, the medial umbilical fold represents the obliterated umbilical vein and the lateral umbilical fold is the site of the inferior epigastric vessels

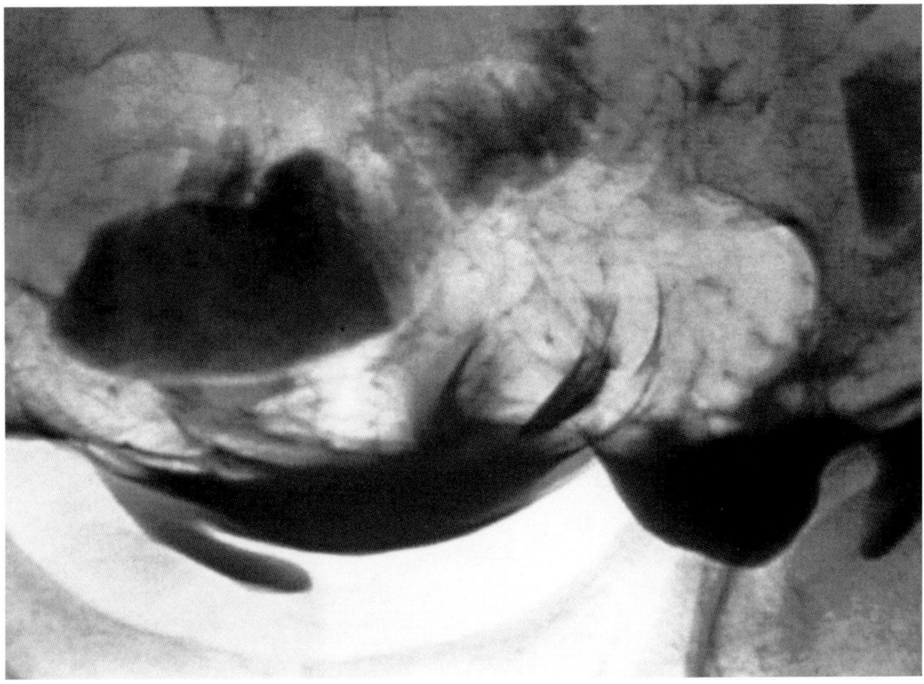

Figure 8. Position of some of the more common groin hernias as seen on a herniogram. The normal radiographic anatomical landmarks are also shown

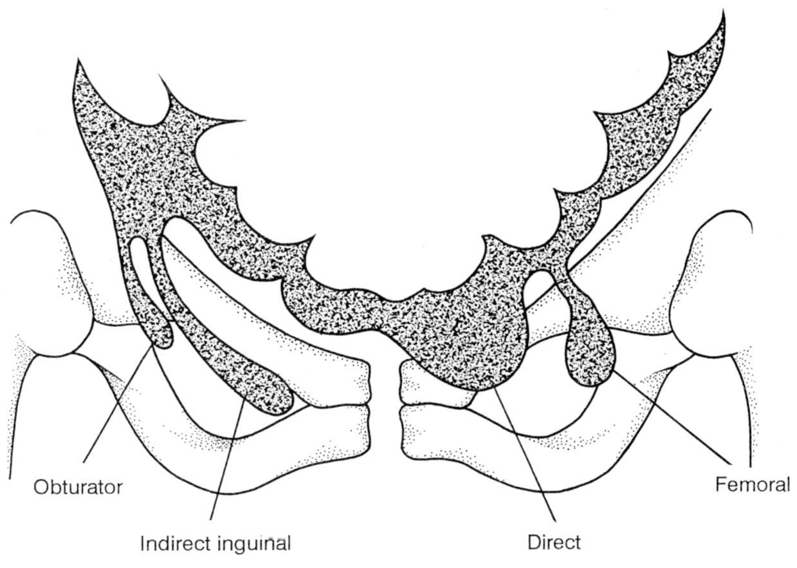

Figure 9. Diagrammatic representation of the common abnormalities found at herniography

Type of pain	No. of patients	Sex ratio (M:F)	Median age (years)
Continuous pain	28	17:11	55 (20–89)
Pain on exercise	14	12:2	35 (23–47)
Pain and suspected recurrent hernia	10	7:3	54 (39–70)
Total	52	36:16	46 (20–89)

Table 1. Details of patients with groin pain

two sides in the same patient. It is common to see a herniographic cough impulse with direct type bulging of the peritoneum. We do not diagnose a direct inguinal hernia unless this is prominent and clearly extends below the level of the inguinal ligament.

RESULTS

In an initial prospective trial,[7] 52 patients underwent herniography during a 3-year period in our department. All had a history of groin pain with no clinically detectable hernia. Herniography was performed as an outpatient procedure in all cases.

Thirty six men and 16 women aged 20–89 (median 46 years) were studied. In 14 patients the groin pain was exacerbated by exercise and in 10 it began consequent to a previous hernia repair. Persistent groin pain of unknown origin was present in 28 patients (Table 1). Clinical examination revealed no abnormality in 32 patients and a possible cough impulse in 20.

There were no complications following herniography. Two patients, both receiving ionic contrast in the early part of the study, complained of pain during the procedure; this had resolved completely by the end of the examination. Small amounts of contrast material were injected into the anterior abdominal wall in three patients, into the bowel in three, and retroperitoneally in one, with no sequelae.

The results are summarized in Table 2. Herniography identified 19 inguinal, two femoral and one obturator hernia in 18 patients. Diffuse peritoneal bulging was seen in nine patients.

Four patients who complained of symptoms on only one side were found on herniography to have a bilateral hernia. Two of these patients had previously undergone hernia repair while the other two were suffering continuous pain at rest. One of these contralateral hernias become clinically obvious and required repair.

Type of pain	Hernia	No hernia	Total
Continuous pain	13	15	28
Pain on exercise	2	12	14
Pain and suspected recurrent hernia	3	7	10
Total	18[a]	34	52

[a]18 patients had 22 hernias; the contralateral asymptomatic hernia is excluded.

Table 2. Herniographic findings

Only seven of the hernias identified were associated with a 'possible' cough impulse, while the remaining 15 showed no clinical abnormality. Only two of the 14 patients presenting with pain after or during exercise were shown to have a positive herniogram.

Positive herniographic findings were confirmed at operation in 16 patients. In keeping with other studies there were no false-positive herniographic diagnoses. Two patients declined surgery. One patient presenting with a possible cough impulse and a negative herniogram subsequently underwent surgical exploration which revealed a lipoma of the spermatic cord and no evidence of a hernia sac. At follow-up all 16 patients who underwent hernia repair were pain free.

None of the 34 patients with a negative herniogram has developed a hernia. At subsequent review with follow-up of between 6 months and 3 years, pain has settled spontaneously in 29 of these 34 patients. None of these patients was given specific advice regarding straining or exercise. The remaining five patients were believed to be suffering from musculoskeletal pain and were referred to a pain clinic for further management; four responded to local anaesthetic injection and one suffered persistent pain despite several modes of treatment.

This initial study, in addition to demonstrating the sensitivity of herniography, highlighted the poor correlation between a possible cough impulse (that is clinical uncertainty) and an underlying hernia. It also demonstrated the safety of the procedure – with the three patients suffering inadvertent puncture of the bowel wall suffering no untoward sequelae – and the importance of using nonionic contrast material.

A subsequent review of a further 100 patients undergoing herniography confirmed the findings of the initial trial. In these patients no clinically detectable hernia was present, and again operative and clinical outcomes were assessed. Side-effects were again found to be of a minimal nature with no significant sequelae. Contrast was injected into bowel or anterior abdominal wall in 7% of cases. In 11% of cases, loculation of contrast within the bowel mesentery occurred. Thirty one hernias were identified in 26 patients and subsequently confirmed at operation in 17 patients. A variety of hernias was found, with 5 patients showing bilateral hernias. Fourteen of these patients undergoing hernia repair were found to be pain free at review. Five patients with negative herniograms underwent surgery; small direct inguinal hernias were found in two patients whose groin pain resolved following treatment. In the other three patients, lipomata of the cord were found, but the groin pain persisted.

In the patients with a negative herniogram who did not undergo operation, 42% showed a spontaneous resolution of the pain with a median follow-up interval of 3 years. Of the remaining 33 patients, four have been found to have other pathologies; 13 patients are now attending a pain clinic.

CONCLUSIONS

Herniography is useful as an adjunct to clinical assessment of selected patients with groin pain. It is simple and safe, though interpretation requires careful consideration of groin anatomy. Selection of patients for herniography is of paramount importance; if properly applied, positive results will correlate well with operative findings.

REFERENCES

1 Ekberg O. Inguinal herniography in adults: technique, normal anatomy and diagnostic criteria for hernias. *Radiology* 1981; **138**(1):31–6.
2 Gullmo A. Herniography. *World J Surg* 1989; **13**(5):560–8.
3 Hall C, Hall PN, Wingate JP, Neoptolemos JP. Evaluation of herniography in the diagnosis of an occult abdominal wall hernia in symptomatic adults. *Br J Surg* 1990; 77(8):902–6.
4 Ducharme JC, Bertrand R, Chacar R. Is it possible to diagnose inguinal hernia by x-ray? A preliminary report on herniography. *J Can Assoc Radiol* 1967; **18**:448–51.
5 Leape LL. Herniograms – a commentary (editorial). *Surgery* 1978; **83**(3):361–2.
6 Ekberg O, Fritzdorf J, Blomquist P. Herniographic appearance of contralateral inguinal hernia. *Acta Radiol Diag* 1984; **25**(2):125–8.
7 Eames NW, Deans GT, Lawson JT, Irwin ST. Herniography for occult hernia and groin pain. *Br J Surg* 1994; **81**(10):1529–30.
8 Binswanger RO, Togendorff J, Hansson JE, Hegglin J. Imaging of abdominal hernias by herniography. Imaging technique, results and tolerance in 67 patients. *Swiss Surg* 1995; **6**:279–84.
9 van den Berg JC, Strijk SP. Groin hernia: role of herniography. *Radiology* 1992; **184**(1):191–4.
10 Magnusson J, Gustafson T, Gullstrand P, Holmin T. Herniography – a useful diagnostic method in patients with obscure groin pain. *Ann Chir Gynaecol* 1984; **73**(2):91–4.
11 Smedberg SG, Broome AE, Elmer O, Gullmo A. Herniography in the diagnosis of obscure groin pain. *Acta Chir Scand* 1985; **151**(8):663–7.
12 Van Ginderachter P, Steyaert L, Pattyn G *et al.* Herniography in adults: review and personal studies. *J Belge Radiol* 1990; **73**(3):181–8.
13 Ekberg O, Abrahamsson PA, Kesek P. Inguinal hernia in urological patients: the value of herniography. *J Urol* 1988; **139**(6):1253–5.
14 Gilmore OJA. Gilmore's groin: ten years experience of groin disruption – a previously

unresolved problem in sportsmen. In MacLeod DAD, Maughan RJ, Williams C *et al.*, eds. *Intermittent high intensity exercise – preparation, stresses and damage limitation.* London: E & FN Spon 1983; 477–86.

15 Ekberg O, Persson NH, Abrahamsson PA, Westlin NE, Lilja B. Longstanding groin pain in athletes. A multidisciplinary approach. *Sports Med* 1988; **6**(1):56–61.

16 Yilmazlar T, Kizil A, Zorluoglu A, Ozguc H. The value of herniography in football players with obscure groin pain. *Acta Chir Belg* 1996; **96**(3):115–18.

17 Smedberg SG, Broome AE, Gullmo A, Roos H. Herniography in athletes with groin pain. *Am J Surg* 1985; **149**(3):378–82.

18 Magnusson J, Gustafson T, Gullstand P, Holmin T. Preoperative herniography in clinically manifest groin hernias. *Ann Chir Gynaecol* 1985; **74**(4):172–5.

19 Lancet Editorial. Herniography. *Lancet* 1980; **ii**:1065.

20 Smedberg SG, Broome AE, Elmer O, Gullmo A. Herniography: a diagnostic tool in groin symptoms following hernial surgery. *Acta Chir Scand* 1986; **152**:273–7.

21 Hamlin JA, Kahn AM. Herniography in symptomatic patients following inguinal hernia repair. *Western J Med* 1995; **162**(1):28–31.

22 Smedberg SG, Broome AE, Gullmo A. Ligation of the hernial sac? *Surg Clin North Am* 1984; **64**(2):299–306.

23 Kahn AM, Hamlin JA. Herniography following indirect hernioplasty using the Marlex "mesh plug" technique. *Am Surgeon* 1995; **61**(11):947–8.

24 Ralphs DNL, Brian AJL, Grundy DJ *et al.* How accurately can direct and indirect inguinal hernias be distinguished? *BMJ* 1980; **280**:1039.

25 Ekberg O, Fork FT, Fritzdorf J. Herniography in atypical hernia. *Br J Radiol* 1984; **57**(684):1077–82.

26 Bergenfeldt M, Ekberg O, Kesek P, Lasson A. Femoral hernia: clinical significance of radiologic diagnosis. *Eur J Radiol* 1990; **10**(3):177–80.

27 Ratcliffe JF, Doig C, Stassen L. Herniography in an uncommon inguinal hernia. *J R Coll Surg Edin* 1986; **31**(3):188–9.

28 Ekberg O, Nordblom I, Fork FT, Gullmo A. Herniography of femoral, obturator and perineal hernias. *ROFO: Fortschr Geb Rontgenstr Nuklearmed* 1985; **143**(2):193–9.

29 Persson NH, Bergqvist D, Ekberg O. Obturator hernia – clinical significance of radiologic diagnosis. *Acta Chir Scand* 1987; **153**(5–6):361–4.

30 Svahn T, Spangen L. Peritoneography in spiegelian hernias. *Acta Radiol Diag* 1976; **1F**(1):97–100.

31 Harrison LA, Keesling CA, Martin NL, Lee KR, Wetzel LH. Abdominal wall hernias: a review of herniography and correlation with cross-sectional imaging. *Radiographics* 1995; **15**(2):315–32.

32 Ekberg O, Nilsson PE. Herniography: comparison of morbidity and image quality after use of high and low osmolality contrast media. *Invest Radiol* 1986; **21**(5):404–7.

14 TRANSABDOMINAL PREPERITONEAL LAPAROSCOPIC INGUINAL HERNIA REPAIR

Liam F Horgan and James M Wellwood

INTRODUCTION

Several factors have now combined to fuel the explosion of interest in laparoscopic inguinal hernia repair. Since the first laparoscopy was performed by Ott[1] in 1901, rapid technological developments, including rod lens systems, insufflation devices, fibre optics, laparoscopic instrumentation and the video camera,[2–4] lead to the first laparoscopic cholecystectomy in 1987 by Mouret.[5] Most cholecystectomies are now performed laparoscopically, and surgeons with their new skills have turned their attention to laparoscopic inguinal hernia repair.

The use of mesh for the primary repair of inguinal hernias was first published by Usher and colleagues in 1959[6,7] and more recently has been popularized by Lichtenstein.[8] The placement of a tension-free mesh in the primary repair of inguinal hernias is now generally accepted.

The first description of the open preperitoneal repair of an inguinal hernia was by Annandale in 1876[9] and was subsequently popularized by Nyhus.[10] The placement of a mesh in the preperitoneal plane was later advocated by Rignault and others[11–14] with good results. Placing the mesh in the preperitoneal plane as opposed to beneath the external oblique[15] has been shown to produce a stronger repair.[16]

LAPAROSCOPIC METHODS OF REPAIR

The first published report of a laparoscopic inguinal hernia repair was that of a transabdominal procedure performed by Ger in 1979.[17] Since then, various methods of laparoscopic inguinal hernia repair have been advocated[18] and are mentioned briefly.

Simple closure

The simplest method of repair involved ligation of the neck of the sac[17,19] with or without sutured closure of the deep ring.[19,20] This method is practised by a few surgeons for type 1 (Nyhus) hernias but has been abandoned by most because of high recurrence rates.

Plug and patch

The next development was the plug and patch technique, which involved placing a wedge of rolled up mesh into the hernial defect with or without an overlaid small mesh before closing the peritoneum.[21–23] The small mesh was not fixed and subsequent mesh migration, particularly into the scrotum, was noted. The results were disappointing and again the technique has been discarded.

Intraperitoneal onlay mesh (IPOM)

The simple concept of placing a mesh directly over the defect and stapling it to the peritoneum was developed by Fitzgibbons and co-workers.[24] This intraperitoneal onlay mesh (IPOM) repair requires little dissection and is quick to complete. However, fixation can be difficult, particularly in large medial defects, and Fitzgibbons does not recommend it for direct or sliding hernias.[25,26] The risk of adhesion development to the exposed mesh is a major objection. Using mesh with a lower propensity to develop adhesions may overcome this objection and other authors favour developing this approach.[27–29]

Transabdominal preperitoneal (TAPP)

The transabdominal preperitoneal (TAPP) laparoscopic inguinal hernia repair[30] is the most commonly performed at present,[31] and many personal series have been reported in the literature.[32–34] The authors embarked on the TAPP repair in 1992 and have preferred to develop this technique. The TAPP repair is theoretically the same as the open preperitoneal repair using a prosthetic mesh placed in the preperitoneal plane but the surgical approach to that plane is different. The advantages or disadvantages should therefore be as a result of the approach and any alterations to the technique. The technique is relatively easy to learn and is described in detail later. The main disadvantage of the TAPP repair is that the peritoneal cavity is breached in four places (three ports and a peritoneal incision) with a consequent risk of adhesion formation. In common with other transabdominal inguinal hernia repairs, damage to intra-abdominal structures with subsequent morbidity is a recognized complication. Trials of the TAPP repair versus open repairs are now appearing in the literature[35–38] and suggest that the TAPP repair can be carried out safely, with reduced postoperative pain and a quicker return to work. In particular, it is an attractive approach for the repair of recurrent and bilateral inguinal hernias.

Totally extraperitoneal (TEP)

Over the past few years the totally extraperitoneal (TEP) laparoscopic inguinal hernia repair has gained in popularity. McKernan was one of the first to develop this approach.[39] Its main advantage is that the peritoneum is not breached and this negates the arguments against the TAPP repair.[40] However, the anatomy and the technique are more difficult to learn. Balloon dissection is commonly used to develop the preperitoneal plane and a mesh is inserted to cover the defect. It may be stapled or merely left in place. Large indirect inguinal hernias can be difficult to deal with using this approach. TEP has a higher conversion rate back to TAPP or open repair than for other laparoscopic inguinal hernia repairs[39,40] and recurrence rates are similar to TAPP repair.

Both TAPP and TEP repairs currently have their own followers, but data from long-term follow-up on morbidity and recurrence rates may alter this situation. The indications for the different procedures may be refined and determined by the type of inguinal hernia involved.

THE TECHNIQUE OF TRANSABDOMINAL PREPERITONEAL REPAIR (TAPP)

TAPP is performed under a general anaesthetic. The patient is positioned supine on the operating table with the arms by the side. The authors catheterized the first 50 patients but now avoid this by asking the patient to void urine immediately preoperatively. Nasogastric intubation is not used. The abdomen is prepared from the ziphisternum to the upper thighs and the patient is draped.

For all inguinal hernia repairs the surgeon stands on the left of the patient with the assistant on the right side holding the camera. The scrub nurse is positioned on the left of the surgeon at the level of the patient's knees. The authors usually use one monitor placed at the patient's feet. If two monitors are available then one is placed at each foot. The diathermy and insufflation/suction machines are placed in a convenient space within view of the surgeon.

The scrub nurse immediately passes a dish containing a swab, a scalpel, a Verres needle and a syringe of saline to the surgeon. While the surgeon makes the infra-umbilical incision, the scrub nurse connects the insufflation line. The incision may be above or below the umbilicus and either vertical or transverse depending on the shape of the patient. It is large enough to allow passage of a 10-mm port. The Verres needle is checked for free flow of saline and then advanced through the abdominal wall into the peritoneal cavity. Correct position of the needle is confirmed by the easy introduction of saline and the drop test. Insufflation of a carbon dioxide pneumoperitoneum is commenced. During insufflation, the scrub nurse and assistant ready the other leads and the camera is adjusted if needed. Once the intra-abdominal pressure rises to 10 mmHg and the abdomen is adequately distended, a 10-mm port is introduced. A zero degree laparoscope is introduced and laparoscopy performed. A 12-mm port is inserted at the lateral border of the rectus abdominis on the right at the level of the umbilicus. A 5-mm port is placed in a similar position on the left (Fig. 1). The patient is now placed in the Trendelenburg position with as much head down as possible to keep the bowel away from the operation field. A grasper is inserted through the 5-mm port and dissecting scissors with diathermy attached through the 12-mm port.

The anatomy of the inguinal region is defined and the presence of a hernia established (Fig. 2). The relationship of the hernial orifice to the inferior epigastric vessels indicates whether the hernia is direct or indirect or a combination of both. The dissection begins by incising the peritoneum above the hernial orifice and continuing the incision laterally to the anterior superior iliac spine, which is confirmed by external digital indentation (Fig. 3). The peritoneum below the incision is then fully mobilized to develop a pocket in the preperitoneal plane deep enough to accommodate the mesh (Fig. 4). The incision is then extended medially across the inferior epigastric vessels towards the midline to allow exposure of the symphysis pubis. The medial part of the incision is now developed to create a second pocket extending just beyond the symphysis pubis and exposing the pubic ramus to at least the midline. The final stage of this part of the dissection involves the freeing of the peritoneum or the indirect inguinal hernia sac from the structures at the internal ring, notably the vas deferens and the testicular vessels (Fig. 5). This is the most difficult part of the dissection and care to avoid injury to the vas and vessels and to maintain good haemostasis at this stage is important. An indirect sac is withdrawn into the abdominal cavity unless it is large, in which case it is transected with the distal end left *in situ.* Direct sacs are usually fully withdrawn into the peritoneal cavity. The pocket must be sufficiently large to amply accommodate the mesh. The size of the mesh is important. Recurrence is likely if it is too small. The authors now use a minimum size 14 × 10 cm for a unilateral hernia.

The mesh is introduced into the abdominal cavity through the 12-mm port on the right by grasping it at a corner and rolling it around the instrument. Once within the abdomen the mesh is unfolded and placed over the inguinal area. The mesh is manipulated until it is laying flat and orientated correctly. The superior edge of the mesh must overlap the superior edge of the defect by at least 2 cm. The medial edge of the mesh must reach or overlap the symphysis pubis. This ensures that both direct and indirect defects are covered. The mesh is not slit and is not placed behind the inferior epigastric vessels or the cord. Once in place the medial edge is stapled to the pubic bone with two or three staples using an EMS stapling gun (Ethicon EndoSurgery,

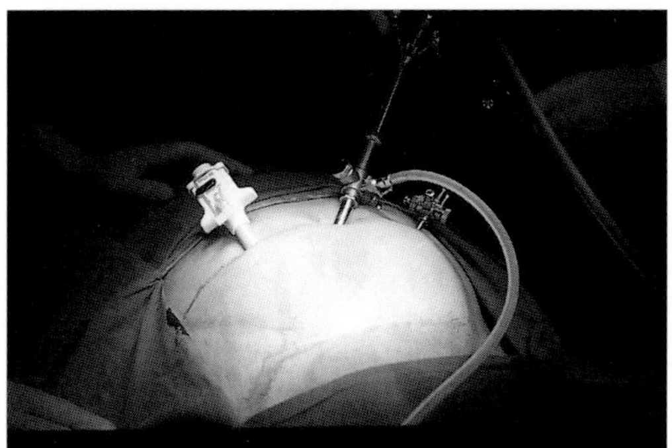

Figure 1. Port position for TAPP

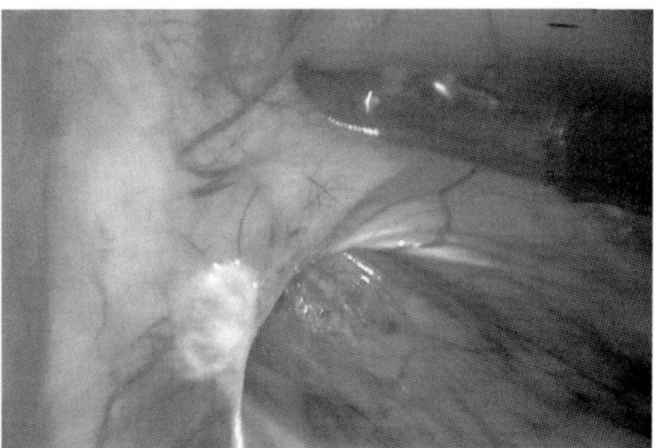

Figure 2. Right indirect inguinal hernia. Instrument points to inferior epigastric vessels

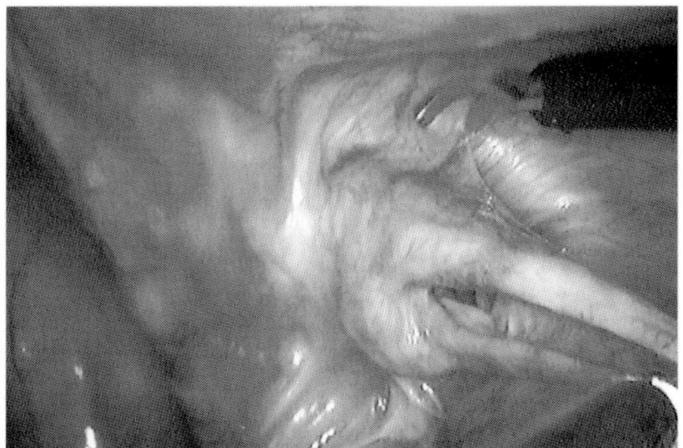

Figure 3. Indirect sac is reduced and peritoneum is about to be incised

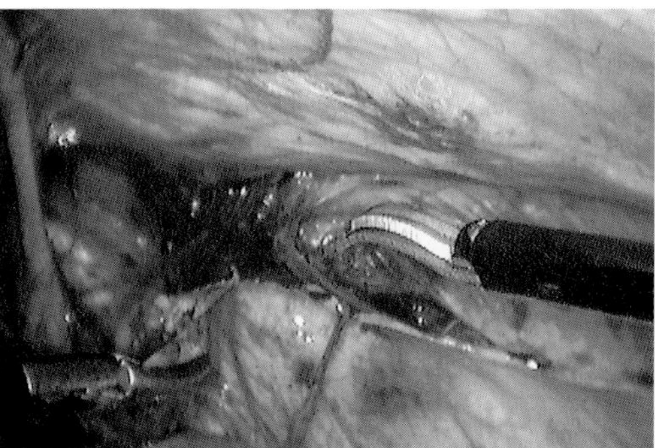

Figure 4. Space lateral to cord and hernia is developed

Edinburgh, UK) through the 12-mm port. The superior edge of the mesh is then stapled at intervals of 2 cm taking care to avoid damage to the inferior epigastric vessels. Counter pressure from the hand externally ensures that the tissue is at right angles to the stapler head (Fig. 6). No staples are placed lower than the superior border of the mesh to avoid nerve injury (Fig. 7).

When the mesh has been adequately secured the peritoneum is lifted back to cover the mesh and exclude it from the peritoneal cavity. At this point the inferior edge of the mesh can easily roll up to expose the hernial defect. This must be corrected as it may lead to recurrence.[41] The peritoneum is stapled in position using the EMS gun (Fig. 8). Any holes in the peritoneum are closed using staples to avoid herniation of the small bowel into the preperitoneal space. When the operation has been completed

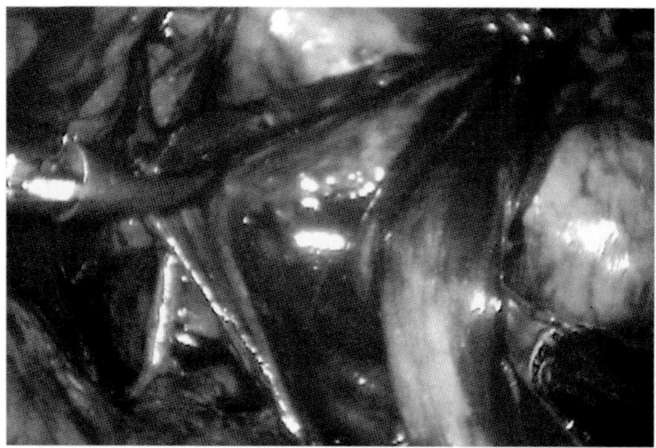

Figure 5. Vas deferens and testicular vessels displayed

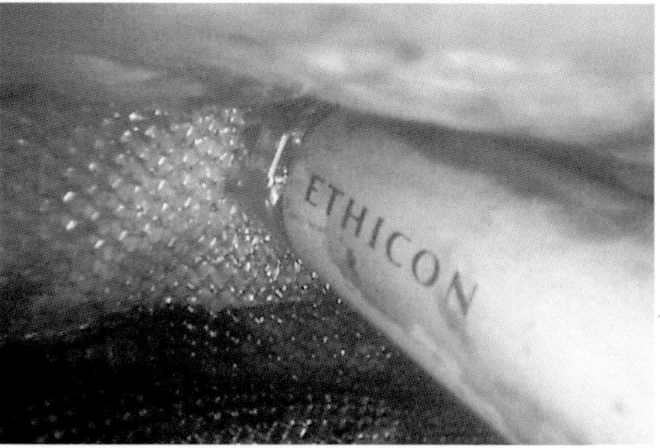

Figure 6. Hand applying external counter pressure to staple head

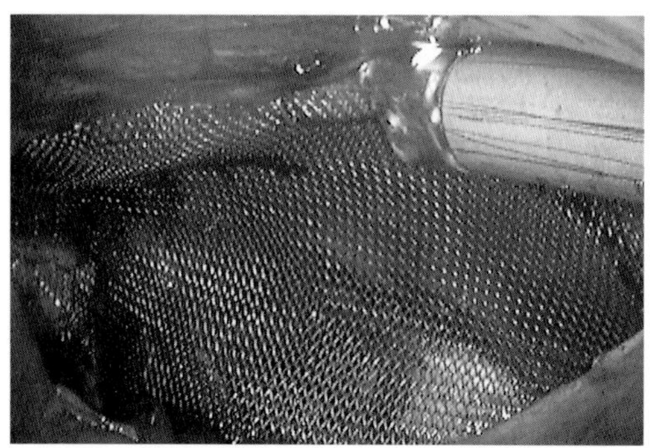

Figure 7. Stapling superior border of mesh

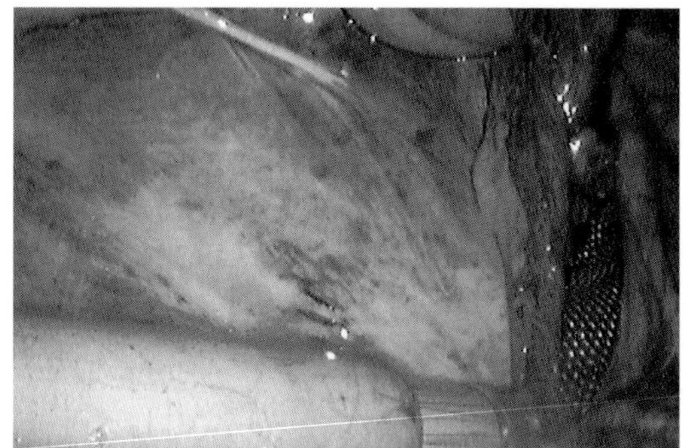

Figure 8. Peritoneum stapled closed to exclude mesh

the lateral ports are inspected to check for bleeding and the pneumoperitoneum released. The laparoscope and other ports are then withdrawn to reduce the possibility of an immediate port site hernia. Port sites of 10 mm or greater are closed. Local anaesthetic is used to infiltrate the port sites to reduce postoperative discomfort. A single skin stitch is inserted at each port site.

When bilateral hernias are being repaired the dissection described above is performed on both sides and the medial pockets are joined across the midline so that a single large pocket passing from right to left superior iliac spine is produced. A 28 × 10 cm mesh is then inserted in one piece, making sure that it does not twist as it passes behind the bladder.

All the patients are treated as day cases if possible and with few exceptions are expected to be discharged on the same day as the operation.

WHIPP'S CROSS TRIALS

Trial 1

Laparoscopic versus open inguinal hernia repair: randomized prospective trial[35]

Between 1992 and 1993 the TAPP technique was developed by the senior author (JW) at Whipp's Cross Hospital. As no reliable results were available,[42] and the Royal College of Surgeons was advising against performing laparoscopic inguinal hernia repair except within properly structured trials,[43] it was decided to design a randomized trial comparing TAPP with a conventional repair. Between 1993 and 1994 all patients presenting to the outpatient department at Whipp's Cross Hospital were invited to enter a randomized trial comparing laparoscopic TAPP with an open Maloney darn. The Maloney darn had been the senior author's (JW) standard method of hernia repair since 1980 with an estimated recurrence rate of 5%.

One hundred and fifty patients were recruited with a total of 167 hernias (Table 1). The main findings were that length of hospital stay was similar, but that the laparoscopic inguinal hernia repair group had less pain, returned to work earlier and had fewer

Characteristic	Operation	
	Open	**Laparoscopic**
Patient characteristics		
Number of patients	75	75
Age (Years)	60 (45–71)	59 (45–68)
Sex (M/F)	72/3	71/4
Hernias		
Total number	84	83
Unilateral	66	67
Bilateral	9	8
Operation time (min)		
Unilateral	35	50 min $P<0.001$
Bilateral	60	92 min $P=0.04$
Overall mean pain score	3.1	1.8 $P<0.001$
Cost		+£168

Table 1. Group characteristics and data (Trial 1)

	Operation	
Complications	**Open**	**Laparoscopic**
Atelectasis	0	1
Pus from wound	5	1
Persistent wound pain	6	3
Primary wound haemorrhage	1	0
Symptomatic haematoma	3	1
Acute retention of urine	1	0
Total number of complications	16(21%)	6(8%) $P<0.005$

Table 2. Complications (Trial 1)

complications than the open group (Table 2). The laparoscopic inguinal hernia repair took longer. The median operation time for the first 20 laparoscopic inguinal hernia repairs at the start of the trial was 60 min. This dropped to 30 min for the last 20 operations. The laparoscopic inguinal hernia repair was more expensive by £168. The costing was based on disposable staplers and scissors, with reusable ports. The trial was completed within 1 year.

Three-year follow-up of Trial 1

In 1996, 3 years after completing the trial, a follow-up study was implemented. Each patient in the trial was contacted over the telephone and by letter and asked to attend Whipp's Cross Hospital for an examination. Because of the unreliability of postal questionnaires, only patients who attended were reported. The response rate was 66% in the TAPP group and 62% in the open group. The patients were asked to complete an SF-36 as a quality of life measure, questioned about problems and examined.

The only statistical difference found in this study was in the number of patients who complained of chronic groin pain (Table 3). The laparoscopic group fared better. It is also sobering to realize that of the 99 patients who responded, 32 (33%) had some element of groin pain 3 years after their operation. Although there were five complaints of groin numbness in the open group, with none in the laparoscopic group, this did not reach significance with these patient numbers. There were four recurrences in the open group and none in the laparoscopic group (not significant).

	Operation	
	Open	Laparoscopic
Number of patients	48	51
Recurrent hernia	4	0
Testicular atrophy	0	0
Testicular pain	2	2
Port site hernia	0	2
Groin pain	21	11 $P<0.05$
Groin numbness	5	0

Table 3. Complications (Trial 1, 3-year follow-up)

This trial is regarded as the first properly constructed study to compare open and laparoscopic inguinal hernia repairs. However, there were two important criticisms. Firstly, the method of repair chosen for the open group (Maloney darn) is now seen as outdated. The open mesh repair (Lichtenstein) with its published low recurrence rates[44] is now regarded as the gold standard against which any new methods should be compared.[45] Secondly, the open repair can be performed under local anaesthesia which the proponents of the open repair consider a major factor.[46]

Trial 2

Prospective randomized trial comparing laparoscopic TAPP repair with local anaesthetic Lichtenstein repair

A second trial was designed to address the above criticisms. It compared laparoscopic inguinal hernia repair (TAPP) with the open mesh repair (Lichtenstein) performed under local anaesthetic. This trial was funded by the Medical Research Council and was carried out at Whipp's Cross Hospital by the senior author (JW) in conjunction with Mr David Stoker at the North Middlesex Hospital. Two hundred patients have been randomized to the laparoscopic group and 200 to the open Lichtenstein under local anaesthetic group. Patient accrual ceased in December 1996. The data will be published in 1998.

Outcomes being measured include satisfaction, quality of life studies, analgesia requirements, pain scores, length of hospital stay, time to return to normal activity and work, operation costing, income lost, complications and recurrences.

Early results of Trial 2

Preliminary assessment of the data indicates an equal proportion of patients in each group leaving hospital the same day as the operation (over 90%). There has been no injury to visceral structures in either group so far. There has been one death from myocardial infarction 28 days after local anaesthetic open repair. Four patients randomized to the local anaesthetic open repair (2%) had to be given a general anaesthetic because they would not tolerate being awake during the operation. One patient (0.5%) had to be converted from TAPP to an open operation due to failure to obtain an adequate pneumoperitoneum.

There is evidence from analysis of the first 100 patients that return to normal activities has been quicker in the laparoscopic group and that the cost to the patient in terms of lost income has been lower in the laparoscopic group. Patient satisfaction with the operation appears to have been good for both procedures but scores were slightly higher in the laparoscopic group. Purulent wound discharge and groin pain appear higher in the open group. None of these results have been analysed for statistical significance. Full details of the trial will be published during 1998.

LEARNING CURVE OF LAPAROSCOPIC INGUINAL HERNIA REPAIR

Seven hundred hernia patients, including those in both trials, have now been treated laparoscopically under the care of the authors. There has been no procedure-related death. There have been seven recurrences (recurrence rate = 1%), five of which were in the first 200 repairs. Initially a mesh size of 8 × 6 cm was used for unilateral hernias and this appears to have been the main cause for the recurrences in the early stages of the technique.[16,41] Experimental work on laparoscopic inguinal hernia repair by one author (LH) has pointed out that the repair is weak medially and that adequate coverage of the mesh to the midline is crucial here.[16] This finding has been confirmed in the clinical situation by others.[41] A mesh size of 14 or 15 × 10 cm is now used and there have been no recurrences of unilateral hernias using this size of mesh. Two of the recurrences were in laparoscopic bilateral inguinal hernia repairs. Initially bilateral hernia repairs were performed using two separate meshes; since adopting a single 28 × 10 cm mesh there have been no recurrences.

The learning curve of the senior author (JW) can be demonstrated by the measurement of the time taken to do the repair. The average time required for the first 20 unilateral repairs was 54 minutes whereas that taken for the 20 unilateral repairs numbered 251–270 was 33 minutes. There has been no small bowel obstruction and the only injury to an intra-abdominal viscus was a small bladder hole that responded to conservative treatment by catheterization only. There have been no major vascular injuries nor any injuries to the femoral, genitofemoral or lateral cutaneous nerves.

DISCUSSION

The laparoscopic TAPP repair has now been improved as a result of enlarging the size of the mesh and placing it medially at least as far as the midline.[16] The recurrence rate is comparable to that quoted by surgeons using the Lichtenstein repair (1%).[47] Further evolution of the technique, which was not possible during the conduct of these trials, could include the cheaper options of fixing the mesh with sutures and closing the peritoneum with sutures. This would eliminate the cost of the stapling device and make the theatre costs of the two procedures more comparable.

In the authors' practice at present, a laparoscopic repair is advised in patients with bilateral inguinal hernias, in patients with recurrent inguinal hernias and in any patient in whom a rapid return to work is a high priority. The laparoscopic or open mesh repair is offered to all patients with primary inguinal hernias. The open mesh under local anaesthetic is used for those patients who are unfit for a general anaesthetic or who are anticoagulated.

We concede that laparoscopic hernia repair is technically more difficult than open Lichtenstein repair and furthermore that there is a longer learning curve for this procedure than for the open Lichtenstein repair. However, it is a safe procedure in experienced hands and we believe that most surgical trainees can readily learn it if taught properly. Trial data currently being analysed will inform the debate concerning the ultimate role of laparoscopic inguinal hernia repair. The authors feel that laparoscopic techniques for inguinal hernia repair represent an important addition to the armamentarium of the fully trained surgeon with a particular interest in inguinal hernia repair.

REFERENCES

1 Ott D. Illumination of the abdomen (ventroscopia) [Russian]. *J Akush Zhensk* 1901; **15**:1045.

2 Marlow J. History of laparoscopy, optics, fibreoptics and instrumentation. *Clin Obstet Gynaecol* 1976; **19**:261–75.

3 Semm K. History. In Sanfilippo JS, Levine RL, eds. *Operative gynaecological endoscopy*. Edinburgh: Livingstone 1989.

4 Paraskeva PA, Nduka CC, Darzi A. The evolution of laparoscopic surgery. *MIT* 1994; **3**:69–75.

5 Dubois F, Berthelot G, Levard H. Laparoscopic cholecystectomy: historical perspective and personal experience. *Surg Laparosc Endosc* 1991; **1**:52–7.

6 Usher FC, Fries JG, Ochsner JL, Tuttle LLD. Marlex mesh, a new plastic mesh for replacing tissue defects. 2: Clinical studies. *Arch Surg* 1959; **78**:138–45.

7 Usher FC. Further observations on the use of Marlex Mesh: a new technique for the repair of inguinal hernias. *Am Surge* 1959; **25**:792–5.

8 Lichtenstein IL, Shulman AG, Amid PK, Montllor MM. The tension-free hernioplasty. *Am J Surg* 1989; **157**:188–93.

9 Annandale T. Case in which a reducible oblique and direct inguinal hernia existed on the same side and were successfully treated by operation. *Edinburgh Med J* 1876; **21**:1087–91.

10 Nyhus LM, Condon RE, Harkins HW. Clinical experience with pre-peritoneal hernia repair for all types of hernia of the groin. *Am J Surg* 1960; **100**:234–44.

11 Rignault DP. Preperitoneal prosthetic inguinal hernioplasty through a Pfannenstiel approach. *Surg Gynecol Obstet* 1986; **163**:465–8.

12 Nyhus LM, Pollak R, Bombeck CT, Donahue PE. The preperitoneal approach and prosthetic buttress repair for recurrent hernia. The evolution of a technique. *Ann Surg* 1988; **208**:733–7.

13 Stoppa R, Petit J, Henry X. Unsutured Dacron prosthesis in groin hernias. *Int Surg* 1975; **60**:411–12.

14 Rives J. Surgical treatment of the inguinal hernia with dacron patch. *Int Surg* 1967; **47**:360–1.

15 Amid PK, Shulman AG, Lichtenstein IL. Open 'tension-free' repair of inguinal hernias: the Lichtenstein technique. *Eur J Surg* 1996; **162**:447–53.

16 Horgan LF, Shelton J, O'Riordan DC, Moore D, Winslet M, Davidson B. Strengths and weakness of laparoscopic and open mesh inguinal hernia repair: a randomised controlled experimental study. *Br J Surg* 1996; **83**:1463–7.

17 Ger R. The management of certain abdominal hernias by intra abdominal closure of the neck. *Ann R Coll Surg Engl* 1982; **64**:342–4.

18 Macintyre IM, Miles WFA. Critical appraisal and current position of laparoscopic hernia repair. *J R Coll Surg Edinburgh* 1995; **40**:331–6.

19 Rosin RD. A rational approach to laparoscopic hernia repair with particular emphasis on herniotomy and/or ring closure. In Arregui ME, Nagan RF, eds. *Inguinal hernia. Advances or controversies?* Oxford: Radcliffe Medical Press 1994; 229–32.

20 Dion YM. Laparoscopic inguinal herniorraphy: an individualized approach. *Surg Laparosc Endosc* 1993; **3**:451–5.

21 Schultz L, Graber J, Pietrafitta J, Hickok D. Laser laparoscopic herniorraphy: a clinical trial preliminary results. *J Laparoendoscopic Surg* 1990; **1**:41–5.

22 Corbitt JD Jr. Laparoscopic herniorraphy. *Surg Laparosc Endosc* 1991; **1**:23–5.

23 Diaco JF, Wright TE, Diaco DS, Brannan AN. Laparoscopic herniorraphy: a review of 401 tension-free repairs. *Int Surg* 1994; **79**:290–2.

24 Salerno GM, Fitzgibbons RJ Jr, Filipi CJ. Laparoscopic inguinal hernia repair. In Zucker KA, Reddick EJ, Bailey R, eds. *Surgical laparoscopy.* St Louis: Quality Medical Publishing 1990; 281–93.

25 Salerno GM, Fitzgibbons RJ Jr, Corbitt JD Jr, Hart RO, Filipi CJ. Laparoscopic inguinal hernia repair. In Zucker KA, Reddick EJ, Bailey R, eds. *Surgical laparoscopy.* St Louis: Quality Medical Publishing 1992; 373–394.

26 Fitzgibbons RJ Jr, Salerno GM, Filipi CJ, Hunter WJ, Watson P. A laparoscopic intraperitoneal onlay mesh technique for the repair of an indirect inguinal hernia. *Ann Surg* 1994; **219**:144–56.

27 Toy FK, Smoot RT Jr. Toy–Smoot laparoscopic hernioplasty. *Delaware Med J* 1992; **64**:23–8.

28 Spaw ST, Ennis BW, Spaw LP. Laparoscopic hernia repair: the anatomic basis. *J Laparoendoscopic Surg* 1991; **1**:269–77.

29 Vogt DM, Curet MJ, Pitcher DE, Martin DT, Zucker KA. Preliminary results of a prospective randomized trial of laparoscopic onlay versus conventional inguinal herniorraphy. *Am J Surg* 1995; **169**:84–9; discussion 89–90.

30 Arregui ME, Davis CJ, Yucel O, Nagan RF. Laparoscopic mesh repair of inguinal hernia using a preperitoneal approach: a preliminary report. *Surg Laparosc Endosc* 1992; **2**:53–8.

31 Phillips EH, Arregui ME, Carroll BJ *et al.* Incidence of complications following laparoscopic hernioplasty. *Surg Endosc* 1995; **9**:16–21.

32 Geis WP, Grafton WB, Novak MJ. Laparoscopic herniorraphy: results and technical aspects in 450 consecutive procedures. *Surgery* 1993; **114**:765–74.

33 Sandblicher P, Gstier H, Baumgartner C, Furtschegger A, Egender G, Steiner E. Laparoskopische Leistenherniaoperation durch transperitoneale implantation eines kunstoffnetzes: Technik und Fruhergebnisse. *Chirurg* 1994; **65**:64–7.

34 Milkins RC, Brough WA, Royston CMS. Laparoscopic hernia repair: a prospective study of 409 cases. *MIT* 1993; **2**:237–42.

35 Stoker DL, Spiegelhalter DJ, Singh R, Wellwood JM. Laparoscopic versus open inguinal hernia repair: randomised prospective trial. *Lancet* 1994; **343**:1243–5.

36 Lawrence K, McWhinnie D, Goodwin A *et al.* Randomised controlled trial of laparoscopic versus open repair of inguinal hernia: early results. *BMJ* 1995; **311**:981–5.

37 Himpens J, Cadiere GB, Bruyns J, Verroken R. Totally preperitoneal laparoscopic approach combined with minianterior dissection in the treatment of indirect inguinal hernias. *Surg Laparosc Endosc* 1995; **5**:450–2.

38 Payne JH Jr, Grininger LM, Izawa MT, Podoll EF, Lindahl PJ, Balfour J. Laparoscopic or open inguinal herniorraphy? A randomized prospective trial. *Arch Surg* 1994; **129**:973–9; discussion 979–81.

39 McKernan JB, Laws HL. Laparoscopic repair of inguinal hernias using a totally extraperitoneal prosthetic approach. *Surg Endosc* 1993; **7**:26–8.

40 Ferzli GS, Massad A, Albert P. Extraperitoneal endoscopic inguinal hernia repair. *J Laparoendoscopic Surg* 1992; **2**:281–6.

41 Deans GT, Wilson MS, Royston CMS, Brough WA. Recurrent inguinal hernia after laparoscopic repair: possible cause and prevention. *Br J Surg* 1995; **82**:539–41.

42 Watson DI, Johnson AG. Randomised trials for laparoscopic surgery. *Aust NZ J Surg* 1994; **64**:813–14.

43 Royal College of Surgeons of England. *Clinical Guidelines on the Management of Groin Hernias in Adults.* London: RCS 1993.

44 Shulman AG, Amid PK, Lichtenstein IL. A survery of non-expert surgeons using the open tension free mesh patch repair for primary inguinal hernias. *Int Surg* 1995; **80**:35–6.

45 Amid PK, Shulman AG, Lichtenstein IL. A critical comparison of laparoscopic hernia repair with Lichtenstein tension-free hernioplasty. *Med J Aust* 1994; **161**:239–41.

46 Notaras MJ. Minimally invasive surgery. No benefit in hernia repair. . . [letter]. *BMJ* 1994; **308**:199.

47 Shulman AG, Amid PK, Lichtenstein IL. The safety of mesh repair for primary inguinal hernias: results of 3,019 operations from five diverse surgical sources. *Am Surg* 1992; **58**:255–7.

15 RECURRENT INGUINAL HERNIA: ANTERIOR APPROACH

Martin Kurzer, Philip A Belsham and Allan E Kark

The reported incidence of recurrent inguinal hernia from specialised clinics, individual surgeons or groups of surgeons with a particular interest in hernia surgery is well under 5%.[1-3] Nevertheless we know that amongst the large reported series of hernia repairs the proportion of operations for recurrent compared with primary hernia is at least 10%.[4-7] Apart from this rough approximation, which is probably an underestimate, the true *overall* incidence of recurrence after primary inguinal hernia repair from non-specialized centres is very difficult to establish.

The difficulties in establishing the recurrence rate after primary inguinal hernia repair are magnified when dealing with recurrent hernias. The assessment that up to 19% of recurrent hernias re-recur[8] probably underestimates the problem, while it is likely that the risk of repeated recurrence increases with each subsequent repair.[9] Recurrence rates of over 30% have been reported even by surgeons with a special interest in hernia repair.[10-13]

The data presented here are from one particular study – a consecutive series of recurrent hernias seen at one institution and operated on by specialist surgeons (surgeons with a special interest in hernias). Over 95% were carried out under local anaesthetic and prosthetic mesh was used routinely in all cases. At the time of this study all groin hernias, primary or recurrent, were operated on via an anterior approach. We now believe that using one type of operation to deal with all recurrent groin hernias is probably incorrect, and we currently favour a preperitoneal technique for recurrent groin hernias.

PATIENTS

Over a 3-year period 223 patients with 232 recurrent inguinal hernias were operated on at the British Hernia Centre (BHC). The follow-up period was between 9 and 46 months (mean follow-up 25 months). All the recurrent inguinal hernias were repaired as day cases using local anaesthetic. The total number of hernias repaired at the BHC over this time was 2139, so that 9% of all hernias seen were recurrent ones.

Seventeen patients were seen who had previous hernia repairs elsewhere and who complained of discomfort or pain in the inguinal region, either convinced that they had

	Patients	Recurrent hernias
Left side only	84	84
Right side only	115	115
Bilateral recurrent	9	18
Bilateral: one recurrent and one primary	15	15

Table 1.   Details of 223 patients with 232 recurrent inguinal hernias

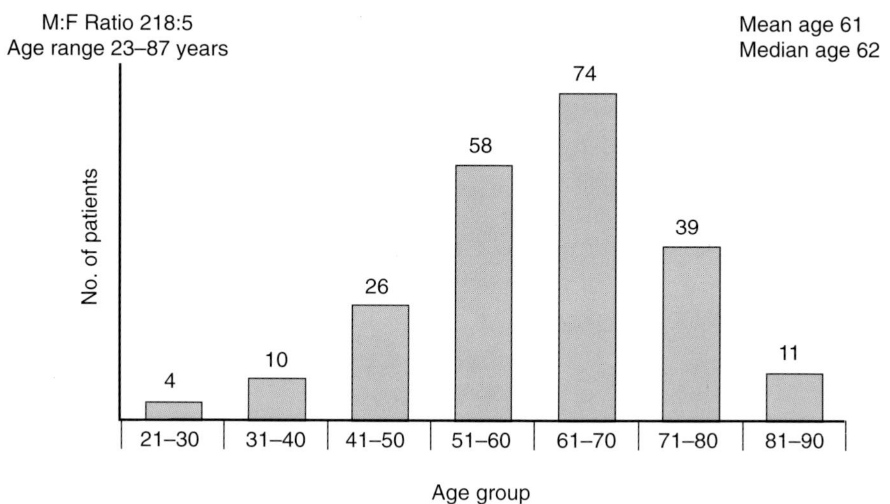

Figure 1.   Age distribution of patients

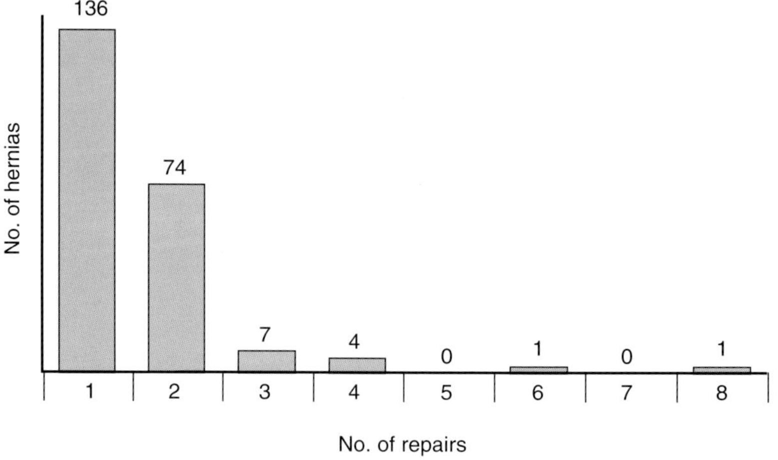

Figure 2.   Number of previous repairs for patients

a recurrent hernia or wanting reassurance. If there was no clinical evidence of a recurrent bulge or cough impulse the option of a herniagram was discussed with the patient. In all these doubtful cases the patients opted for a 'wait and see' approach and no further investigations were carried out. Four patients with recurrent hernia required a general anaesthetic (obesity, anticipated technical problems, anxiety, patient preference); 199 patients had unilateral hernias, 84 left-sided, 115 right-sided, and 24 patients had bilateral inguinal hernias. In 15 of these latter patients one side was recurrent (eight left and seven right) and the contralateral side was primary. In nine patients both sides were recurrent (18 recurrent hernias) and all were repaired at the same operation (Table 1).

The mean age of the patients was 61 years (range 23–87), the median age 62, and there were five women. The age distribution is shown in Fig. 1 and the number of previous repairs in Fig. 2. There were 136 patients who had one previous repair and 13 patients who had three or more.

METHODS

The local anaesthetic used was a combination of bupivacaine 0.25% without adrenaline and lignocaine 0.5% without adrenaline. The site of the recurrent bulge was marked on the skin with an indelible marker pen immediately preoperatively, after shaving and with the patient standing (Fig. 3). In cases where a discrete defect could be easily

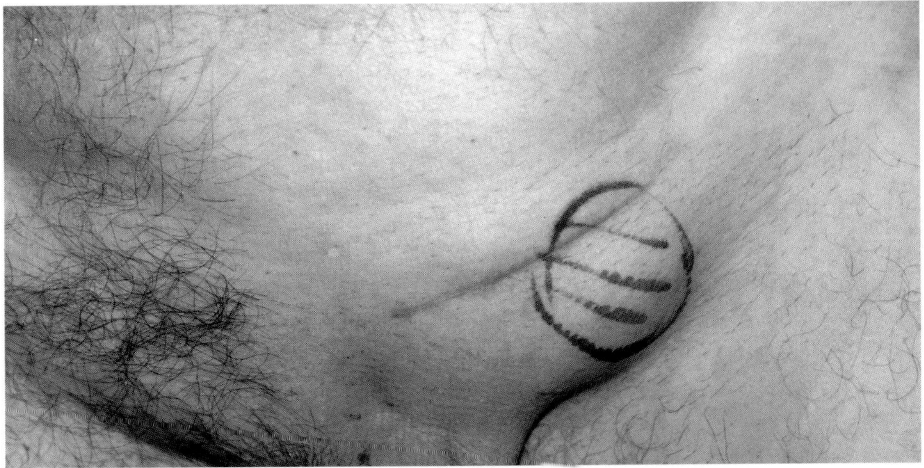

Figure 3. Bulge of a recurrent left inguinal hernia marked on the skin preoperatively with the patient standing

189

palpated preoperatively the skin incision was limited and the dissection directed towards the neck of the recurrent sac. This was found to be easiest in slim patients, and indeed obesity was the biggest technical intraoperative problem encountered. The technique of local infiltration was essentially the same as that employed in our primary repairs (see Chapter 9). We did not use a regional block, preferring to infiltrate the tissues as the incision was deepened. This is perhaps even more useful when operating on recurrent hernias as a technique of 'hydro-dissection' can be employed, separating the tissue planes by infiltration of dilute anaesthetic fluid.

A broad spectrum antibiotic, Co-amoxyclav (or erythromycin in cases of penicillin allergy), was given by mouth 1 h preoperatively. Midazolam, administered by the operator, was used for sedation, up to a maximum of 10 mg. In 71 patients (32%) an anaesthetist was present to administer the sedation and monitor the patient; this included patients with cardiopulmonary disease, patients aged over 65 and all patients with bilateral hernias.

It can be surprisingly difficult to locate a recurrent sac or defect while dissecting through rigid scar tissue and distorted anatomy, with the ever present worry of damage to the spermatic cord. The factors that were most helpful in overcoming this were the preoperative skin marking and the ability to ask the patient, because of using local anaesthetic, to cough or strain intraoperatively.

OPERATIVE FINDINGS AND TREATMENT

Recurrences were classified at operation as either lateral or medial, corresponding approximately to indirect and direct recurrences, respectively. The medial defects were further subdivided into three groups according to whether their diameter was less than 2.5 cm, between 2.5 and 4 cm, or greater than 4 cm. With lateral or indirect recurrences it was inevitably found that a complete re-dissection of the canal was required. The sac was mobilized and inverted or excised whichever seemed appropriate. No formal repair of the inguinal ring was attempted. A standard onlay mesh repair was then carried out as for primary repairs. Small medial recurrences (less than 2.5 cm) were treated by freeing the margins of the sac from the surrounding scar tissue and then inverting the sac and placing a rolled up plug of mesh into the defect (Figs 4 and 5). The plug was then sutured to the margins of the defect using interrupted or continuous nonabsorbable sutures (2/0 prolene) (Fig. 6). In these cases only as much dissection as was necessary to identify the margins of the sac was carried out, the inguinal canal was not laid open completely and plug insertion was the sole method of repair.

A similar procedure was used for medial or direct defects between 2.5 and 4 cm diameter; in these the cord structures required mobilization to allow an onlay patch of mesh to be placed over the posterior wall of the inguinal canal. With medial defects greater than 4 cm in diameter a patch of prosthetic mesh was inserted beneath the scarred transversalis fascia in the preperitoneal space (see Chapter 8) whenever possible, and an onlay patch was then used to reinforce the posterior wall of the canal. The

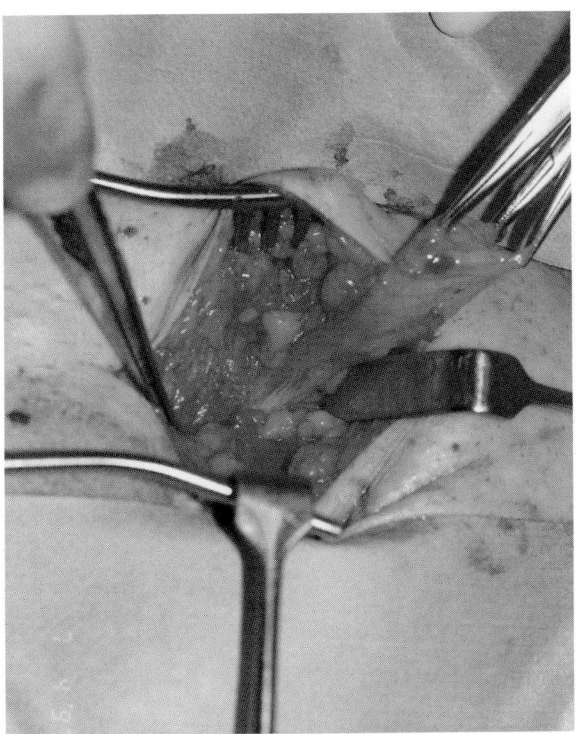

Figure 4. Sac of a recurrent inguinal hernia dissected out from the surrounding tissues, down to the scarred transversalis fascia. The full anatomy of the inguinal canal has not been exposed

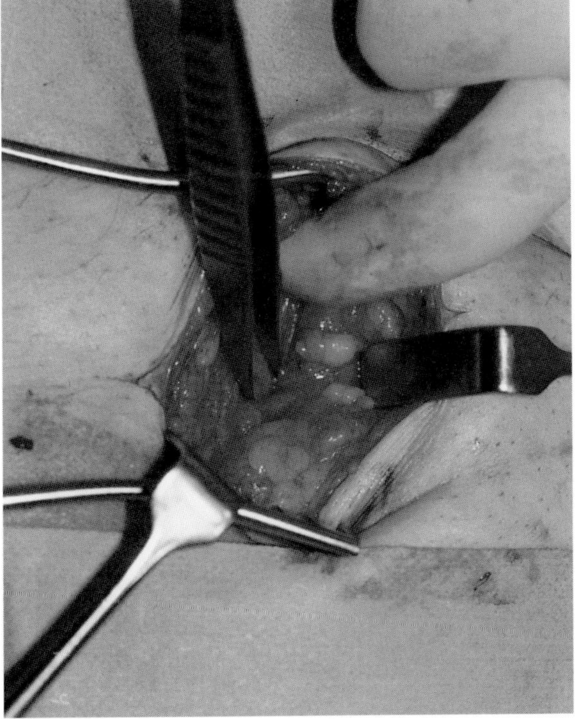

Figure 5. The sac has been inverted – simply pushed back through the defect in the transversalis fascia

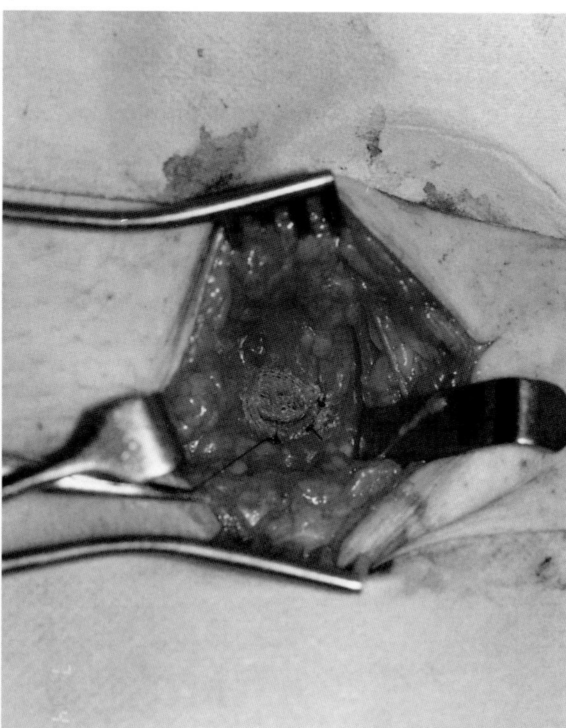

Figure 6. Mesh plug inserted into the defect. Interrupted nonabsorbable sutures are inserted circumferentially

wound was closed with absorbable sutures and subcuticular Dexon was used for the skin. Drains were not used routinely.

Postoperatively a diclofenac suppository was administered (unless contraindicated) and patients were walked back to a recovery area where they remained in a reclining chair for 1.5–2 h. Before leaving they were asked to empty their bladders and were all accompanied by a responsible adult on leaving the clinic. They were also given a detailed postoperative instruction sheet. An initial follow-up visit took place between 10 days and 4 weeks postoperatively. If there had been no complications, the next examination took place 12–18 months later, and yearly thereafter.

RESULTS

Early postoperative results (Table 2)

Seven patients developed haematomas, three in the wound and four in the scrotum, all of which settled without surgical intervention or the need for drainage. Prophylactic antibiotics (apart from the routine preoperative dose) were not used in these situations and none of the haematomas became infected.

	No. patients	%
Haematoma	7	3.0
Testicular swelling	6	2.7
Wound infection	2	1.0
Prolonged pain and discomfort (pain >14 days)	6	2.7
Cardiopulmonary	0	0
Urinary retention	0	0
Recurrence	11	5.0

Table 2. Complications of repair of recurrent inguinal hernia: 223 patients

Testicular swelling was noted in six patients, occurring between 5 and 20 days. Closer follow-up of these six patients showed that in five cases the testicular swelling settled with no residual abnormality, but in two cases the testes were noted to be smaller than at the preoperative assessment.

There were no cardiopulmonary complications, no cases of deep venous thrombosis, and no patients developed urinary retention.

Two patients (1%) developed a wound infection with redness, swelling and wound tenderness which responded to antibiotic treatment. There were three cases of chronic infection or sinus formation.

Postoperative pain was thought, anecdotally, by the surgeon to be more pronounced than after a primary tension-free mesh repair. However, none of these patients had had a mesh repair before, and almost all thought that the amount and length of time of pain and discomfort was less than with their previous repairs. Nevertheless, six patients complained of pain requiring oral analgesics for more than 14 days, though all of these had settled by 3 months postoperatively.

Recurrences (Table 3)

There were 11 recurrences in this group of 232 recurrent repairs (5%). In six cases we have suggested a possible reason for failure of the repair, but in the remaining five we have no explanation. Four of these patients (1, 7, 10, 11) have subsequently had a large patch of mesh placed in the preperitoneal space (GPRVS – giant prosthetic reinforcement of the visceral sac, see Chapters 16 and 17) and their repairs have remained sound to date (Fig. 7).

Two patients (5 and 6), in whom the re-recurrence was assessed as being small and discrete underwent a further operation under local anaesthetic at which the dissection was limited to the region of the defect and a prolene plug was inserted. In patient 4

Patient	Age	No. of previous recurrences	BHC recurrence	Time following BHC mesh repair to recurrence (months)	Reason for failure	Treatment	Current status
1	66	2	1	6	Absent inguinal ligament	GPRVS GA	NSR at 14 months
2	62	1	1	25	Very large defect	No treatment	Asymptomatic bulge
3	70	1	1	2	?	Bulge – truss	Wears a truss
4	70	2	2	4	Plug extruded	Patch	
				9	Recurrence lateral to 2nd mesh	Patch over lateral bulge LA	NSR 24 months
5	71	2	1	24	Recurrence lateral to edge of mesh	Plug LA	NSR
6	56	2	1	15	Recurrence inferior to mesh	Plug LA	NSR
7	44	3	1	7	?	GPRVS GA	NSR
8	52	3	2	14	Recurrence lateral to mesh	Patch LA	No treatment
				12	?	Advise GPRVS	
9	56	2	1	13	?	Advise GPRVS	No treatment
10	71	1	1	8	?	GPRVS LA	NSR
11	62	2	1	6	?	GPRVS LA	NSR

Abbreviations: GPRVS, giant prosthetic reinforcement of the visceral sac; NSR, no sign of recurrence; LA, local anaesthetic; GA, general anaesthetic.

Table 3. British Hernia Centre (BHC) recurrent recurrences

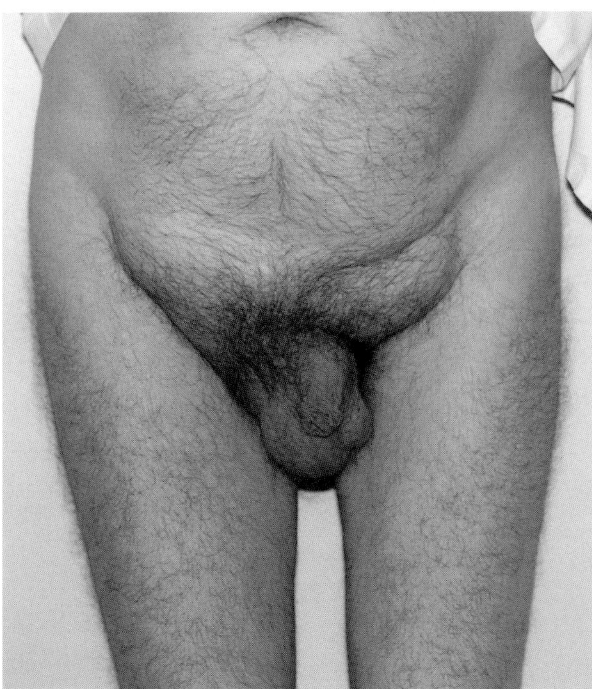

Figure 7. Patient 1 with bilateral recurrent inguinal hernias. An attempt to repair the left side under LA using an onlay patch led to an early recurrence. Both inguinal ligaments were absent (note the loss of the normal groin skin crease) with loss of tissue from the previous operations. He subsequently underwent a successful bilateral GPRVS (Stoppa) procedure, with no sign of recurrence at 14 months

the recurrence was a vague bulge lateral to the lateral extent of the mesh patch, and under local anaesthetic a further piece of mesh was inserted lateral to the deep ring beneath the external oblique. The remaining four patients have chosen to live with their re-recurrences for the time being rather than undergo further surgery, and in fact one of them had not noticed the recurrence until it was pointed out to him by the surgeon.

DISCUSSION

Specialized clinics or surgeons with a particular interest in hernia surgery report recurrence rates after primary inguinal hernia repair of well under 5%.[1-3] However, the true incidence of recurrence after primary inguinal hernia repair is probably between 10 and 15%.[5] The difficulty in establishing exact figures from one particular centre is partly due to problems with follow-up. Most busy general surgeons either do not have the time or wherewithal to establish long-term follow-up programmes to look at the medium- and long-term results of their primary hernia repairs; and many patients with failed hernia repairs are reluctant to return to their original surgeon. An unknown number are probably reluctant to seek further surgery anywhere and in addition there are an unknown number of patients who do not even realize that they have a recurrence.

Sweden has tackled this problem by instituting a nationwide audit programme whereby all participating hospitals have to report the results of hernia repair, including recurrences, to a central body (see Chapter 2). Even with a short follow-up, their results to date show a recurrence rate of 16–17%.

There are even greater difficulties in establishing the recurrence rate for recurrent hernias. General surgical units probably deal with too few recurrences to establish an effective protocol for dealing with this difficult surgical problem, and further failures make it even less likely that the patient will return for yet another operation to the same surgeon. Specialized units may attract patients with recurrent hernias from elsewhere, but their results will inevitably not reflect those obtained by general surgeons. There are few reports in the literature that have looked only at the results of repair of recurrent hernia and the data are usually included with those of primary repairs because most surgeons see and operate on too few recurrent hernias in a year to be able to draw any meaningful conclusions from their results.

Historical papers invariably spent much time analysing the aetiology of recurrences and recurrent recurrences, looking at surgical factors, as well as patient profiles (age, body weight, occupation, time of return to work, etc.)[1,2,14–19] They all had their own views as to the best technique to use for the recurrent repair, e.g. Shouldice, McVay, Halstead, cord transposition or transection, fascia lata grafts or various synthetic prostheses, etc.

Non-mesh classical repairs (Table 4)

Marsden's 1958 paper[19] was a detailed analysis of the possible aetiology of recurrent herniation, and an attempt to determine the best method of repair; 1000 primary inguinal hernia repairs were followed up for 3 years: 54 were recurrent hernias and 12 had recurred at the end of the follow-up period – a 22% three-year recurrence rate. Thirty years later he reported his personal series of 287 recurrent inguinal hernias repairs.[15] In fact he examined 238 of the cases, 11 being lost to follow-up and 38 having died without review. Of these, 27 recurrent repairs (10%) had failed over a follow-up period of 10–15 years, a result that he found disappointing. He used a variety of methods of repair, and in 43 cases he closed the inguinal canal, a euphemism for division of the spermatic cord. He considered this radical step justified as he felt that these 43 cases were at high risk of re-recurrence and only two of the patients thus treated developed a subsequent recurrence. Like many surgeons of his time he admitted to a prejudice against the use of nylon mesh, citing a high incidence of infection and chronic sinus formation, but said that he regretted not using it in more cases.

A smaller, though carefully followed-up, personal series of recurrent repairs was reported by Quillinan in 1969.[20] He did not transect the cord and was also most reluctant to 'resort to the use of prosthetic devices'. He did so in three cases, using tantalum

Author	Year	No. of cases	Follow-up (years)	Number of recurrences	Recurrences (%)
Clear[13]	1951	59	10	23	39.0
Ryan[14]	1953	369	1–10	3	0.8
Glassow[1]	1973	2912	3–20	28	1.0
Quillinan[20]	1969	44	2–10	4	10.0
Thieme[12]	1971	166	6–9	46	28.0
Halverson[2]	1970	135	1–22	4	3.0
Marsden[15]	1988	287	10–15	27	9.0
Ijzermans[11]	1991	163	4.5	37	23.0
Shulman[24]	1990	1402 (mesh)	3–21	21	1.5

Table 4. Results of open repair of recurrent inguinal hernia

mesh. The follow-up period ranged from 2 to 10 years, and there were four re-recurrences – an overall incidence of 10%.

Ryan's detailed paper from the Shouldice Clinic in 1953[14] looked at the factors involved in the aetiology of recurrent inguinal hernia. Of 369 cases, 13 had had their original operation at the Shouldice Clinic, the remainder elsewhere; 50 of these cases had had more than one previous repair and in over half (66%) of the re-recurrences, the failure had taken place within 1 year. Of the failures, 80% had occurred within 2 years of the recurrent repair. The inescapable conclusion is as valid now as it was then – that in these 'early' failures the hernia was actually overlooked or the repair was grossly inadequate. Just over a decade later, Glassow reviewed almost 3000 recurrent hernias operated on at the Shouldice clinic,[4] finding that 28 had re-recurred – an overall incidence of just under 1%.

Thieme[12] followed 166 recurrent inguinal hernia repairs for 9 years, finding an overall recurrence rate of 33.1%. Similar to Ijzermans[11] he found that 34% of the re-recurrences had appeared within 1 year of the recurrent repair. Another high re-recurrence rate of 39% was reported by Clear[13] in 53 cases of recurrent inguinal hernia followed for 10 years.

The classic paper of Halverson and McVay[2] reviewed a 22-year experience of the senior author in repairing 1200 groin hernias. During this period, 135 recurrent hernias were repaired, four of which subsequently recurred, a recurrence rate of 3%. A 'prosthetic device' was used in 13 of these recurrent repairs but 'only when necessary'.

A detailed clinical and histologic study of 100 recurrent inguinal hernia repairs was reported by Weinstein and Roberts.[17] They were loathe to use any form of synthetic prosthesis so that in patients with extensive tissue destruction and an absent inguinal ligament they used a flap of anterior rectus sheath (25 cases). The overall recurrence rate was 16%, but re-operating on their own re-recurrences their final failure rate was 7%.

Surgeons specializing in and having a large experience of hernia repair are responsible for these very impressive figures. Notwithstanding these outstanding results, failing to use prosthetic mesh in the repair of recurrent hernias is likely to yield poor results. Ijzermans followed up 163 patients who had been operated on for recurrent hernias using an anterior approach.[11] A 'classical hernioplasty' (no prosthetic mesh) with absorbable sutures was used for the repairs and the follow-up period ranged from 2 to 9 years. The cumulative recurrence rate at 5 years was 23%, and most of these recurrences had appeared within the first year. Clearly the combination of an anterior approach, no mesh, absorbable sutures and non-specialist surgeons are not to be recommended when tackling recurrent groin hernias.

Better results could be obtained with some form of prosthetic insert, although the repair of a recurrent inguinal hernia via an anterior approach presents problems even when using extraneous material. There may be extensive scar tissue and fibrosis, and frequently the anatomy is distorted. While damage to the testicular vessels in primary inguinal hernia repair is rare, when operating on a recurrent hernia the risk of testicular damage has been estimated at between 0.8% and 5%.[21,22] In our series six patients developed postoperative testicular swelling, and two (1%) were subsequently found to have a degree of testicular atrophy.

Prosthetic mesh repairs

Law and Ellis[23] used an expanded PTFE patch as an onlay in 52 'difficult' (multiple defects, an excessively large defect or poor tissue quality) recurrent inguinal hernias. With a mean follow-up of 2 years re-recurrences were found in five cases (10%).

The Lichtenstein Hernia Institute took a radically different approach. They reported a large series of 1402 recurrent groin hernias operated over a 20-year period,[24] almost all of which were treated successfully by simply 'plugging' the defect with prosthetic mesh. The follow-up was between 3 and 20 years and the recurrence rate extremely low at 1.6%. The advantages of not re-dissecting out the inguinal canal, and confining attention only to the defect are considerable in terms of ease and morbidity but may not be applicable to every case.

Nyhus,[8] a strong advocate of the preperitoneal approach, reported his experience operating on 203 recurrent groin hernias over 10 years. He felt that the re-recurrence rate was unacceptably high, six out of 115 followed up (5.2%), with suture alone. With an additional mesh buttress to cover the sutured repair the overall re-recurrence rate

Distorted anatomy

Scar tissue

Danger to the spermatic cord

Deficiency of tissue

Risk of haematoma and infection

Table 5. Problems in the repair of recurrent groin hernia

fell to 1.7%. The skin incision for this approach was above the previous incision, thus avoiding a dissection through scar tissue from previous surgery and reducing the risk of damage to the testicular vessels.

Schaap et al[25] used a similar preperitoneal method in 98 recurrent inguinal hernias; 55 were repaired by suture alone, and mesh was used in the remaining 43. Unfortunately in their hands both techniques had a high re-recurrence rate over a follow-up period of 45 months – 27% in unilateral hernias and 59% in bilateral hernias. This group admitted technical shortcomings as a likely explanation for these disappointing figures, but also found a large number of asymptomatic recurrences on routine examination.

Mozingo and his colleagues[26] used preperitoneal mesh repair in 100 recurrent inguinal hernias with only three re-recurrences over a follow-up period ranging from 6 months to 5 years. Interestingly all three recurrences occurred within the first 6 months postoperatively, suggesting technical failure as the reason.

Schumpelick[27] (see Chapter 8) also inserted the mesh preperitoneally, but did this through the inguinal canal. Placing the mesh in this position theoretically gives a better repair than a simple onlay, but the transinguinal approach still carries the disadvantage of a potentially difficult dissection through scar tissue and the risk of damage to the testicular vessels.

Stoppa[28] (see Chapter 16) and Wantz (see Chapter 17) advocate a preperitoneal approach, but with a very large piece of mesh that envelopes the peritoneum ('visceral sac') in a 'tension-free' technique that does not attempt to close the defect. The results over the medium- and long-term are excellent and the incidence of complications, especially testicular ones, are extremely low. Laparoscopic techniques are also being used in this situation though with a relatively short follow-up to date.[29]

The long-term results of recurrent hernia repair are of paramount importance. However, long-term follow-up may not be necessary to assess recurrence rates when using prosthetic mesh. Once the sac has been appropriately dealt with and the mesh has been placed in the correct position we suspect that late (more than 5 years post-repair) recurrences are unlikely to occur except perhaps when a plug alone was used for a discrete defect. If this is so then as little as 1–2 years may be adequate. Even with non-mesh repairs, in many of the detailed reviews of the results of recurrent repair mentioned above, the high percentage of failures that reveal themselves in the first year of follow-up is noted.

The reader is referred to an excellent comprehensive review of the technical faults that may lead to failure in both open and laparoscopic preperitoneal mesh repair of recurrent groin hernias.[29,30] The factors included surgeon inexperience, inadequate dissection, insufficient size of the prosthesis, haematoma formation (resulting in lifting of the mesh) and missed hernias.

CONCLUSION

This chapter has presented the results of using one technique, an anterior approach with mesh onlay, in an unselected consecutive series of patients with a variety of different types of recurrent inguinal hernia. Out of the 11 failures, five have subsequently had a preperitoneal prosthetic mesh repair with no sign of recurrence to date. In retrospect those 11 patients should probably have been offered a preperitoneal repair originally, although some would argue that using the Rives–Stoppa or unilateral Wantz operation in, say, an elderly slim man with a discrete medial recurrence is excessively complex. The placing of a prosthetic mesh plug under local anaesthetic in these circumstances may be perfectly adequate. In the absence of objective evidence the best solution at present must remain a matter of clinical judgment.

REFERENCES

1 Glassow F. The surgical repair of inguinal and femoral hernias. *Can Med Assoc J* 1973; **108**:308–13.

2 Halverson K, McVay CB. Inguinal and femoral hernioplasty. *Arch Surg* 1970; **101**:127–35.

3 Bendavid R. The Shouldice repair. In Nyhus LM, Condon RE, eds. *Hernia*, 4th edn. Philadelphia: JB Lippincott 1995.

4 Glassow F. Recurrent inguinal and femoral hernia: 3000 cases. *Can J Surg* 1964; **7**:284–8.

5 RAND Corp. Conceptualization and measurement of physiologic health of adults. Santa Monica, CA: RAND Corp 1983:15.

6 Bendavid R. The need for mesh. In Bendavid R, ed. *Prostheses and abdominal wall hernias*. Austin: RG Landes 1994:116–22.

7 Glassow F. Recurrent inguinal and femoral hernia. *BMJ* 1970; **1**:215–19.

8 Nyhus LM, Pollak R, Bombeck T et al. The preperitoneal approach and prosthetic buttress repair for recurrent hernia. *Ann Surg* 1988; **208**:733–7.

9 Greenburg AG. Revisiting the recurrent groin hernia. *Am J Surg* 1987; **154**:35–40.

10 Berliner S, Burston L, Katz P *et al.* An anterior transversalis fascia repair for adult inguinal hernias. *Am J Surg* 1978; **135**:633–6.

11 Ijzermans JNM, de Wilt H, Hop WCJ. Recurrent inguinal hernia treated by classical hernioplasty. *Arch Surg* 1991; **126**:1097–1100.

12 Thieme ET. Recurrent inguinal hernia. *Arch Surg* 1971; **103**:238–41.

13 Clear JJ. Ten year statistical study of inguinal hernias. *Arch Surg* 1951; **62**:70–8.

14 Ryan EA. Recurrent hernias: an analysis of 369 consecutive cases of recurrent inguinal and femoral hernias. *Surgical Gynecol Obstet.* 1953; **96**:343–54.

15 Marsden AJ. Recurrent inguinal hernia: a personal study. *Br J Surg* 1988; **75**:263–6.

16 Zimmerman LM. Recurrent inguinal hernia. *Surg Clin N Am* 1971; **51**:1317–24.

17 Weinstein M, Roberts M. Recurrent inguinal hernia. Follow-up study of 100 postoperative patients. *Am J Surg* 1975; **129**:564–9.

18 Shuttleworth KED, Davis WH. Treatment of inguinal herniae. *Lancet* 1960; **1**:126–7.

19 Marsden AJ. Inguinal hernia: a three year review of one thousand cases. *Br J Surg* 1958; **46**:234–43.

20 Quillinan R. Repair of recurrent inguinal hernia. *Am J Surg* 1969; **118**:593–5.

21 Wantz GE. Testicular atrophy and chronic residual neuralgia as risks of inguinal hernioplasty. *Surg Clin North Am* 1993; **73**:571–81.

22 Reid I, Devlin HB. Testicular atrophy as a consequence of inguinal hernia repair. *Br J Surg* 1994; **81**:91–3.

23 Law NW, Ellis H. Preliminary results for the repair of difficult recurrent inguinal hernias using expanded PTFE patch. *Act Chir Scand* 1990; **156**:609–12.

24 Shulman AG, Amid PK, Lichtenstein IL. The 'plug' repair of 1402 recurrent inguinal hernias. *Arch Surg* 1990; **125**:265–7.

25 Schaap HM, van de Pavoordt HD, Bast TJ. The preperitoneal approach in the repair of recurrent inguinal hernias. *Surg Gynecol Obstet* 1992; **176**:460–4.

26 Mozingo DW, Walters MJ, Otchy DP et al. Preperitoneal synthetic mesh repair of recurrent inguinal hernias. *Surg Gynecol Obstet* 1992; **174**:33–5.

27 Schumpelick V, Arlt G. Transinguinal preperitoneal mesh prosthesis (TIPP) for repair of inguinal hernia under local anaesthesia. *Chirurgica* 1996; **67**:419–24.

28 Stoppa R, Rives JL, Warlaumont C et al. The use of Dacron in the hernias of the groin. *Surg Clin N Am* 1984; **64**:269–85.

29 Felix EL, Michas C, McKnight RL. Laparoscopic repair of recurrent groin hernias. *Surg Laparosc Endosc* 1994; **4**:200–4.

30 Lowham AS, Filipi CJ, Fitzgibbons RJ Jr et al. Mechanisms of hernia recurrence after preperitoneal mesh repair. Traditional and laparoscopic. *Ann Surg* 1997; **225**:422–31.

16 GROIN HERNIA REPAIR BY BILATERAL EXTRAPERITONEAL MESH PROSTHESIS

Renée Stoppa

The operative repair of inguinal hernias remains controversial mainly because hernias are polymorphous lesions and also because the circumstances of operations for hernias and the features of the patients are diverse. In the past 100 years, with the advent of aseptic surgery and based on the work of Bassini, Marcy, Lotheisen and others, valuable techniques for repairing the deeper inguinal layers have been described. However the high recurrence rate reported in many series makes further discussion essential and stresses the need for further research. We need to develop recurrence-preventing operations, not only for the surgeons' pride, but for economic reasons.

Precise anatomic knowledge is a basic principle for improving operations for hernia. In 1956 Fruchaud[1] proposed a unified concept of groin hernias showing that wherever they might emerge superficially (inguinal, femoral, prevascular, medial or later), they all must pass through the musculopectineal (myopectineal) opening. Thus in that area the transversalis fascia, the inguinal portion of the endoabdominal fascia, is the level or layer at which inguinal hernia repair is best done. The only variably resistant layer is the intra-abdominal pressure-tight layer of the wall.

Behind the transversalis fascia is a wide cleavable cellular space that spreads to the two sides of the infra-umbilical midline the retrofascial preperitoneal and prevesical spaces, which incorporate the anatomical spaces of Retzius and Bogros.

We believe that perfect and permanent tightness of the deep inguinal layer is easily assured by a piece of synthetic mesh and we therefore believe that prostheses must be part of the surgical arsenal in hernia surgery. They are an almost foolproof weapon against recurrences, on the condition that they are used according to the original method that we have described. The preperitoneal approach together with a prosthetic repair are strategically and tactically related in our concept of hernial repair.

The operation of giant prosthetic reinforcement of the visceral sac (GPRVS) has been frequently misunderstood and altered since its inception,[2] and underwent further misinterpretation when proposed as a model for laparoscopic hernia repair. Following Nyhus, Rives, in France, has since 1965 emphasized the posterior approach[3] and since 1969 we have used the Cheatle–Henry preperitoneal sub-umbilical approach.[2] The advantages of the approach are facility of separation of the retrofascial cellular space, direct access to the posterior inguinal structures, clear understanding of hernial lesions, and good exposure of the musculopectineal opening.

USEFULNESS OF THIS METHOD

As we have mentioned, hernial lesions are diverse and therefore call for diverse methods of repair. For simple lesions, a simple (non-prosthetic) technique may be sufficient. For the severest lesions of the inguinal structures and mostly for multiple recurrent hernias (particularly those with Poupart's or Cooper's ligament and the transversalis fascia destroyed), prosthetic repair is a preferable, possibly the only, solution. The best reason for the use of prostheses is their efficacy. They solve the mechanical problem created by the deficiency of the impervious layer of the abdominal wall in hernias caused by weakness because they reinforce the transversalis fascia or replace it. These advantages are counterbalanced by some risks, among which is sepsis.

Familiarity with this approach and with prostheses means we no longer have to distinguish between the different types of groin hernias (inguinal or femoral). The preperitoneal approach is perfectly convenient for even the most difficult hernial repairs, such as those of multirecurrent, prevascular, sliding, enormous, and bilateral hernias. Because one avoids the superficial inguinal nerves and the testicular vessels by using the preperitoneal approach, the number of testicular atrophies and painful sequelae is decreased.

This is different from the anterior approach for preperitoneal prosthetic repair of inguinal hernias. This latter procedure requires dissection of the spermatic cord, inguinal layers, and hernial sac which may be difficult in recurrent hernias. We do know that Rives and associates have been successful, and we have some personal experience with the technique, but have had less consistent results and more septic complications than after the use of our large bilateral prosthesis.

THE IDEAL PROSTHESIS

The ideal prosthetic material should be biologically inert, easy to sterilize, elastic, have immediate and permanent strength, x-ray transparency, availability and low cost. A good prosthetic material must also provoke a moderate inflammatory reaction and have strong fibroblastic activity. Thermohardening resins (silicone, elastomers) are never used because they are impervious and will not fix themselves in position. We have routinely used Dacron mesh,[4] advocated in France by Rives and associates for 20 years. Marlex or Prolene mesh and Rhodergon 8000 can be used, but they are less supple than Dacron and thus less convenient.

PRINCIPLES OF REPAIR

We do not simply place a patch over the defect but insert a large interposition of prosthetic mesh able to hold face to face with the neighbouring layers and to instantly and permanently support the inguinal wall. Wrapping the lower portion of the visceral sac (peritoneum) in nonabsorbable mesh makes the visceral sac inextensible in this area so that herniation can no longer occur and closure of the hernia defect in the abdominal wall is not necessary. For this purpose the prosthesis must extend broadly beyond the weak inguinal area in all directions (Figs 1, 2) so that when the peritoneal sac is replaced, the prosthesis is pressed by intra-abdominal pressure against the inner face of

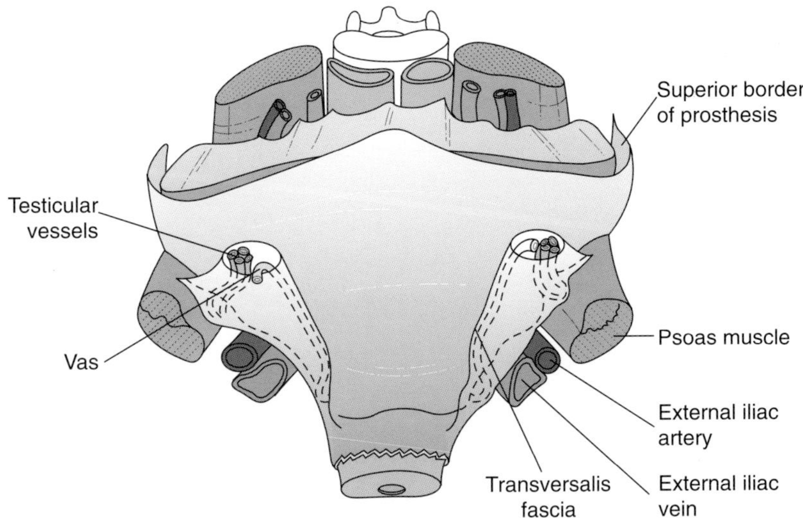

Figure 1. Anterior view of the chevron-shaped Dacron mesh in place with the pelvis and muscles of the lower abdominal wall 'removed'. In this diagram the inferolateral borders of the mesh are covered by the fascia enveloping the vas and the spermatic vessels. The mesh intervenes between the peritoneum and the vas and vessels. The development of this preperitoneal space to separate the vas and vessels from the peritoneal sac, so that the mesh can lie between, is a vital step in the operation to ensure that Fruchaud's myopectineal orifice is completely covered (see Chapter 4)

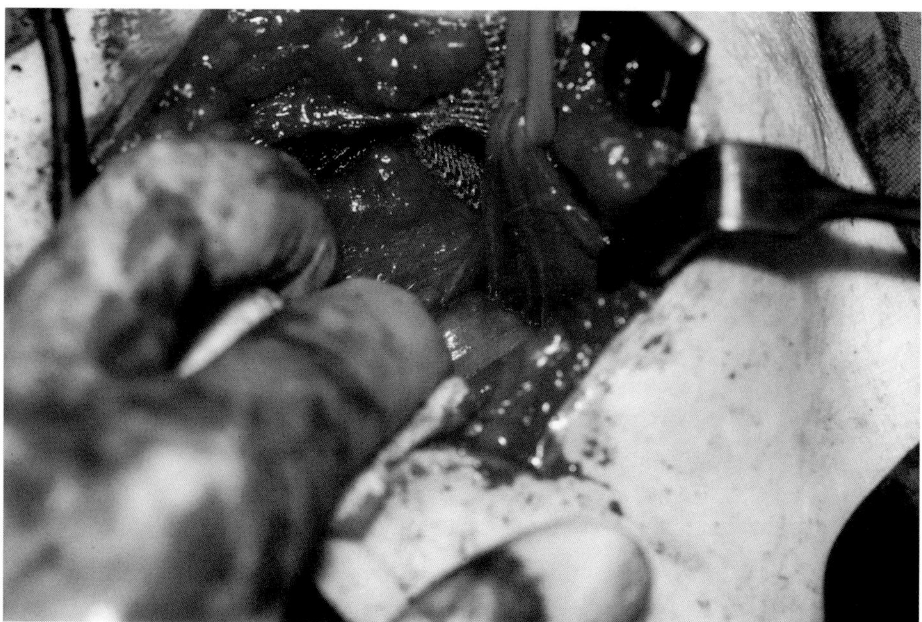

Figure 2. Close up view of the development of the plane between the vas and spermatic vessels (held up in a rubber sling) and the peritoneum or visceral sac

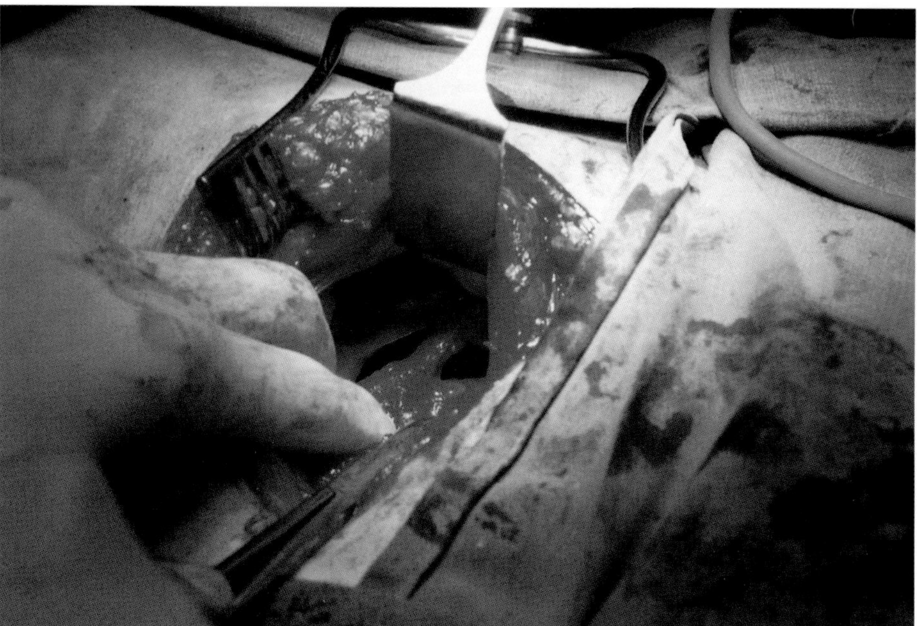

Figure 3. Operator standing on patient's left side; retractor at right edge of transverse (Pfanenstiel) incision. The visceral sac, including the hernia, has been pulled away from the pelvic/abdominal wall. View of the right spermatic cord (vessels and vas) passing towards the back of the inguinal canal

the abdominal wall and quickly attached by the development of the connective tissue through the mesh. This follows Pascal's hydrostatic principle and means that no sutures are required to hold the mesh in place. The central principle of our method is the larger the prosthesis the more efficient the repair. GPRVS was the first method of hernia repair to be both tension-free and sutureless.

TECHNICAL ASPECTS

The skin of the abdomen, scrotum, and perineum must be carefully disinfected; thus prophylactic antibiotic therapy is scarcely used. General anaesthesia (planned for a short duration of 30–40 minutes) is usual, but spinal or epidural anaesthesia is useful in patients at respiratory risk.

The patient is placed in a slight Trendelenberg position (helpful in obese patients). I use the Cheatle–Henry midline subumbilical approach,[5] which ensures that you can operate through undisturbed anatomy in a recurrent repair.[6] The preperitoneal cleavage starts from the lower portion of the wound on the median line in the retropubic space of Retzius. It continues laterally, proceeding behind the epigastric vessels. The dissection advances inferiorly in front of the bladder and then laterally and posteriorly behind the iliopubic ramus in the space of Bogros, thus isolating the hernia pedicle. This dissection does not necessitate a difficult search even in recurrent hernias.

Sacs may be freed by continuous moderate traction followed by incision, resection, and suture of the sac in first-time procedures (Fig. 3). However for multirecurrent indirect or inguinoscrotal hernias with wide defects and parietal sclerosis the surgeon must use a scalpel or scissors.[7–9]

The peritoneum having been closed after resection of the hernial sac, preperitoneal dissection continues rapidly. The cord is seized in its retroparietal course with an Ombredanne forceps or tape, with moderate traction applied, so that the scissors may dissociate the different elements of the cord from the peritoneal sac. This important step is called 'parietalization of cord components'. To perform the retroparietal dissection on the other side, the operator and assistant change sides and proceed in the same manner as for the first side (Fig. 4).

DIMENSIONS OF THE PROSTHESIS

For a large bilateral prosthesis the correct transverse dimension is equal to the distance between the anterosuperior iliac spines minus 2 cm. The height of the prosthesis should be equal to the distance between the umbilicus and the pubis. The mean values are 24 cm transversely and 16 cm vertically.

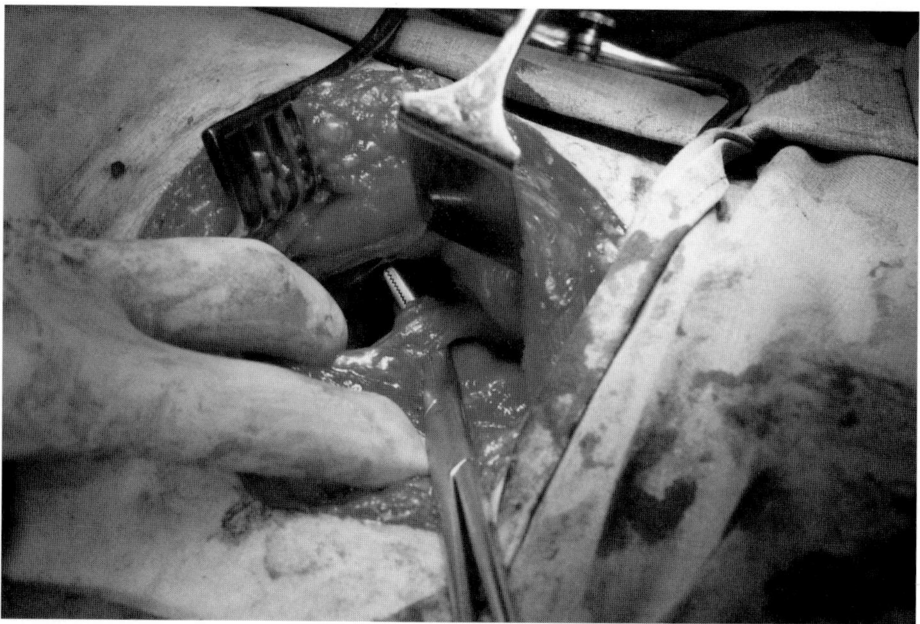

Figure 4.   Rochester forceps passed beneath the right spermatic cord. The operator's fingers are retracting the visceral sac superiorly. The plane between the spermatic cord and the visceral sac must be developed in order to place the prosthesis between the two; the alternative (acceptable occasionally) would be to split the mesh vertically to encircle the spermatic cord at this point

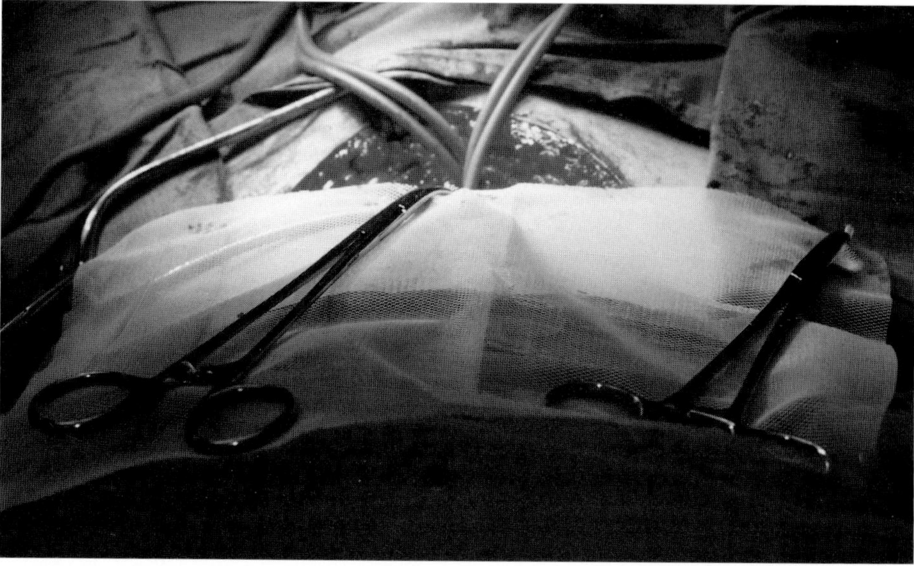

Figure 5.   Chevron-shaped Dacron mesh prosthetic laid on the abdomen prior to insertion. Three Rochester forceps are attached at the inferolateral corners and the centre of the inferior border

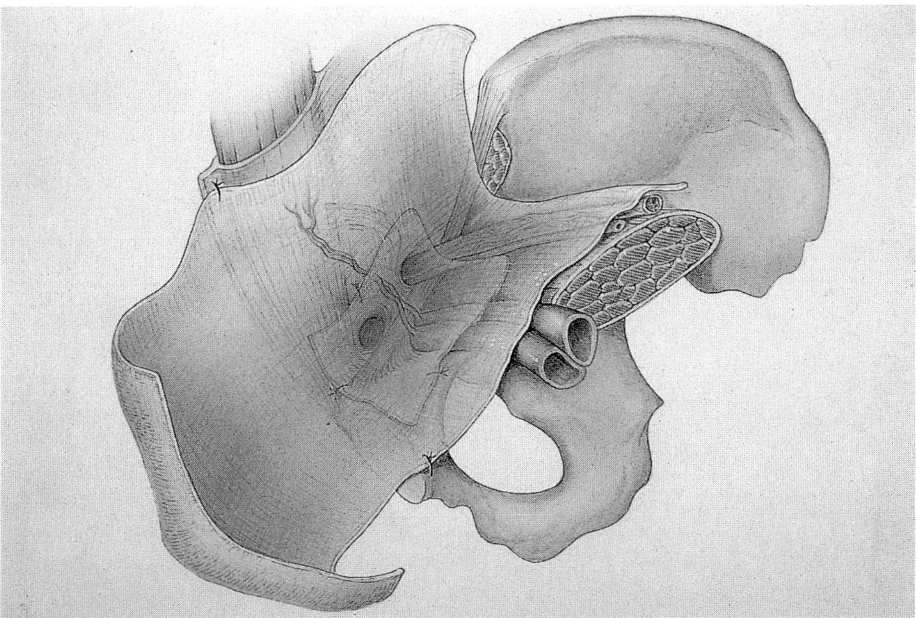

Figure 6. Left oblique view of a 'hemi-pelvis' showing a large piece of mesh positioned for a bilateral repair. (With permission from Gillian Lee Illustrations)

The patch is then seized by all its angles and at the middle of all borders with long forceps that facilitate placement (Fig. 5). The patch is first placed on the side opposite to the operator. The assistant retracts the parietal wall upwards as the operator depresses the peritoneal sac with the left hand, pulling it superiorly at the same time. This opens the parieto-peritoneal cleavage space. The prosthesis is then pushed into this space with the long forceps (Fig. 6). The inferior median forceps is first placed between the pubis and bladder, followed by the inferior angle forceps, median lateral forceps, and superior angle forceps, while pushing them as far as possible. The forceps used to place the prosthesis are then delicately removed at the same angle in which they were placed, while passing along the inner side of the parietal wall. The operator and the assistant again change sides and perform the same manoeuvres on the opposite side. Then the middle of the superior border of the patch is fixed with a catgut or synthetic absorbable suture to the inferior border of the Richet umbilical fascia. No other stitch is used for fixation. The operator and assistant again change sides and proceed in the same manner for the placement of the mesh at the opposite side.

The parietal suture is made with slowly absorbing synthetic suture material; the subcutaneous fat is closed with small catgut sutures, and the skin is sewn with fine nylon. When suction drainage tubes are necessary, they are placed in front of the prosthesis.

POSTOPERATIVE CARE

Recovery of activity is usually not a problem because postoperative discomfort is minimal. Slow-acting heparin is used for a few days. Hospital discharge may occur between the third and the fifth day.

COMPLICATIONS

Septic complications are more disagreeable when they occur after prosthetic repair than after non-prosthetic approaches. Thus extreme vigilance before, during, and after the operation is imperative. Superficial skin inflammation requires an early and generous opening of the skin incision. In the case of a deep infection related to the prosthesis, fortunately a rare occurrence, the wound must be opened widely, although the prosthesis must not be removed immediately. When the drainage is done correctly, the prosthesis can be penetrated and covered by the connective tissue so that healing can take place. Exceptionally, however, a partial resection of the prosthesis is necessary.

Testicular problems are rare, and in our series there were no cases of testicular atrophy. Similarly, chronic post-hernia neuralgia is not seen.

Recurrences after GPRVS are usually due to prostheses that are too small or that have been split.

INDICATIONS FOR GPRVS

1 One may be tempted to use a unilateral patch in unilateral hernias, but for patients older than 50 years we routinely insert a large bilateral prosthesis because of the frequent later appearance of a contralateral hernia.
2 When the hernias are bilateral (primary), elderly patients do profit from a large prosthetic repair which can be done quickly.
3 Certain complicated primary hernias such as huge, sliding or bilateral hernias are more easily treated by a preperitoneal prosthetic repair than by a standard herniorrhaphy.
4 The preperitoneal approach also avoids the difficult dissection by the inguinal approach of modified groin structures (recurrent hernias).
5 When the hernia has recurred after repair by an inguinal patch.
6 When Poupart's or Cooper's ligaments have been destroyed.
7 Obesity, advanced age, and cirrhotic disorders are conditions in which this approach may be helpful.

Straightforward postoperative course	91.1%
Septic complications	2.1%
Global recurrent rate	1.1%
Recurrences:	
Primary groin hernia	0.56%
Recurrent groin hernia	1.3%

Table 1. Personal series of 1992 GPRVS procedures carried out – reviewed up to 1990

CONTRAINDICATIONS TO PROSTHETIC REPAIR

Absolute contraindications:
1   when the risk of sepsis cannot be controlled;

Relative contraindications:
2   one must be extremely selective in using prostheses in emergency operations or to treat strangulated hernias;
3   when general or spinal anaesthesia cannot be used;
4   midline subumbilical scar;
5   iliocaval veins thrombosis history.

RESULTS

The results of GPRVS procedures carried out up to 1990 are given in Table 1.

No recurrences occurred after the first postoperative year. There were no testicular complications and no cases of chronic neuralgia (courtesy of the posterior approach). The 16 recurrences in our series occurred because the prostheses used were too small. Thus the recurrent sac made its way through the insufficient fascia under the lower (11 cases) or the lateral (5 cases) edge.

CONCLUSION

Prosthetic repairs are an important development because of their excellent results. We have not found prosthetic repair of groin hernias by the preperitoneal route to be a risky or complex procedure. The midline preperitoneal approach allows one to reach the deep hernial orifice quickly and easily and with a wide exposure, while also managing a deep cleaved site for the placement of a large bilateral prosthesis. Large prostheses are kept in place by intra-abdominal pressure; they need not be fixed nor should an attempt be made to repair the abdominal wall defect. We have used this technique for more than 25 years without any attempt at repair (closure) of the hernial orifices or fixation of the mesh.

REFERENCES

1   Fruchaud H. *Anatomie chirurgicale des hernies de l'aine.* Paris: Doin 1956.
2   Stoppa R, Quintin M. Les deficiences de la paroi abdominale chez le sûjet agé – colloque avec le praticien. *Sem Hop Paris* 1969; **45**:2182–5.
3   Rives J, Nicaise H. A propos des hernies de l'aineet de leurs recidives. *Sem Hop Paris* 1966; **31**:1932.
4   Stoppa RE, Rives JL, Warlaumont CR et al. The use of Dacron in the repair of hernias of the groin. *Surg Clin North Am* 1984; **64**:269–89.
5   Henry AK. Operation for femoral hernia by a midline extraperitoneal approach. *Lancet* 1936; **iv**:680.
6   Stoppa R. The preperitoneal approach and prosthetic repair of groin hernia. In Nyhus LM, Condon RE, eds. *Hernia,* 4th edn. Philadelphia: JB Lippincott 1995; 188–210.
7   Stoppa R. Hernia of the abdominal wall. In Chevrel JP, ed. *Hernias and Surgery,* 2nd edn, Paris: Springer 1998; 171–277.
8   Ravitch MM. *Repair of Hernias.* Chicago: Year Book 1969.
9   Wantz GE. Giant reinforcement of the visceral sac. *Surg Gynecol Obstet* 1989; **169**:408.

COMMENT ON THE STOPPA OPERATION BY GEORGE E WANTZ

Stoppa's revolutionary and innovative hernioplasty cures all the hernias of the groin without using sutures or staples, or mending the parietal defect in the abdominal wall. He deserves the credit for devising the first truly tension-free and sutureless hernioplasty as far back as 1969. The operation focuses on the mesh retaining the peritoneum. The mesh substitutes for the transversal fascia, adheres to the visceral sac rendering it inextensible, and thereby prevents peritoneal protrusion. It is incorrect, as many surgeons do, to call a properitoneal hernioplasty in which a large piece of mesh is fixed to the posterior abdominal wall 'the Stoppa operation', because fixing the mesh to the abdominal wall changes the focus of the operation. This reasoning may be pedantic but it explains why the operation is called by the descriptive term giant prosthetic reinforcement of the visceral sac (GPRVS) which distinguishes it from other properitoneal prosthetic repairs.

For success of this hernioplasty the prosthesis must be supple, elastic, flexible, conforming, integrated quickly, and have a texture which grips the tissues to prevent wandering of the unfixed mesh. The only commercially available prosthetic mesh having these properties is Mersilene which is composed of the polyfilamented polyester Dacron. Other prosthetic meshes will not do. Unsutured meshes of polypropylene are semi-rigid and will not conform to the complex curves of the pelvis. GoreTex is unsuitable because it is too inert and does not become integrated, but instead is encapsulated by a process that may take more than 30 days.

For reasons that are not totally clear, surgeons in the USA are wary of repairing hernias with meshes made of Dacron although they do not hesitate to use Dacron aortic prostheses. This distrust has resulted in unnecessary recurrences because the popular semi-stiff polypropylene meshes are not a suitable substitute for Mersilene.

Stoppa prefers a midline access incision; it is quick and affords excellent exposure. The operation, however, can also be done via a short and more cosmetic Pfannenstiel incision. When previous groin incisions are present the Pfannenstiel incision may be positioned more cephalad to avoid the dissection of the previous surgeons. In either case the operation in the USA is now done routinely in day surgery. The patients report that they are pleased that they do not have to stay in the hospital overnight, and that the postoperative discomfort is completely tolerable.

As a result of previous groin hernioplasties the deep ring may become repositioned laterally and superiorly toward the anterior iliac spine. In these instances the surgeon may experience difficulty ensuring that the mesh adequately embraces the visceral sac. To make doubly sure of a successful repair, a 3–4 cm swatch of polypropylene, part-way slit, may be slipped around the elements of the cord at the level of the deep ring before implanting the Mersilene.

Correct placement of the Mersilene is important; the surgeon should bear in mind that the mesh is to envelope the peritoneum and is not merely being placed against the inside of the anterior abdominal wall and pelvis. To enable this, the long clamps grasping the mesh are first pushed down and then up behind the visceral sac. The mesh should lay smoothly over the peritoneum. Wrinkling indicates that the mesh may be incorrectly positioned or that the dissection was insufficient to contain the spread-out prosthesis. When a midline incision is used the prosthesis should be fixed with a permanent suture to the umbilical fascia to ensure that the mesh will also act as protection preventing later herniation through the access incision.

Soiling of the properitoneal space, for example by a radical supra pubic prostatectomy, may sometimes be a contraindication for this operation. Bladder diverticula also pose a potential hazard and may be inadvertently entered. In the absence of a frank urinary tract infection, bladder urine is normally sterile and it is usually safe to proceed should the bladder be entered. If the surgeon predicts that an unintentional cystostomy may occur, the prudent strategy would be to preoperatively sterilize the urinary tract with appropriate antimicrobial drugs.

When indicated, the principles of GPRVS may be applied unilaterally to cure a single hernia of the groin through either a transverse abdominal, anterior groin, or anterior groin subinguinal incision. Often in these instances the repair may be done with the aid of local anaesthesia. The reader is referred to the appropriate chapters concerning these techniques.

Stoppa's innovative operation should be a part of every surgeon's armamentarium. It is the best operation to deal with all complex hernias of the groin.

17 UNILATERAL GIANT PROSTHETIC REINFORCEMENT OF THE VISCERAL SAC

George E Wantz

UNILATERAL GPRVS

Unilateral giant prosthetic reinforcement of the visceral sac (GPRVS) is the descriptive term for a properitoneal* hernioplasty with a large unfixed piece of the polyester mesh Mersilene. It is the Stoppa procedure applied to a single groin. Originally it was developed for the treatment of complex hernias of the groin (e.g. recurrent hernias) in an ambulatory setting, with local anesthesia and a minimal chance of the complications, testicular atrophy and chronic neuralgia.[1] Currently, the chief indication for unilateral GPRVS is when the Stoppa operation is unnecessary or inapplicable and when a complex hernia is encountered during an hernioplasty with an anterior groin incision. The properitoneal mesh in unilateral GPRVS may be implanted through a lower quadrant transverse abdominal incision or through an anterior groin incision either transinguinally or subinguinally.[2]

Permanent prostheses for unilateral GPRVS

The permanent prosthesis for unilateral GPRVS must conform to the complex curves of the pelvis and, therefore, should be soft, elastic, supple, and pliable. Also it must become integrated rapidly, be tolerant of infection, have a surface texture that will grip the tissues, and be available in large pieces. To date the only prosthetic mesh meeting these criteria is Mersilene mesh which is composed of multifilamented fibers of the polyester Dacron.[3] Other materials used as mesh are not suitable substitutes. Types of polypropylene meshes are semi-rigid, buckle when bent in two directions, and are not conforming. Furthermore, intra-abdominal pressure is insufficient to hold the unfixed polypropylene mesh in place in the properitoneal space. Gore-tex is conforming but

*Editors' note: the prefix *pro-*, meaning before or in front of, derives from Greek; *pre-* is the Latin equivalent. As the word 'peritoneum' derives from both languages, either prefix may be used in this context.

intolerant of early infection, and, rather than being rapidly integrated, is only slowly encapsulated in the tissues.

Techniques of unilateral GPRVS

Transverse abdominal incision[4]

The properitoneal space is reached by a transverse incision extending from the midline laterally for 8–9 cm. It is made 2–3 cm below the level of the anterior superior iliac spines and should be well above the deep ring and any hernias that might present (Fig. 1). The rectus sheath and oblique abdominal muscles (fascia) are incised the length of the skin incision. The rectus muscle is bluntly dissected from the rectus sheath and the lower abdominal wall retracted medially (Fig. 2). The transversalis fascia will be easily

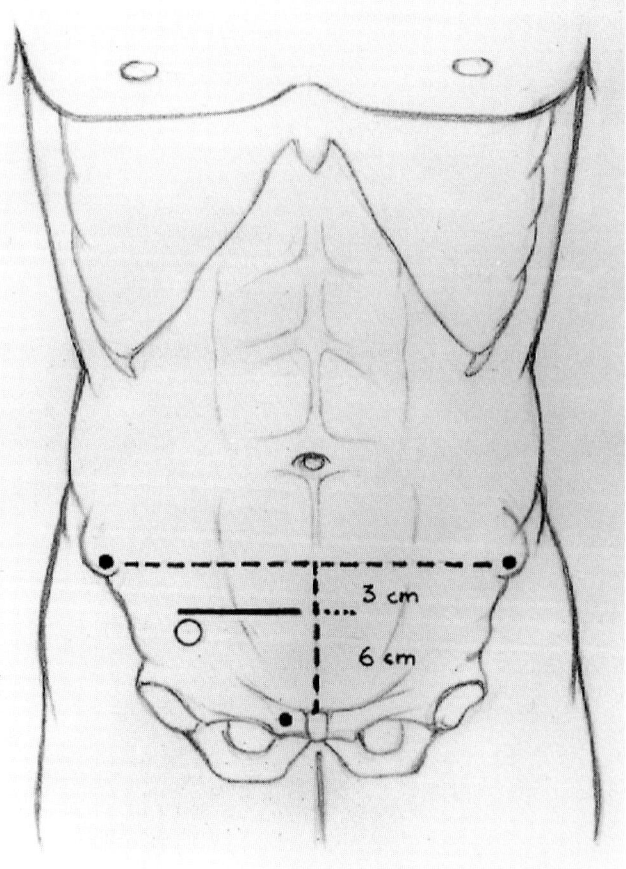

Figure 1. The location of the abdominal incision for properitoneal unilateral (right side) GPRVS. (With permission from Schumpelick and Wantz[2])

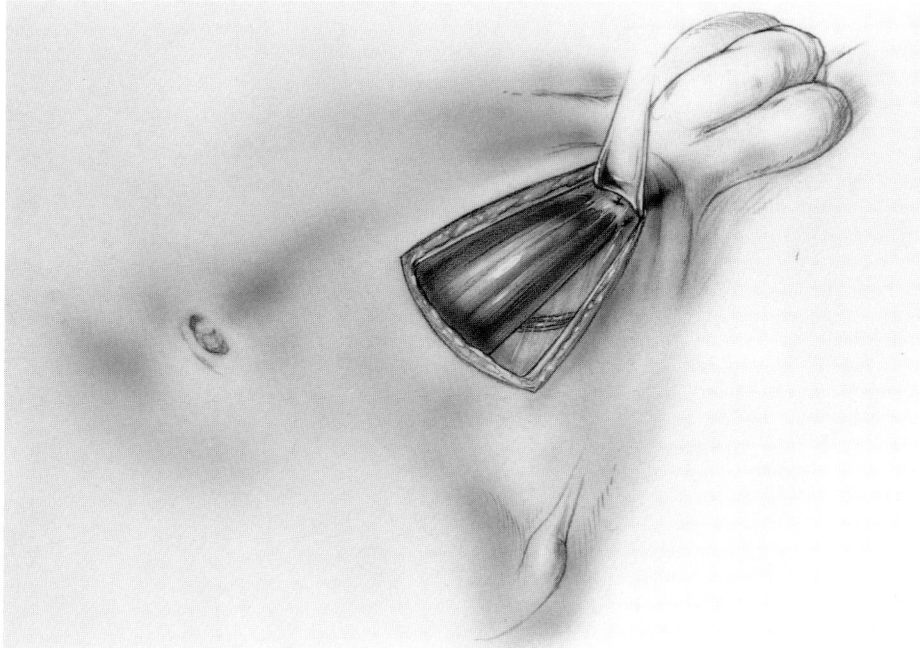

Figure 2. The rectus sheath has been dissected from the rectus muscle and the inferior edge of the wound retracted revealing the rectus muscle and, lateral to it, the thin transversalis fascia covering the inferior epigastric vessels and properitoneal fat. (With permission from Schumpelick and Wantz[2])

identified at the lateral border of the rectus muscle. It is thin, covers the inferior epigastric vessels and the yellow properitoneal fat, and passes deep to the rectus muscle. Incising the transversalis fascia along the border of the rectus muscle frees the muscle, permits entrance into the properitoneal space and exposes the inferior epigastric vessels which do not necessarily require division.

The properitoneal space is cleaved in all directions, medially, laterally and superiorly, behind the rectus muscle and the oblique muscle of the abdominal wall, and inferiorly and deeply, into the pelvis exposing the space of Retzius, the superior ramus of the pubis, the obturator foramen, iliac vessels and iliopsoas muscle.

Hernia sacs are dealt with in conventional ways. The sacs of direct, femoral or other rare hernias, such as obturator, are easily identified and teased from adjacent tissues. If the sacs are large, they are amputated or inverted beneath a purse-string suture in order to smooth the external surface of the visceral sac. The pedicle of simple indirect inguinal hernias is divided and the proximal peritoneum oversewn. The distal peritoneal sac is left in place, undissected and attached to the cord. Of course, all sliding indirect hernia sacs will require dissection from the cord. An incision in the anterior inguinal canal may be required to release voluminous incarcerated hernias.

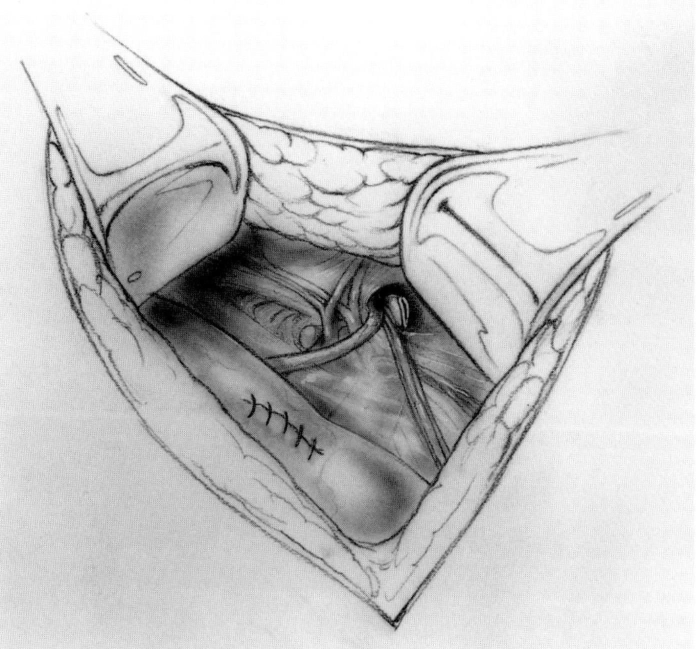

Figure 3. The complete dissection of the properitoneal space showing parietalization of the vas deferens, passing inferomedially from the deep ring, and testicular vessels passing from the deep ring inferolaterally towards the right. (With permission from Wantz[5])

The vas deferens and the testicular vessels enveloped in the parietal lamina all dissected from the visceral peritoneum starting at the level of the deep ring proximally for at least 10 cm. This technique, first described by Stoppa, is called parietalization of the elements of the spermatic cord (Fig. 3).

The hernia defects in the abdominal wall are not closed but the dead space created by the hernia sac should be eliminated by inverting the transversalis fascia (which enveloped the peritoneal sac in the abdominal wall) and suturing it to the abdominal wall. Surplus properitoneal fat should be cleared away from the abdominal wall. Be careful not to withdraw the spermatic cord in the process.

The Mersilene is arranged so that the material stretches transversely. In the developmental stages of the operation, the mesh was shaped as a square or rectangle and was considerably smaller than is used nowadays. Experience (recurrence) showed that the mesh was incorrectly shaped and too small. Currently the prosthesis is shaped like a diamond (Fig. 4). It is important that the bottom edge is wider than the top and that the lateral side is longer than the medial side. The width of the superior edge of the prosthesis equals the distance from the midline to the anterior superior iliac spine minus 1 cm and the vertical length of the medial edge is 14 cm. The inferior border

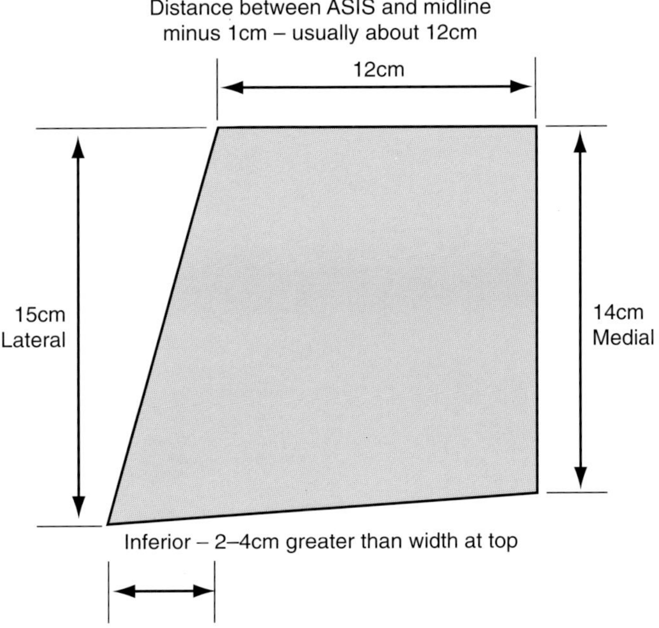

Figure 4. The dimensions of the Mersilene mesh for unilateral GPRVS, via an abdominal approach

is extended 2–4 cm laterally and the lateral border is extended at least 1 cm inferiorly (see Fig. 4). Thus, elongating the inferolateral corner of the mesh ensures a solid prosthetic grip on the lateral visceral sac.

The prosthesis is placed under the rectus muscle and the superior abdominal wall by three synthetic absorbable sutures appropriately placed along the upper border of the mesh (Fig. 5). The sutures secure the mesh to the abdominal wall 2–3 cm above the incision. The superomedial corner suture is near the linea alba, the middle suture is in the semilunar line of Spieghel and the superolateral corner suture passes through the oblique abdominal muscles near the anterior superior iliac spine. A Reverdin suture needle facilitates the placement of the sutures, but lacking this instrument very large curved needles can be used.

The inferior portion of the mesh is implanted with the aid of three long clamps, which grasp the two corners and the middle of the lower edge (Fig. 6). Retracting the abdominal wall opens the properitoneal space, enabling the clamps to unfold the mesh and slide it into place. The clamp grasping the lower medial corner is placed into the space of Retzius and unfolds the mesh behind the rectus muscle and symphisis pubis and in front of the bladder. It is steadied by an assistant. Next, the clamp that grasps

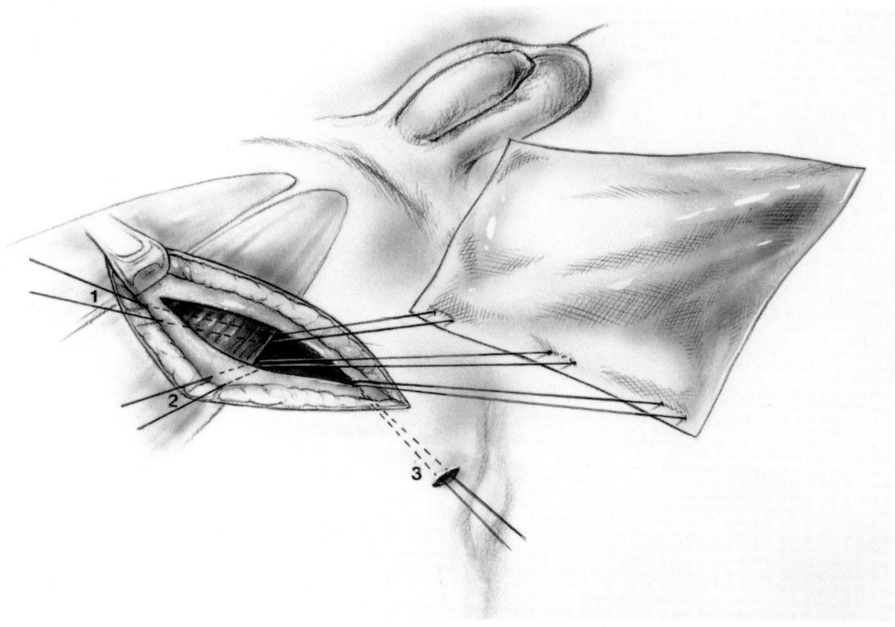

Figure 5. The mesh in unilateral GPRVS is fixed to the anterior abdominal wall 2–3 cm above the access incision with three successive sutures placed along its superior border: 1, superomedial corner suture; 2, middle suture; 3, superolateral corner suture. (With permission from Wantz[5])

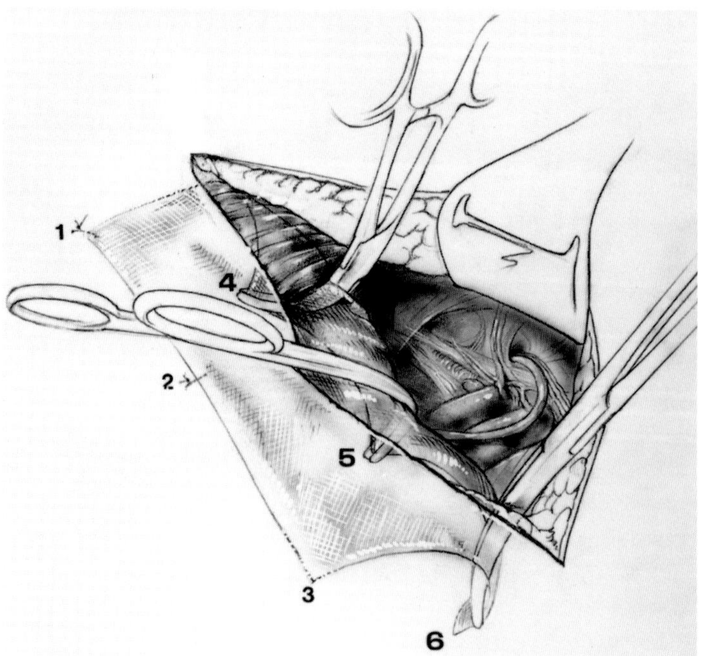

Figure 6. The distal mesh is implanted with three long clamps, which clasp the two corners (4,6) and the middle (5) of the lower edge. The mesh envelops the visceral sac. (With permission from Wantz[5])

the middle of the inferior edge is pushed deeply into the wound to unfold the mesh over the peritoneum facing the superior and inferior rami of the pubis, the obturator foramen and the iliac vessels. It is also steadied by an assistant. Finally, the clamp grasping the lower lateral corner of the mesh slides the prosthesis dorsal and cephalad into the iliac fossa to cover the peritoneum adjacent to the deep ring, the parietalized spermatic cord and the iliopsoas muscle. This is steadied by the surgeon. The retractors are removed and the clamps are released and carefully withdrawn. Wrinkling and folding of the mesh may occur with removal of the clamps if the properitoneal space is insufficiently cleaved. Closed suction drainage is used when hemostasis is incomplete or there remains a large distal indirect hernia sac. The access incision is loosely closed with continuous absorbable suture.

The important feature of GPRVS via a transverse abdominal incision is that dissection or re-dissection of the inguinal canal and its contents are avoided, thereby, eliminating trauma to the spermatic cord and sensory inguinal nerves. Furthermore, the procedure may be accomplished using local anaesthesia if necessary. Anesthetizing the peritoneum adjacent to the pelvic wall, the vas deferens, and the testicular vessels may be difficult and incomplete. Local anesthesia may be supplemented by additional sedation administered by the anesthesiologist. However, drugs which may increase use of abdominal muscles for breathing, such as fentanyl, can severely restrict exposure and should not be used.

Transinguinal GPRVS

Trans-inguinal GPRVS is similar to the Rives hernioplasty but differs from it in that the mesh is not sutured circumferentially and the vas deferens and testicular vessel are parietalized.[5,6] Its main indication is for unexpectedly complex hernias of the groin.

The properitoneal space is reached by division of the posterior wall of the inguinal canal (Fig. 7) in exactly the same way as in the classical hernioplasties. Division of the cremaster muscle, cremaster vessels and genital nerve assists exposure but is not essential. Wide cleavage of the properitoneal space is easily accomplished bluntly with the index finger or sponge stick in all directions. Division of the inferior epigastric vessels facilitates this dissection and the implantation of the prosthesis, but is not always necessary.

The spermatic cord and the testicualr vessels are perietalized as described above. If parietalization is not carried out the operation can be completed as Rives does. A lateral slit is made in the mesh to accommodate the cord. The lateral bisected tails of the mesh are sutured around the cord, and circumferentially to Cooper's ligament and the abdominal wall.

The Mersilene prosthesis should be as large as possible and not less than 10 × 10 cm. It should be arranged so that it stretches transversely. The prosthesis is drawn into the properitoneal space underneath the transversalis muscle by three to five permanent or slowly absorbable synthetic sutures (see Fig. 7). The sutures that suspend the prosthesis are placed medially, superiorly and laterally far beyond the borders of Fruchaud's myopectineal orifice. The sutures not only expedite the correct

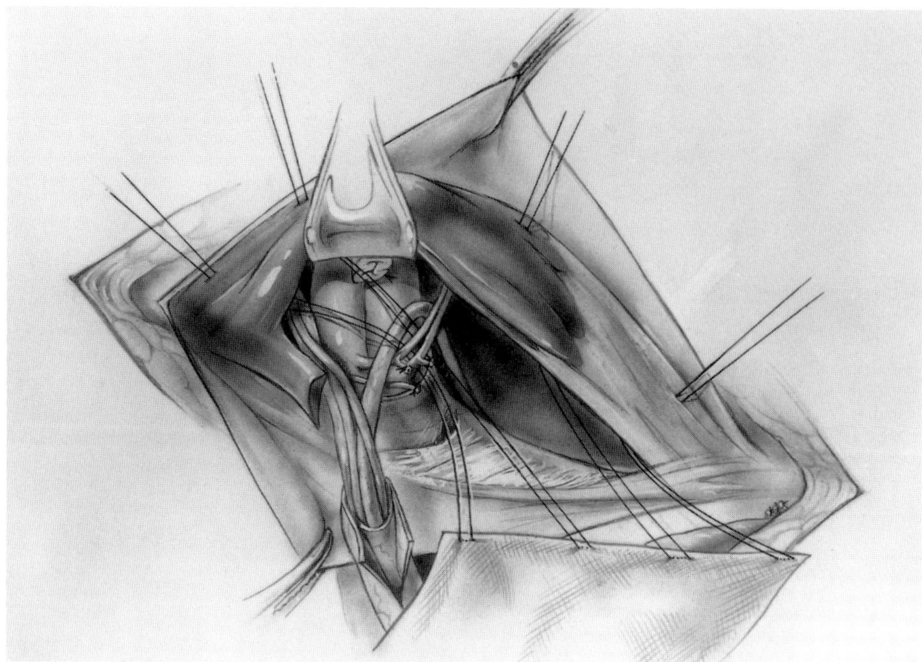

Figure 7. Unilateral GPRVS can be done through an anterior groin incision. In this case, the floor of the inguinal canal is completely incised, the properitoneal space is bluntly dissected, and the cord parietalized. The mesh is fixed to the anterior abdominal wall with three or four sutures. (By permission of *Surgery, Gynecology & Obstetrics*, now known as the *Journal of the American College of Surgeons*)

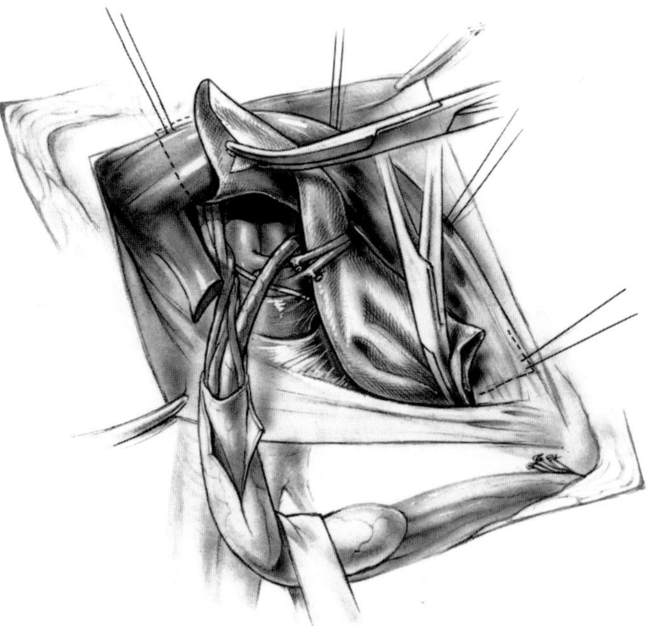

Figure 8. The distal mesh in transinguinal GPRVS is implanted with long clamps to envelop the visceral sac. (By permission of *Surgery, Gynecology & Obstetrics*, now known as the *Journal of the American College of Surgeons*)

placement of the prosthesis superiorly, but ensures its position during the manipulation required to insert the inferior portion of the prosthesis. The inferior border of the prosthesis is implanted with long curved clamps (Wiley or Rochester Pean) that grasp the prosthesis on the corners and in the middle of the distal edge (Fig. 8). The long curved clamps place the prosthesis medially deep into the space of Retzius and laterally far up into the iliac fossa. The clamp in the middle edge aids implantation of the prosthesis over the peritoneum facing the obturator canal. The clamps are then carefully removed and the position of the prosthesis checked to make sure that it has not been dislodged (Fig. 9). The posterior wall of the inguinal canal is closed without tension and with a nonabsorbable monofilament synthetic suture. A formal hernioplasty is not essential, and the wound is closed in a conventional way.

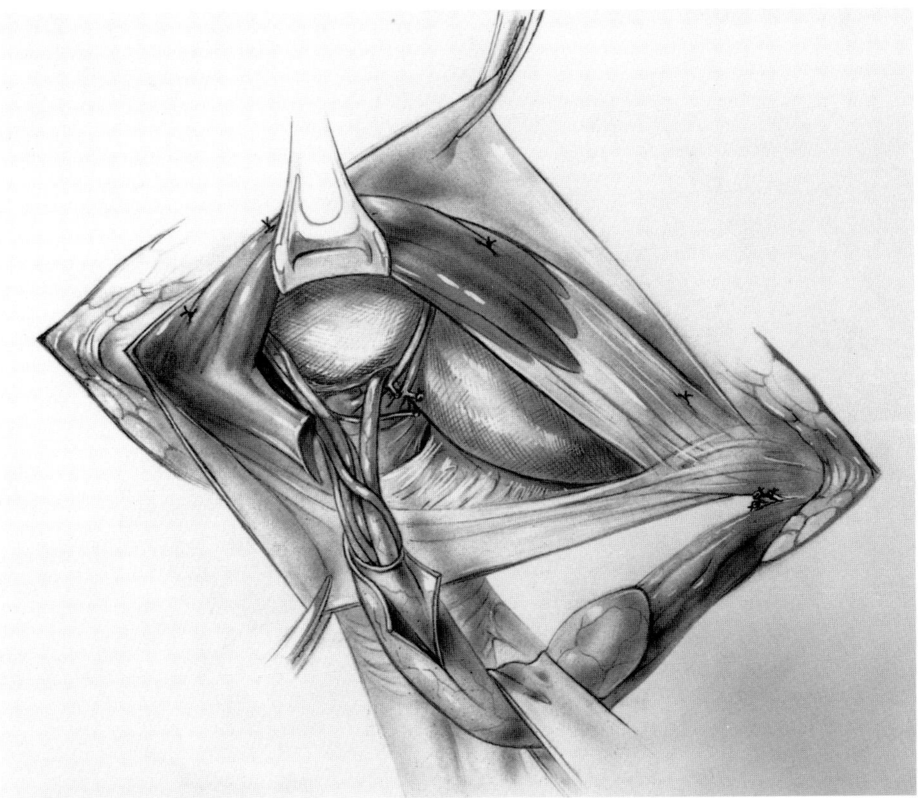

Figure 9. The appearance of the implanted mesh in transinguinal GPRVS. The transversalis fascia and aponeurosis are loosely approximated to complete the procedure. (By permission of *Surgery, Gynecology & Obstetrics*, now known as the *Journal of the American College of Surgeons*)

Subinguinal GPRVS

Subinguinal GPRVS is used when unanticipated perivascular femoral hernias are encountered in elderly frail women during femoral hernioplasty and in patients with perivascular femoral hernias following successful (anterior approach) prosthetic inguinal hernioplasty. It is easily done with unassisted local anesthesia. The need for subinguinal GPRVS is rare, yet knowing the technique is important.

The technique of subinguinal GPRVS resembles the other methods of unilateral GPRVS. The femoral region is reached through an anterior groin incision. The femoral hernia sac is dissected from adjacent tissues and from the edge of the parietal defect. The sac may be ligated and amputated or merely inverted if empty. The properitoneal space is entered through the parietal defect and cleaved by gentle blunt finger dissection in all directions. The dissection, however, is limited on the anterior surface of the iliac vessels by the origin of the inferior epigastric vessels. A square of Mersilene mesh approximately 6×8 cm is arranged so that the stretch is transverse. A larger piece of mesh is not needed because the parietal defect is relatively small compared to the size of the mesh. It is placed in the properitoneal space and secured to the anterior abdominal wall 3 cm above the inguinal ligament with three sutures (Fig. 10). A demitasse spoon is a useful instrument to retain and protect the peritoneum during suturing. Reverdin needles facilitate the placement of the sutures. These sutures, which need not be permanent, are very useful because they assure the position of the superior portion of the mesh during the implantation of the distal border. The distal mesh is implanted with two long clamps which grasp the far edge of the mesh at the corners. The clamps push the mesh in place, medially deep in the space of Retzius and laterally up into the iliac fossa (Fig. 11). The inferior epigastric vessels prevent deep implantation of the midportion of the mesh though injury of these vessels does not occur because the Mersilene is elastic and pliant and can bunch up around them. Closure of the parietal defect is not necessary (Fig. 12).

Recurrence after unilateral GPRVS

As recurrent herniations after GPRVS are due to technical errors, the following pitfalls of the procedure must be avoided for successful repair:

- inadequate cleavage of the properitoneal space
- closure of the defect in the abdominal wall (which should not be done)
- incorrect sizing, shaping and placement of the mesh.

Buckling of the mesh indicates inadequate cleavage or poor placement of the mesh. Hematomas and seromas prevent rapid integration, may displace the mesh and provide a rich medium for bacterial growth. They can be minimized by closed suction drainage when hemostasis is incomplete. *When implanting the mesh the surgeon should picture the mesh enveloping and retaining the peritoneum rather than being applied to the defective abdominal wall.* The most common cause of recurrence is probably too small a piece of mesh being used.

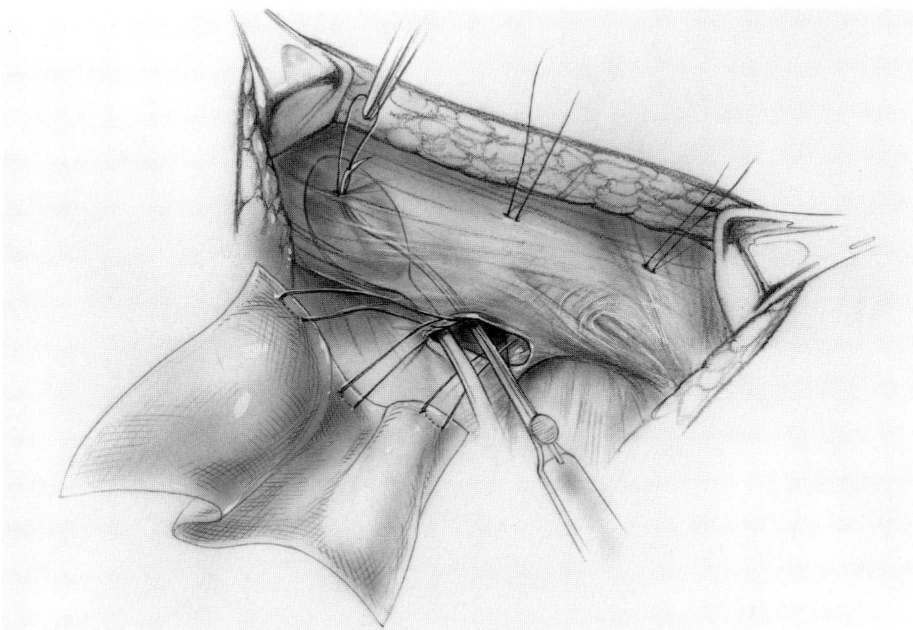

Figure 10.   Subinguinal GPRVS to repair the parietal defect of femoral hernias. The mesh is fixed to the anterior abdominal wall with three sutures. (By permission of the *Journal of the American College of Surgeons*)

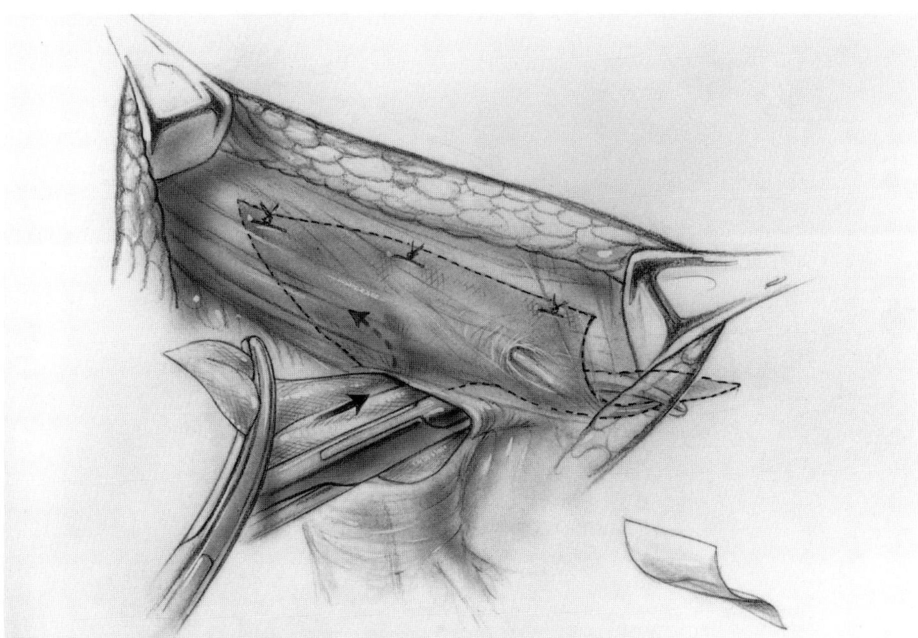

Figure 11.   Subinguinal GPRVS. The distal mesh is implanted with two long clamps. The medial clamp places the mesh in the space of Retzius and the lateral clamp puts the mesh deep into the iliac fossa. (By permission of the *Journal of the American College of Surgeons*)

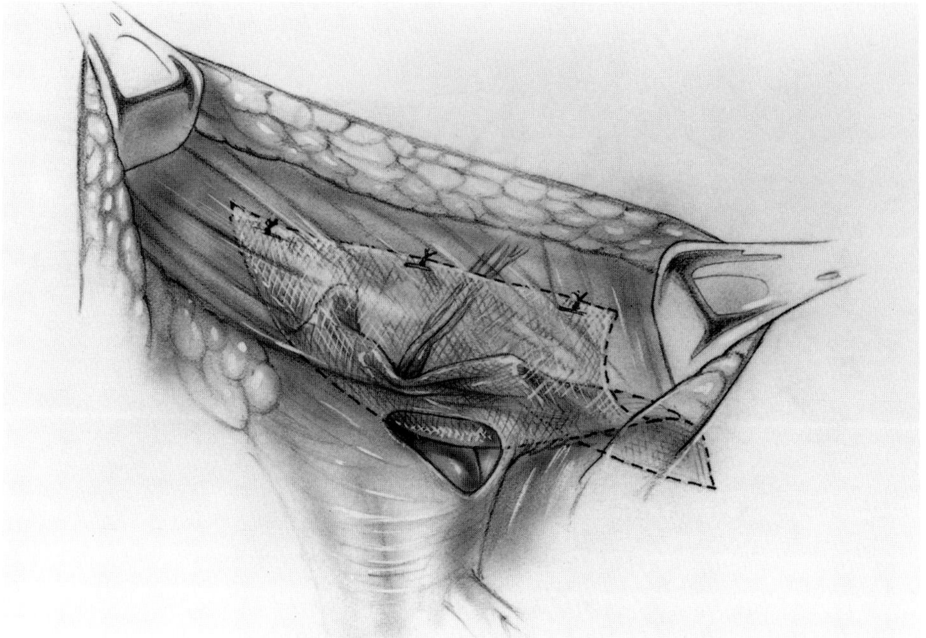

Figure 12. The soft pliable Mersilene mesh bunches up around the inferior epigastric vessels. (By permission of the *Journal of the American College of Surgeons*)

REFERENCES

1   Munshi IA, Wantz GE. Management of recurrent and perivascular femoral hernias by giant prosthetic reinforcement of the visceral sac. *J Am Coll Surg* 1996; **182**:417–22.
2   Schumpelick V, Wantz GE. *Inguinal hernia repair*. Basel: Karger 1995.
3   Stoppa RE, Rives JL, Warlaumont CR et al. The use of Dacron in the repair of hernias of the groin. *Surg Clin North Am* 1984; **64**:269–85.
4   Wantz GE. Giant prosthetic reinforcement of the visceral sac. *Surg Gynecol Obstet* 1989; **169**:408–17.
5   Wantz GE. *Atlas of hernia surgery*. New York: Raven Press 1991.
6   Wantz GE. The technique of giant prosthetic reinforcement of the visceral sac performed through an anterior groin incision. *Surg Gynecol Obstet* 1993; **176**:497–500.

18 MASSIVE MULTIRECURRENT INCISIONAL HERNIA PROSTHETIC REPAIR

*Jean-Bernard Flament, Jean-Pierre Palot, Claude Avisse, Alain Burde and Jean-Pierre Conce**

INTRODUCTION

Our experience with modern procedures for the repair of incisional hernias dates back to 1964. Since then we have observed and treated 1018 cases of incisional hernia, some of which would be considered by many surgeons to be beyond the scope of a surgical cure. Indeed, some cases have 'frightened' surgeons, and many patients have come to us having been told that nothing can be done for them. We have taken on these cases, have tried to do something for them, and now have an experience of over 1000 cases. The results of 478 major incisional hernias treated between 1991 and 1995 are discussed below. Of these hernias, 31 were operated on as an emergency (strangulated hernia), and 447 were elective procedures. These 478 cases have been selected for presentation as they constitute a homogeneous series with respect to both the type of surgical procedure performed and the surgical team who performed the operation (five full-time surgeons).

We focus our presentation on the 332 cases of incisional hernias treated by nonabsorbable mesh.

PATIENTS AND METHODS

Patients

Between 1991 and 1995 we operated on 478 patients: 375 had a midline hernia (79%) and 103 had a lateral hernia (21%). Of the 478 cases, 131 were giant multirecurrent incisional hernias which had undergone at least one previous repair attempt elsewhere; 20

* With the collaboration of Claude Marcus and Viviane Ladam-Marcus

patients had been operated on twice before; six had been operated on three times; two patients had had seven previous attempts at repair; one unfortunate patient had undergone 10 previous operations; and 52 patients had already had some form of mesh inserted.

According to the local conditions, we have used the following techniques:

1 Nonprosthetic repair was undertaken in 98 patients (20.5%); our indications for nonprosthetic repair were:
   - cases of emergency surgery, e.g. strangulation or intestinal obstruction
   - in the presence of overt sepsis or when the bowel is opened
   - in the treatment of small incisional hernias.

2 Nonabsorbable prosthetic repair was carried out in 332 patients (69.5%). In most (322) patients there was no associated risk of sepsis. However, in 20 patients there was an intraoperative risk of sepsis as follows:
   - associated intestinal surgery (five patients)
   - incidental visceral wound (three patients)
   - trophic skin ulcer (two patients).

   All of our subsequent superficial and deep wound infections occurred in this latter group of 10 patients.

3 Absorbable mesh was used in 45 patients.

Concept and principles of the operation of retromuscular prefascial prosthetic repair of incisional hernia

A large inlay of prosthesis is inserted behind the muscle (Pascal principle) and extraperitoneally. It is firmly fixed to avoid folding and slipping. This technique is known as the prefascial retromuscular prosthesis. This procedure was described in 1973 and many papers have been published on this topic.[1–10] Most French surgeons[11] and some Americans have also used this technique.[12]

The ideal prosthetic material should be as light, flexible and as solid as possible, with a certain degree of elasticity. It is also important that the material have a fairly open mesh structure so that the reactive connective tissue is able to invest the prosthesis, thereby facilitating its incorporation. We have chosen to use Dacron (Mersuture or ligalene-tulle) over the past two decades since, in our opinion, it is the best (or least inappropriate) material commercially available that satisfies the above conditions.

We always try to place the prosthesis deep to the muscles, on the posterior rectus sheath above the arcuate line and in the preperitoneal space below the arcuate line. The peritoneal cavity must be closed prior to implantation of the prosthesis. In most cases, suture of the peritoneal margins can be achieved when the peritoneum has been correctly and widely freed, and in the midline the peritoneal layer is much thicker since it is covered by the posterior lamina of the rectus sheath in the region above the arcuate line. However, when a primary peritoneal closure cannot be achieved, a resorbable mesh (such as Vicryl) should be attached to the edges of the peritoneal defect.

228

In cases of midline incisional hernia, the prosthesis is positioned in contact with the posterior surface of the rectus abdominis muscle. The space for implantation may differ for the upper and lower parts of the prosthesis. Thus, the prosthesis is implanted in the rectus sheath above the arcuate line and in the preperitoneal space below it. The upper part of the prosthesis is placed between the rectus abdominis anteriorly and the thorax and internal oblique muscle posteriorly. For subumbilical hernias, the lower part of the prosthesis should be fixed to Cooper's ligament in order to prevent its detachment. In cases of incisional hernias in the inguinal region, it is necessary to position the prosthesis so that it envelops the peritoneum and extends into the iliac fossa and pelvis. The prosthesis is sutured above to the deep surface of the muscles and below to Cooper's ligament or the iliac crest. The patch of mesh should extend well beyond the area of the defect (in all directions) in the preperitoneal space.

In cases of lateral incisional hernia, the abdominal muscles may be seen only along the part of the circumference of the hernial orifice. Thus, with subchondral hernias it is often necessary to position the upper part of the mesh beneath the diaphragm and attach it to the rib cage using transfixing costodiaphragmatic sutures.

The area of insertion of the prosthesis must be as large as possible. Accordingly, the mesh should extend well beyond the myoaponeurotic hernial orifice, with intra-abdominal pressure being used to maintain its position. The force of abdominal pressure holds the prosthesis against the deep surface of the muscles thereby achieving a sort of 'suture of apposition' as pointed out by Rives *et al.*[7] However, this pressure-induced apposition may not be sufficient to maintain the prosthesis in the correct position during the first few postoperative weeks, so solid peripheral suturing of the prosthetic material is required. Traction sutures (resorbable or nonresorbable) are placed through the edge (folded or not) of the mesh. Each end of the suture is passed through the abdominal wall, then through a buttonhole skin incision. For midline incisional hernias, the semilunar line of the edge of the rectus muscle (Spiegel's line) is used as the site for peripheral attachment of the prosthesis.

The closure of the abdominal wall anterior to the prosthesis is possible in most cases because of the tension of the prosthesis. We place two closed suction drains on top of the prosthesis, underlying the abdominal wall, and usually two drains in the subcutaneous space. The skin is then closed with staples.

The conditions for these surgical procedures should obey the basic rules of prosthetic implantation. The risk of infection can be minimized by operating under conditions of scrupulous asepsis (prophylactic antibiotics, skin disinfection, removal of all granulomas, perfect haemostasis, prosthesis soaked in Betadine, closed suction drainage).

RESULTS

Our personal experience with 332 patients with complex multirecurrent incisional hernia repaired with prosthetic mesh is reported (Figs 1 and 2).

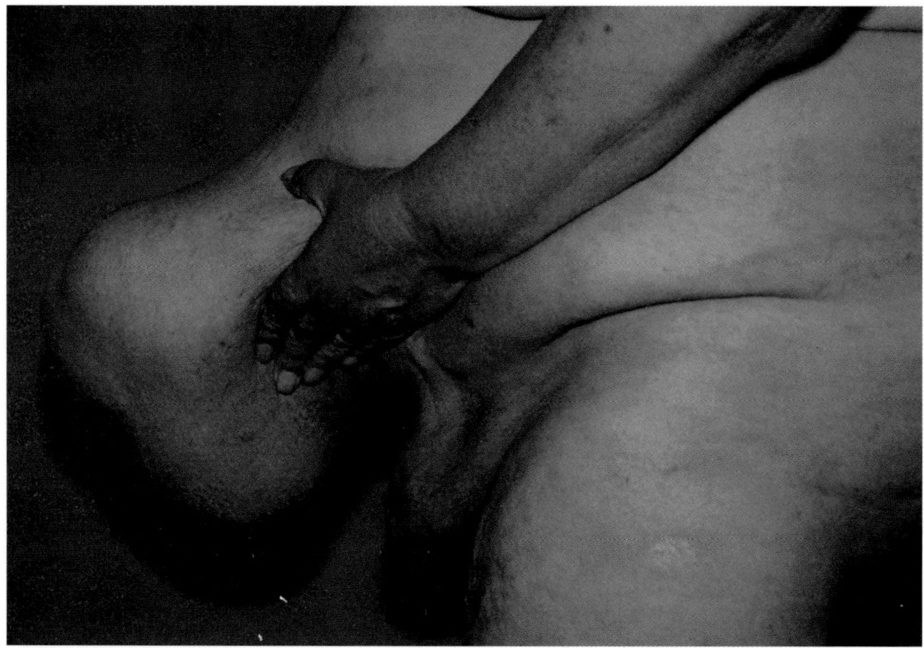

(a)

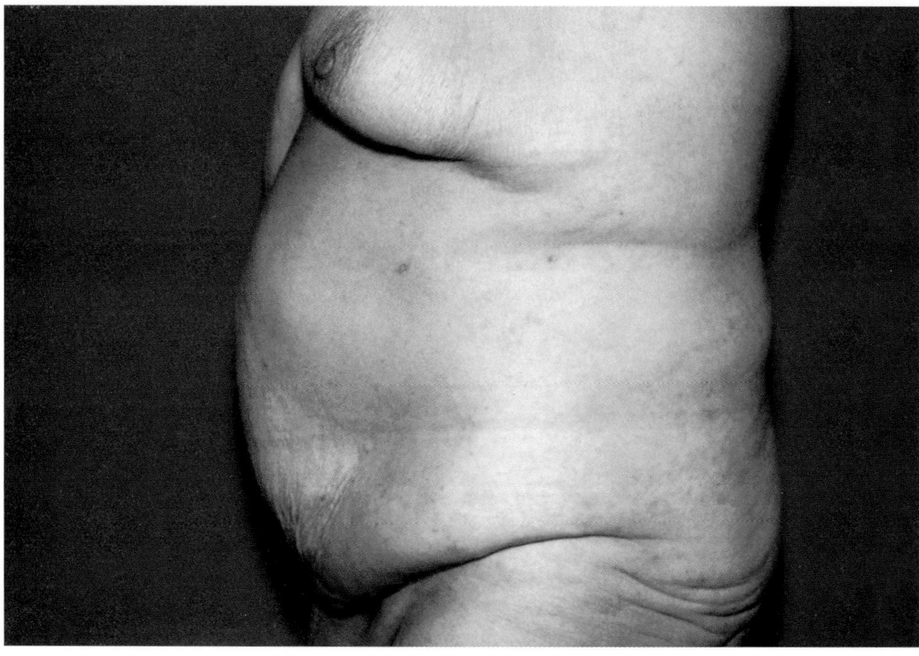

(b)

Figure 1.   (a) In a 58-year-old patient, a subumbilical incisional hernia after weight reduction to 115 Kg (from 170 Kg). (b) Result after prosthetic cure and dermolipectomy

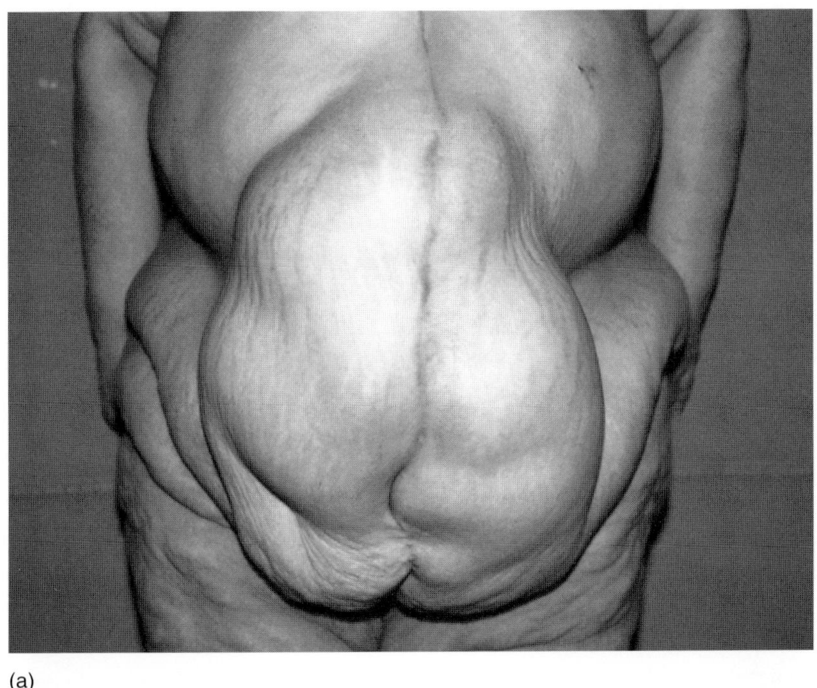

(a)

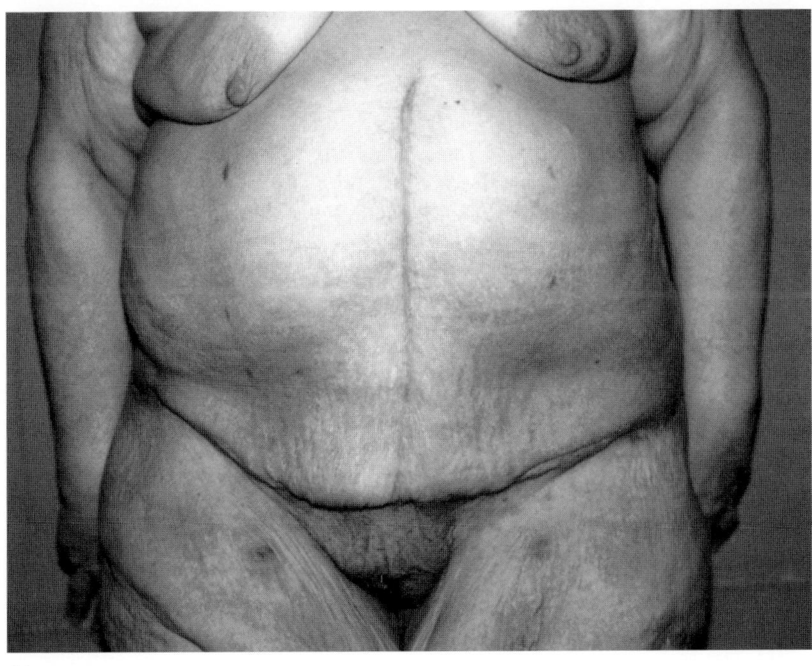

(b)

Figure 2. (a) In a 68-year-old patient, a total midline incisional hernia. (b) Result after prosthetic cure and dermolipectomy

Complications (morbidity and mortality)

In this group of 332 patients, there were three postoperative deaths (0.9%):

- male, 73 years, necrotizing enteritis (autopsy confirmation)
- female, 69 years, cardiac arrest in recovery room
- female, 71 years, deep wound infection, septicaemia (*Staphylococcus aureus*).

Local morbidity complications included two superficial and two deep wound infections. The superficial infections occurred around the cutaneous sutures when a large dermolipectomy was carried out at the same procedure or at peripheral sites of attachment of the prosthesis. In these patients the superficial infection was treated and resolved after a few weeks of local treatment. One case of deep wound infection was fatal (*Staphylococcus aureus* septicaemia). One case of postoperative peritonitis caused by inadvertent small bowel puncture was also observed. After reoperation the patient did well without recurrence.

General morbidity complications included a chest infection and venous thrombosis.

Recurrent herniation in the absence of any septic complications was seen in 5.2% of our patients (16 of 304 cases). In 13 of these patients, definitive repair was achieved by reoperation. In another case, reoperation was not done because of the minor degree of the recurrent hernia.

Some of the 332 patients presented with enormous strangulated hernias and were bedridden, while others were cases of visceral emergency associated with major incisional hernia. All complications in our series were seen in unprepared patients, demonstrating the importance of adequate local and general preparation and the precautions that should be taken to avoid septic complications.

Long-term results

Long-term results were assessed in 304 patients (332 patients operated, three postoperative deaths, 25 lost to follow-up). Excellent long-term results were seen in 98.6% of the patients, with favourable results often seen soon after the operation. In a few cases (4.2%), the definitive result was seen after treating a superficial infection or reoperating for a small lateral recurrence (13 patients). Final good results were obtained in 300 patients. The inconvenience of these complementary procedures, and of the sensory disturbances reported in some cases, is fully erased by the satisfaction of having alleviated a major lesion (sometimes of monstrous dimensions) which had often previously been considered irremediable.

DISCUSSION

Assessment of the hernia

We use CT (computed tomography) scans preoperatively in many of these patients to assess the loss of abdominal wall muscle and to see the amount of bowel present within the hernia that needed replacing within the abdomen during the procedure (Fig. 3).

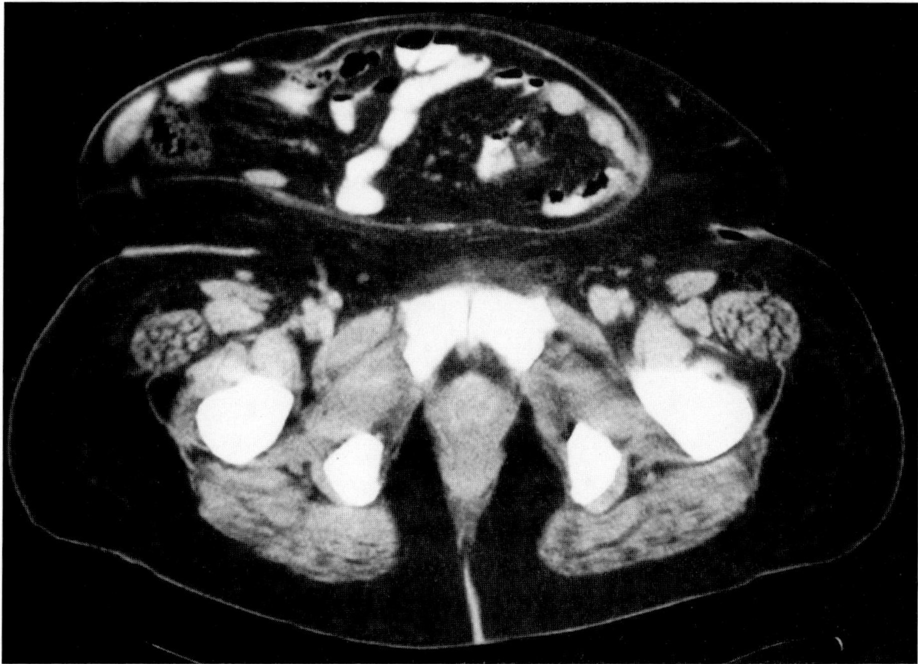

Figure 3. Typical CT scan of a patient with a massive incisional hernia showing the defect in the abdominal wall and the 'second abdominal cavity'

Evaluation of the operative risk, preoperative assessment and preoperative preparation

A multirecurrent incisional hernia is not simply a defect in the abdominal wall that has to be closed. It should be considered a systemic disease – as we have shown in previous publications[4,7] – and these patients need careful assessment and preoperative preparation. We take particular note of respiratory function, and routinely measure the minute respiratory volume and the ratio of the maximum expiratory flow rate to the vital capacity. Blood gas measurement is also carried out, giving the Po_2, Pco_2, pH and percentage oxygen saturation of arterial blood (Table 1).

We can thus evaluate ventilatory efficiency and identify latent respiratory problems. This assessment is made not only on admission but also at regular intervals during respiratory preparation of the patients.

Based on the results of these tests the patients can be classified into 3 groups:

- *Group 1* – patients with results in the normal range on admission.
- *Group 2* – those for whom operation can be considered if ventilatory function can be improved after a few weeks, or even months, of physiotherapy (Tables 2 and 3).

(a) Spirometry		(b) Blood gas measurements		
VC (l)	80	PO_2	95 Torr	40 years
RV	40		90 Torr	50 years
RV/TLC	30		85 Torr	60 years
FEV/VC	75	SaO_2	70%	
		PCO_2	40±5% Torr	
		pH	7.40±0.05	

FEV, forced expiratory volume; RV, residual volume; SaO_2, oxygen saturation of arterial blood; TLC, total lung capacity; VC, vital capacity.

Table 1. Minimum acceptable preoperative values expressed (a) as a percentage of normal lung function and (b) in absolute terms of arterial blood gas

VC (l)	2.79	97% of normal
FEV	2.33	91%
FEV/VC	83	
PO_2	99 Torr	
PCO_2	38 Torr	

Table 2. Preoperative ventilatory function results in a 40-year-old woman (height 161 cm, weight 95 kg), presenting with a major subumbilical incisional hernia following a caesarian section. Postoperative course was uneventful; discharge was 10 days later

	Start	Start + 3 months	Start + 1 year
VC (l)	1.65	2.13	1.88
FEV	0.7	1.26	0.72
FEV/VC	45	51	51
PO_2	53 Torr	55 Torr	57 Torr
PCO_2	44	42	50

Table 3. Typical respiratory function results of an overweight unfit patient improved after physiotherapy

- *Group 3* – patients with poor lung function that will not improve despite physiotherapy and who are unsuitable for surgery (Table 4).

As well as noting the patient's preoperative respiratory state it must be remembered that there will be further compromise in the early postoperative period secondary to a rise in intra-abdominal pressure and marked diaphragm immobilization (Table 5). Conversely, marginal respiratory disturbance associated with gross obesity is often masked or even improved somewhat by the mere existence of an incisional hernia.

One study of 90 obese patients[7] revealed an increased vital capacity (VC) and an increased ratio of residual volume to total lung capacity (RV/TC). We found that the common respiratory disturbances associated with obesity could be compensated for or masked by the presence of a major incisional hernia. Surgical correction of the hernia deprives the patient of this respiratory advantage and exposes them to a degree of respiratory embarrassment which could not have been predicted from the preoperative lung function tests.

	Initial	After preparation
VC (l)	2.35	2.45
FEV	1.05	1
FEV/VC	44	40.8
PO_2	60	61
PCO_2	45	47

Table 4. Respiratory function results in a 68-year-old alcoholic woman (height 160 cm, weight 95 kg): unsuitable for operation because of disturbed alveolocapillary diffusion of O_2 and CO_2 (confirmed by the CO_2 compliance test)

	Obesity without herniation	Obesity plus herniation	Significance
VC (l)	90.8±16.4	116.1±19.3	*P*<0.001
TLC	97.4±30.2	110.7±17.3	NS
RV/TLC	38.1±5.8	30.2±7.9	*P*<0.001
MEFR/VC	68.9±13.1	68.9±11.8	NS

MEFR, maximum expiratory flow rate

Table 5. Results of lung function studies in obese patients with and without an incisional hernia. The incisional hernia compensates for the respiratory dysfunction associated with obesity. Values shown are the mean of measurements made in 90 cases of incisional hernia

Preoperative preparation

Careful preoperative preparation may take weeks or even months and is at least as important as the actual surgery.

1 Weight loss is mandatory.
2 Respiratory preparation consists of:
   * cessation of smoking
   * prescription of a mucolytic agent
   * respiratory physiotherapy including intercostal muscle and diaphragm exercises
   * assisted coughing by clapping exercises
   * postural drainage where appropriate
   * instrumental physiotherapy using a pressure-related breathing apparatus (this may be used in the patient's home) (Fig. 4).
3 For preoperative pneumoperitoneum, we use the excellent and universally accepted technique of I. Goni-Moreno.[13]
4 Disinfection of skin folds and treatment of associated fungal infections or other skin lesions is required. In cases with trophic ulceration (Fig. 5), resection and primary closure of the ulcerated skin prior to attempting repair of the hernia may be advisable.
5 Associated diseases such as cardiac conditions, hypertension and diabetes should be treated and stabilized.

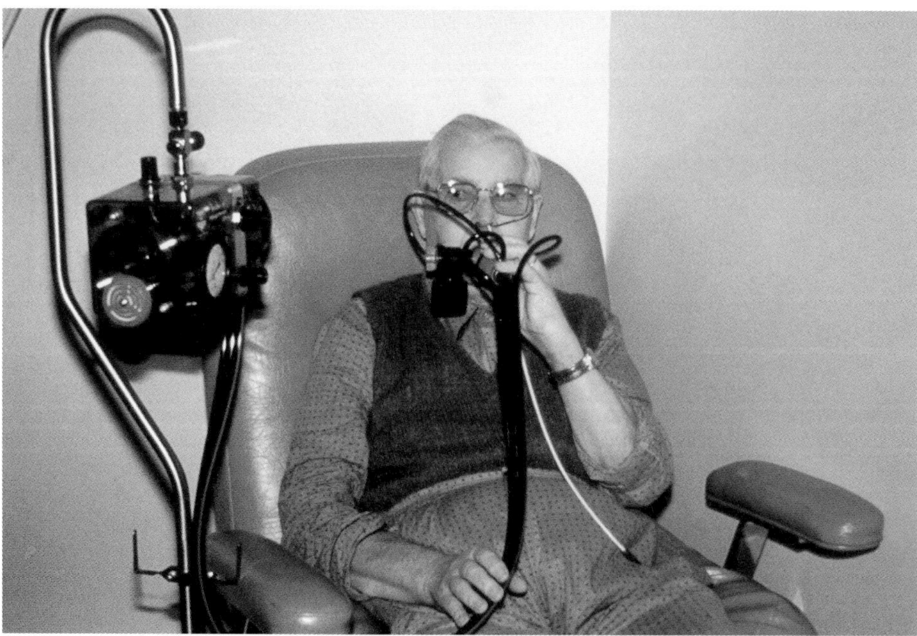

Figure 4. Patient undergoing instrumental physiotherapy using a pressure-related breathing device

236

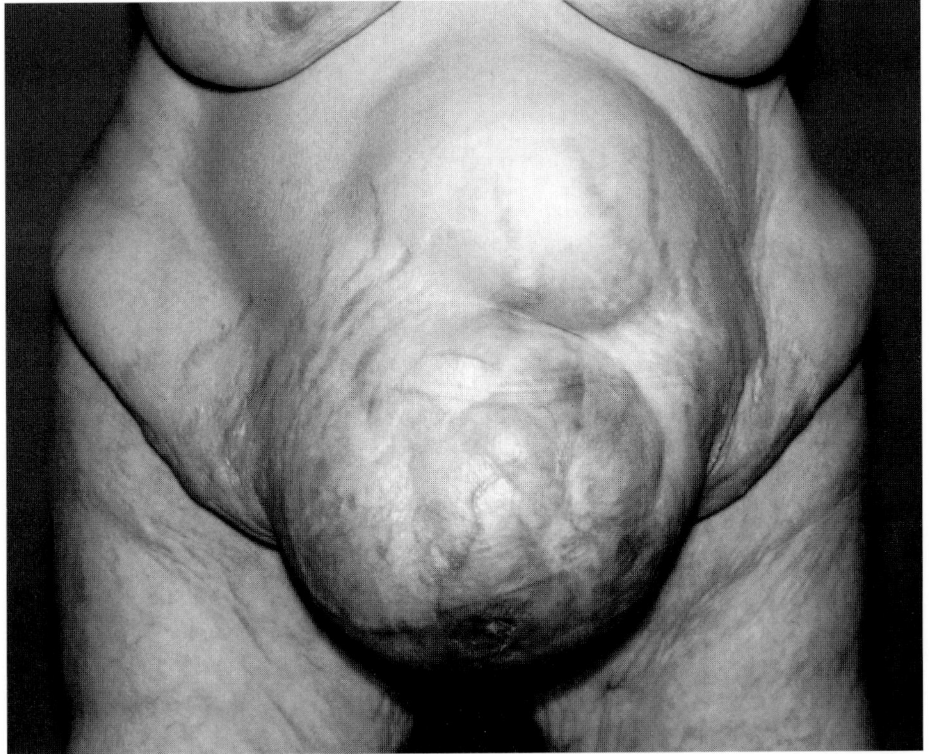

(a)

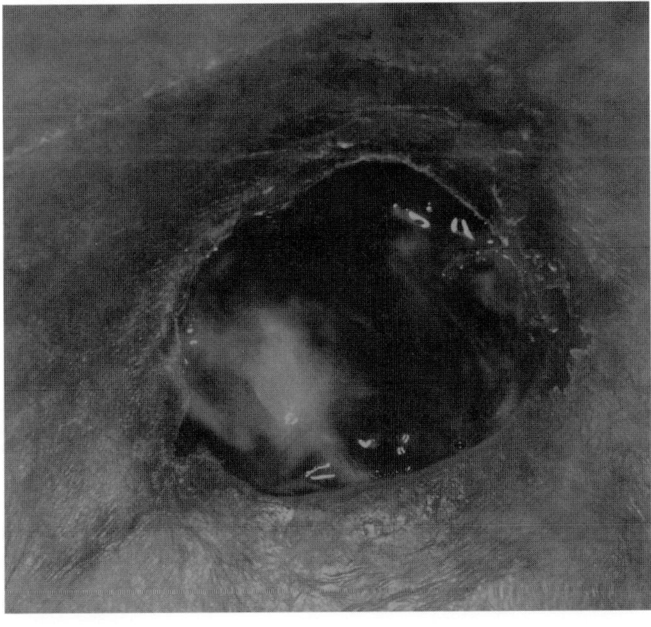

(b)

Figure 5. (a) Trophic ulcer associated with a massive midline incisional hernia. (b) Close-up view

Anaesthesia and postoperative care

Anaesthesia is facilitated by artificial preoperative ventilation. Operative analgesia is obtained by administration of a morphinomimetic drug and anaesthesia is induced by a narcotic drug. Muscle relaxation is done with a curarimimetic. Immediate paralysis must not be sought. Artificial ventilation must be maintained until there is complete recovery of muscular power and respiratory function, with active physiotherapy started immediately afterwards.

Finally, postoperative analgesia must not be overlooked; we frequently use the technique of 'patient controlled analgesia'. The first signs of respiratory insufficiency must be detected. Blood gas monitoring is particularly useful for detecting modifications of blood gas, especially hypercapnia associated with normal Po_2.

Alternative surgical procedures for hernia defect repair

As described earlier, out preference in most cases is for prosthetic repair of large multi-recurrent incisional hernias, placing the mesh in the retromuscular prefascial position. Other techniques have been described; the most important are listed below.

The classical methods of repair are based on aponeurotic or muscular reconstructive surgery using the anatomical structure of the abdominal wall:

1 Simple suturing of the edges of the defect after replacement of the herniated viscera into the abdominal cavity, and closure of the hernia sac. This is possible when the defect is small or 'narrow', e.g. a hernia at a drain site. With wider defects, relaxing incisions of the anterior rectus sheath may be used (Fig. 6) as proposed by Gibson[14] and Trivellini.[15]

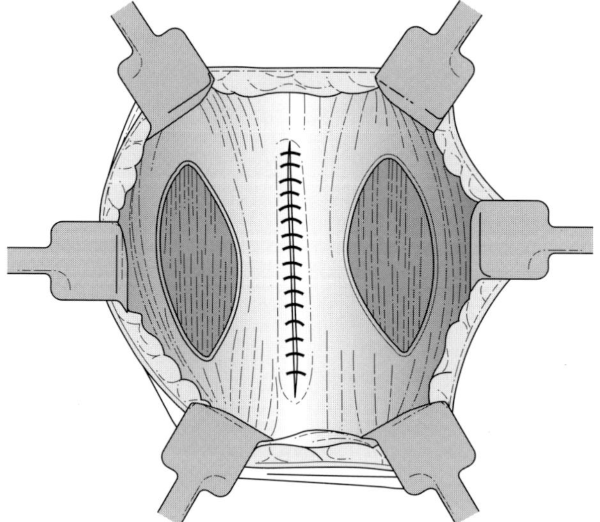

Figure 6. Gibson procedure: lateral anterior rectus sheath relaxing incisions

2 Suturing by Judd's technique[16] requires that the aponeuroses be solid and that the margins of the orifice be brought into apposition without difficulty. This technique is mainly applicable to the treatment of lateral incisional hernia, although it can be used in cases of midline hernia.

3 The procedure of Welti and Eudel[17] is used in France for midline repair and consists of making two lateral incisions (parallel to the midline) through the anterior rectus sheath. The two resulting aponeurotic flaps are then sutured together over the midline defect. Finally, the muscular margins of the recti abdominis are sutured medially over the aponeurotic repair.

In conjunction with a period of postoperative pneumoperitoneum, the procedures described above can be used to treat relatively simple incisional hernia when there is no loss of abdominal tissue, or a sclerotic retraction of the muscle edges. However the high rate of recurrence is rather discouraging. Nevertheless, nonprosthetic repair is the only alternative when there is an obvious risk of septic contamination. Of all the above, our preference is for the Welti–Eudel procedure.

Other methods include the use of prosthetic mesh to repair complex hernias and to treat formidable lesions previously considered to be beyond the scope of surgical repair. Our preference is to place the prosthesis in the retromuscular prefascial plane, but other sites have been described:

1 Intraperitoneal placement of the prosthesis. The advantage is that peritoneum rapidly envelopes the prosthesis, thus offering a good defence against infection without haematoma formation. However, fibroblastic invasion of the prosthesis is accompanied by adhesion of the bowel loops with potentially dire consequences. We have personally seen two cases of intraintestinal migration of intraperitoneally placed mesh. If intraperitoneal placement cannot be avoided, it is preferable to put the mesh on a bed of omentum to prevent direct contact with loops of the bowel.

2 Premuscular positioning of mesh (onlay mesh). Our personal experience[1] has now been extended to include over 200 cases. The initial steps of the procedure are similar to the Welti–Eudel procedure and are followed by implantation of a large prosthesis (we use Mersilene) over the sutured area. Although precautions must be taken when this procedure is used, especially in cases where cutaneous cover is less than satisfactory, its major advantage over a deeper implantation is the reduced risk of septic complications for patients with infection.[18]

CONCLUSION

Treatment of complex incisional hernias of the abdominal wall requires the co-operation of surgeons, anaesthetists and physiotherapists. Careful preoperative assessment, preoperative preparation and postoperative care are as important as the actual surgery.

Consideration must also be given to the operability of the lesion and the most suitable choice of technique in each individual case. This includes correction of preoperative respiratory insufficiency, use of pneumoperitoneum and meticulous skin preparation.

The decision to use a prosthetic or not for repair will depend on the experience of the surgeon, recent progress in prosthetic materials and the presence or absence of sepsis. It would be as unwise to never use a prosthesis as to use one in every case.

We feel that with the above points in mind, it is possible to cure almost 99% of complex multirecurrent incisional hernias.

REFERENCES

1 Chevrel JP, Flament JB. Les éventrations de la paroi abdominale. In *Rapport au 92ème Congrès Français de Chirurgie, 1997*, Paris: Masson.

2 Chevrel JP, Flament JB. Traitement des éventrations de la paroi abdominale. In Techniques Chirurgicales, Appareil digestif. *Encycl. Méd. Chir.* 40–165. Paris: Editions Techniques, 1995.

3 Flament JB, Palot JP. Prostheses and major incisional hernia. In Bendavid R, ed. *Prostheses and major incisional hernias.* Austin: Landes Biomedical 1994.

4 Flament JB, Palot JP, Burde A, Delattre JF, Avisse C. Treatment of major incisional hernias. *Prob Gen Surg* 1995; **12**:151–8.

5 Palot JP, Flament JB, Avisse C, Greffier D, Burde A. Utilisation des prostheses dans les conditions de la chirurgie d'urgence. Etude retrospective de 204 hernies de l'aine étranglées. *Chirurgie* 1996; **121**:48–50.

6 Pire JC, Body C, Flament JB. La capacité vitale, un piège dans le bilan des grandes éventrations. *Nouv Presse Med* 1977; **6**:3641.

7 Rives J, Lardennois B, Pire JC, Hibon J. Les grandes éventrations. Importance du 'volet abdominal' et des troubles respiratoires qui lui ont secondaires. *Chirurgie* 1973; **99**:547–63.

8 Rives J, Pire JC, Flament JB, Convers G. Traitement des éventrations. *Encycl. Méd. Chir.*, Paris: Editions Techniques, 1977, 4.0.07, 40–165.

9 Rives J, Pire JC, Flament JB, Palot JP, Body C. Le traitement des grandes éventrations. Nouvelles indications thérapeutiques à propos de 322 cas. *Chirurgie* 1985; **3**:215–25.

10 Rives J, Pire JC, Palot JP, Flament JB. Major incisional hernias. In Chevrel JP, ed. *Surgery of the abdominal wall.* Berlin, Heidelberg: Springer Verlag, 1987.

11 Stoppa R, Moungar F, Verhaeghe P. Traitement chirurgical des éventrations médianes sous ombilicales. *J Chir* 1991; **172**:129–37.

12 Wantz GE. Incisional hernioplasty with mersilene. *Surgery* 1991; **172**:129–37.

13 Goni-Moreno I. Le pneumopéritoine dans la réparation pré-opérative des grandes éventrations. *Chirurgie* 1970; **9**: 581–5.

14 Gibson CL. Operation for cure of large ventral hernias. *Ann Surg* 1920; **72**:214.

15 Trivellini G, Danelli PG. Use of two prostheses in the surgical repair of recurrent hernia. *Postgraduate General Surgery Hernias* 1992; **4**:136–9.

16 Judd ES. The prevention and treatment of ventral hernia. *Surg Gynecol Obstet* 1912; **15**: 175–82.

17 Welti H, Eudel F. Un procédé de cure radicale des éventrations post-opératives par auto-étalement des muscles grand droits, après incision du feuillet antérieur de leurs gaines. *Mem Acad Chir* 1941; **28**:791–8.

18 Godquin B. Une technique sûre de réparation des éventrations abdominales post-operatives: plastie aponévrotique associée à une prosthèse. A propos de 38 observations. *Chirugie* 1979; **105**: 721–4

19

THE CONTRIBUTION OF CLINICAL TRIALS TO THE DEVELOPMENT OF HERNIA SURGERY

Andrew Kingsnorth

The introduction of new biomaterials, laparoscopic technology and the need to make hernia surgery cost-effective has made demands on surgeons to provide evidence-based evaluations of these new alternatives in surgical practice. It is unlikely that new developments will be widely adopted unless they have been proven by the ultimate rigorous test of the randomized controlled trial (RCT). Such an attitude, however, has not been prevalent until the last decade, and this chapter traces the origins of the application of scientific method to the development of hernia surgery.

ASSESSING THE STRENGTH OF THE EVIDENCE

Doran had a lifetime interest in herniology, and in 1972 published the first prospective randomized trial in hernia surgery, which indicated that the addition of a rectus flap did not improve the outcome of a Lytle's repair.[1] In this publication Doran made a plea for the rejection of the simple collection and tabulation of facts and observations (what he called Baconian empiricism), such as the annual publication of recurrence rates that still appear frequently in the literature even to this day. He stated that surgical work should be evaluated by properly constructed trials, a fact of which we are aware today. By randomly allocating 155 patients to receive either a Lytle's operation or a Lytle's operation with a rectus flap, he showed that both methods were of equal value and that the rectus flap was superfluous. In this series of 155 cases undergoing herniorraphy in a scientific trial, he claimed that more valid information was obtained than could be concluded from 2000 cases mechanically collected and tabulated in accordance with the rules of Baconian empiricism.

Surgical practice must evolve on the basis of scientific evidence (Table 1) which ranges from case series without controls to RCTs with power and end points.[2] The

I	Randomized controlled trials with power and end points
II-1	Other clinical trials
II-2	Prospective cohort trials with controls
II-3	Case-control (retrospective) studies
III	Observational studies, with literature controls
IV	Case series without controls

Table 1. Assessing the strength of the evidence

evaluation of any new healthcare advance or health technology should be based on the quality of the evidence which it provides. Properly qualified evaluation groups, led preferably by clinically based academic institutes, are capable of bridging the gap between clinical practice and research findings and can consign to each study one of the five qualities of evidence shown in Table 1. It is likely that future health commissioning will be based upon the quality of evidence from clinical trials to ensure appropriateness and cost-effectiveness and to maximize healthcare benefits to the patient population. This perspective is particularly relevant at a time when healthcare costs are proportionately escalating in relation to gross national product.[3] The value of any indicated treatment is directly proportional to treatment outcome and inversely proportional to treatment cost. The valuation of both the numerator (outcome quality) and the denominator (cost) of this equation is subject to many methodological limitations. Value depends on whether it is viewed from the perspective of the patient, surgeon, hospital, employer, provider or industry.

HISTORICAL BACKGROUND

Bassini, the father of modern hernia surgery, studied under the great Theodor Billroth for a year during 1873.[4,5] Billroth was perhaps the first surgeon to report on a case of self-audit in hernia surgery which can provide a (low) measure of evidence-based practice. Billroth's first operation was a herniotomy, performed in 1852 while he was a senior medical student on vacation in Staffelde near Berlin, trying unsuccessfully to save the life of a local shepherdess with a strangulated hernia. A day later he performed her autopsy to be certain that he had not contributed to her death. In 1890 Bassini set the bench mark with a recurrence rate of 2.7% using his new operation.[6] By the 1920s this recurrence rate had slipped to more than 10% and by 1949 Doran had stated that there was now 'a huge statistical slagheap of Baconian empiricism'.[1]

Date	Author	Findings
1890	Bassini[6]	2.7% recurrence rate in a consecutive series of 251 patients followed for 1–4½ years with 7 recurrences
1920	Taylor[7]	10.9% recurrence rate in a personal series with the Bassini operation
1924	Andrews[8]	A review of the literature revealed a 9–11% recurrence rate with the Bassini operation
1949	Doran[1]	Uncovered 'a huge statistical slagheap of Baconian empiricism'

Table 2. Herniology 1890–1945

Type of evaluation	Authors
Prospective evaluation	Doran[1] and Marsden[9] (Britain) Palumbo[10] and McVay[11] (USA) Glassow (Canada)[12]
Animal experimentation with prosthetic mesh	
Socioeconomic evaluation	

Table 3. Herniology 1945–72

Brandon,[5] reviewing the published work on inguinal hernia in 1945, concluded that far from advancing the science of hernia surgery had swung back 'like a pendulum' into an era in which advancements had not been made for about 50 years (see Table 2). However, after 1945 prospective evaluation (type III evidence) was begun in Britain by Doran[1] and Marsden[9], in the USA by Palumbo[10] and McVay[11] and in Canada by Glassow[12] (Table 3). In addition, socioeconomic evaluation of results was initiated and there was some animal experimentation, particularly in the use of prosthetic mesh. Socioeconomic evaluation was in its infancy, but for most aspects of hernia surgery there was no scientific basis. At this time clinical practice was largely dictated by tradition, personal notions and unsubstantiated opinion.

More recently Baker and Kirk[13] have advocated strengthening the research base of the National Health Service to improve the health of the community as well as caring for the needs of individual people. They have challenged the usefulness of clinical guidelines and consensus conferences, which they argue may not change the culture of health care. Rather this should be done through properly planned research and development seeking for evidence, evaluation and effectiveness. At its simplest level, results of surgery are audited, usually by the surgeon performing the procedures (self-audit) or on a wider basis, co-ordinated at a central level such as takes place in the Royal College of Surgeons of England with its quality assurance groups.

However, the reliability of assessment by the clinician who performed a procedure is open to question.[14] In a systematic review of morbidity and mortality of carotid endarterectomy, 50 RCTs, with a total of 15 956 operations performed since 1980, were assessed by a Cochrane collaboration-style systematic review. Two outcome measures, the risk of stroke and death, were examined in each of these 50 studies. When assessed by a neurologist, a physician, multiple surgeons and a single surgeon, the risks of stroke and death were 7.7%, 6.4%, 5.5% and 2.3%, respectively. This analysis indicates that there is at least a three-fold difference in outcome when the result is assessed by the operating surgeon as opposed to an independent impartial observer such as the neurologist. The reasons for this could be numerous and include scientific fraud, publication bias or case mix and illustrates the potential for selective citation of published work to mislead. Rothwell and Warlow[14] state 'self-audit should be taken with a pinch of salt'. Thus, in the absence of more compelling or higher quality evidence, a single author case series should be largely ignored because it may be impossible to generalize the results.

CLINICAL TRIALS

There is a dual impetus for clinical trials which has become apparent in recent years: an intellectual drive to practise evidence-based medicine and the economic constraints of limited financial resources. Evidence-based medicine involves the integration of clinical expertise on the one hand and the best external evidence (trials, not necessarily randomized).[15] This process should involve clinicians, public health practitioners, purchasers, planners and the public. Critics of this approach claim that the hidden agenda is a drive for cost-cutting and suppression of clinical freedom. Protagonists claim that it is not cook book medicine and that a good husbanding of healthcare resources in one sector will free up resources to be spent in other hard-pressed areas rather than be returned to the exchequer.

Clinical research must be an adequately resourced enterprise and incentives should be given for high quality studies. Currently healthcare systems do not provide such a framework and do not routinely collect information on such important aspects as quality of life and disability. Surgeons in particular are more interested in looking at hard data such as recurrence rates after hernia repair.

It is worth considering the ideal pathway from clinical research to routine application[13] which should involve: basic research, the emergence of a new development,

Research stages	
Basic research	Eureka!
New development	10% inspiration, 90% perspiration
Evaluation	Costs and benefits
Uptake and practical use	Generalizability
Dissemination	Publication, media, workshops

Table 4. The pathway from clinical research to routine application

	Operation type		
Research stages	Shouldice repair	Lichtenstein	Laparoscopic
Basic research	1945	1970	1982
New development	1952	1984	1991
Evaluation	Annual self-audit 1992, RCTs	Self-audit	EAES, 1994
Dissemination	'Plugging the gap between research and findings and clinical practice'		
Uptake and practical use by UK surgeons	15% in 1995	20–35% in 1995	<7% in 1993

EAES, European Association of Endoscopic Surgeons.

Table 5. Clinical research to routine application

evaluation, dissemination, uptake and practical use (Table 4). Such a strategy requires co-ordination. In Britain this will involve partnerships between the Research Councils, charities, industry, the Department of Health and higher education funding councils. Applying these criteria to the three popular surgical techniques of the Shouldice operation, the Lichtenstein tension-free repair and laparoscopic hernia repair (Table 5) it is obvious that the phase of evaluation has been incompletely carried out, dissemination has not occurred to the whole of the surgical community and that generalizability (uptake and practical use) is lacking. It is perhaps astonishing that it took 40 years of repeated annual cycles of self-reported monotonous excellence from the Shouldice hospital, before a properly constructed RCT revealed that the performance of the Shouldice operation outside this institution could not be repeated.[16] Type I evidence is still lacking for the Lichtenstein and laparoscopic procedures.

Surgeons have been slow to adopt RCTs to evaluate surgical operations.[17] Even when RCTs are performed by surgeons the overall quality seems to be inferior in terms of the methodology used to evaluate the effectiveness of surgical procedures. Surgeons appear to place a greater reliance on case series and other less rigorous design of trials. The ideal setting for an RCT is one in which there is no funding limitation, there is adequate methodological expertise and a willingness of all potential investigators to participate. However, surgeons are often confronted with a situation in which the case mix of patients is biased, there are methodological problems such as timing, or the introduction of new technology, or even recent dramatic discoveries such as laparoscopic advancements. Moreover, patient preferences and surgical preferences may act as surrogate and potentially biasing influences. There is a need to educate surgeons in research methodology, to establish clinical research groups and to facilitate the funding of RCTs. When reporting an RCT the manuscript should conform with the CONSORT statement which lists 21 items that should be included in a report.[18]

EVALUATION OF THE SHOULDICE REPAIR

Table 6 shows six clinical trials which have evaluated the Shouldice operation in different institutions.[16, 19–23] Overall, 1354 Shouldice operations were undertaken by trainees in these six trials. During a median follow-up between 24 and 60 months, a total of 86 hernias recurred indicating a predicted overall 5-year recurrence rate of 5.7%. Some of the series selectively allocated patients with direct hernias or primary hernias. Other series included all primary and direct hernias. The patients in the series from Cologne, France and Vienna, although operated on by trainees, had their operations supervised by an accredited surgeon who oversaw all the operations. The conclusion to be drawn from these series is that when the Shouldice operation is exported into the hands of trainees in other institutions, recurrence rates escalate from under 1% to approximately 5%. Surprisingly this 5% recurrence rate is the figure that Barwell achieved in his accumulated uncontrolled series collected over 20 years.[24] For the 2669 hernias he repaired, the recurrence rate was 0.8% in indirect hernias and 2.7% in direct hernias. His well-tutored trainees had recurrence rates of 5.2% and 5.0% in indirect and direct hernias, respectively, during a cumulative experience of 1293 operations. However, a systematic review carried out by Simons *et al.*[25] does not concur with these findings; this study involved a comprehensive search of the medical literature to identify all clinical trials (article or abstract) evaluating the Shouldice repair and after assessment of certain quality criteria had been applied, the best studies were pooled in a meta-analysis. Nine publications were found with 11 study arms and in 10 studies the results of the Shouldice technique were better than the results of the control arm. In spite of possible bias caused by different variables (modification of operative technique, suture material, level of surgeon and outcome measurement) the Shouldice operation was perceived as the best current conventional technique for inguinal hernia repair.

Reference (location)	No. of Shouldice operations	Median follow-up	Recurrence (%)	Selection	Predicted 5 years recurrence (%)
Kingsnorth et al., 1992 (Liverpool)[16]	151	30	4.3	All	6.1
Panos et al., 1992 (Texas)[19]	154	36.4	6.6	Direct only	8.2
Tran et al., 1992 (Cologne)[20]	65	24	10.8	All primary	16.4
Hay et al., 1993 (France)[23]	400	60	3 (SSW) 6 (PP)	14 centres	3 SSW 6 PP
Paul et al., 1994 (Cologne)[21]	119 (290)[a]	40	1.7 (5)	Primary, fit	2.1 6.1
Kux and Fuchsjager, 1994 (Vienna)[22]	185	40	3	All	3.7
Total	1354				5.7 (86)[b]

[a]Excluded, but analysable.
[b]Actual number of recurrences.
SSW, stainless steel wire; PP, polypropylene.

Table 6. Shouldice repair trials (trainees as operators)

However, it is debatable if the nine criteria used for measuring quality were appropriate ones on which to grade the evidence. The Shouldice operation is a difficult procedure, and in the Shouldice Hospital it is a requirement for a new surgeon to assist at 150 operations, then to perform another 50 under the supervision before a first assessment. A second critical assessment is made after 1000 operations indicating that this maybe the length of the learning curve before perfection is achieved. Perhaps the time has come to discard the Shouldice operation as the 'gold standard'.

EVALUATION OF LAPAROSCOPY

Laparoscopic hernia repair has been scrutinized at a consensus development conference in 1994 by the European Association of Endoscopic Surgeons (EAES).[26] Criteria for this technology assessment included feasibility (safety), efficacy (benefit in centres of excellence), effectiveness (reproducibility) and costs. Sixty-one published series were given quality ratings by 11 expert hernia surgeons. Only three of these studies were classified as top quality evidence in terms of being randomized controlled studies with power and relevant clinical end points. Most series were cohort studies or case series without controls. After deliberation, the EAES concluded that laparoscopic hernia repair was feasible if performed by experienced surgeons but not yet effective in general practice, it was efficacious in the short term but its safety had not been sufficiently evaluated. Moreover, analysis of cost-effectiveness and cost benefits were lacking and there was a need for multicentre RCTs. Two recent randomized trials[27,28] comparing laparoscopic versus open inguinal hernia repair indicate reduced pain in the early postoperative period with the laparoscopic operation. However, there were conflicting findings regarding return to normal activity and work, and the Oxford study[28] concluded that the total theatre costs were three times higher with the laparoscopic operation. Barkun *et al.* reached the same conclusion and also highlighted some of the confounding factors that may be an obstacle to generalizable conclusions.[29] These were the relatively poor definition of end points, unclear impacts on quality of life, flawed control over patient selection, preoperative patient expectation and outcome measurement. They recommended that separate randomization boxes should be given to each surgeon to ensure an equal proportion of each of the randomized operations would be undertaken by individual operators and also that pre- and postoperative data should be collected by research assistants and not the surgeons participating in the care of the patients.

EVALUATION OF LICHTENSTEIN TENSION-FREE HERNIOPLASTY

The Lichtenstein tension-free hernioplasty was perfected by 1984 and the definitive operation was reported in the literature in 1989.[30] Four other centres (Table 7) have reported their experience in preliminary cohort studies with some contradictory results.[31–34] Although the recurrence rate of less than 1% achieved in the Lichtenstein Institute was reproduced in three of the centres, the study of Rutten of 130 cases had six recurrences in 12.7 months indicating a faulty application of the technique.[31] Whether this error will be repeated when the operation is disseminated will not be known until the appropriate randomized trials are undertaken. The uptake of new operations before the quality of the evidence (RCTs) is adequate is a cause for concern. Fitzgibbons has stated that the requirements for a successful clinical trial include a

Hospital	No. of cases	Follow-up	Recurrence (%)
Lichtenstein Institute, Los Angeles[30]	1000	1–6 years	4 (0.4)
Clinique Notre-Dame, Brussels[31]	130	12–17 months	6 (4.6)
St Josef Krankenhaus, Vienna[32]	102	12 months	1 (1%)
Royal Liverpool, England[33]	125	3–9 months	0 (0)

Table 7. The tension-free hernioplasty

standardized outcome assessment, independent evaluation and rigorous data collection by designated data managers for which considerable financial support will be required.[35]

FUTURE PROSPECTS

The current challenges for outcome measurement in surgical practice have been clearly stated by Williams *et al.*[36] and include multidisciplinary collaboration between surgeons, epidemiologists, statisticians, health economists and medical psychologists. Much more research is required before the practice of hernia surgery is truly evidence based.

REFERENCES

1 Doran FSA. A clinical trial to determine whether a Lytle's repair of a primary indirect hernia needs the addition of a rectus flap. *Br J Surg* 1972; **59**:339–45.
2 Stevens A, Colin-Jones D, Gabbay J. 'Quick and clean': authoritative health technology assessment for local health care contracting. *Health trends* 1995; **27**:37–42.
3 Millikan KW, Deziel DJ. The management of hernia: consideration in cost-effectiveness. *Surg Clin North Am* 1996; **76**:105–16.
4 Rutledge RH. Theodor Billroth: a century later. *Surgery* 1995; **118**:36–43.
5 Brandon WJM. Inguinal hernia: the house that Bassini built. *Lancet* 1945; **i**:167–71.
6 Bassini E. Uber die Behandlung des Leistenbruches. *Langenbeck Archiv für Klinische Chirurgie.* 1890; **40**:429–76.
7 Taylor AS. *Arch Surg* 1920; **1**:382–6.
8 Andrews E. A method of herniotomy utilising only white fascia. *Ann Surg* 1924; **80**:225–34.

9 Marsden AJ. Inguinal hernia: a three year review of one thousand cases. *Br J Surg* 1958; **46**:234–43.

10 Palumbo LT, Sharp WS. Primary direct inguinal hernioplasty: sixteen year's study of 686 operations. *Am J Surg* 1964; **108**:815–19.

11 McVay CB, Anson BJ. Inguinal and femoral hernioplasty. *Surg Gynecol Obstet* 1949; **88**:473–85.

12 Glassow F. Recurrent inguinal and femoral hernia. *Br Med J* 1970; **i**:215–19.

13 Baker M, Kirk S. *Research and development for the NHS: evidence, evaluation and effectiveness.* Oxford: Radcliffe Medical Press 1996.

14 Rothwell P, Warlow C. Is Self-audit reliable? *Lancet* 1995; **346**:1623.

15 Sackett DL, Rosenberg WMC, Muir Gray JA, Haynes RB, Richardson WS. Evidence based medicine: what it is and what it isn't. *BMJ* 1996; **312**:71–2.

16 Kingsnorth AN, Gray MR, Nott DM. Prospective randomized trial comparing the Shouldice technique and plication darn for inguinal hernia. *Br J Surg* 1992; **79**:1068–70.

17 Solomon MJ, McLeod RS. Should we be performing more randomized controlled trials evaluating surgical operations? *Surgery* 1995; **118**:459–67.

18 CONSORT. Better reporting of randomised controlled trials. *BMJ* 1996; **313**:570–1.

19 Panos RG, Beck DE, Maresh JE, Harford FJ. Preliminary results of a prospective randomized study of Cooper's ligament versus Shouldice herniorrhaphy technique. *Surg Gynecol Obstet* 1992; **175**:315–19.

20 Tran VK, Putz T, Rohde H. A randomized controlled trial for inguinal hernia repair to compare the Shouldice and the Bassini–Kirschner operation. *Int Surg* 1992; **77**:235–7.

21 Paul A, Troidl H, Williams JI, Rixen D, Lamgen R and the Cologne Hernia Study Group. Randomized trial of modified Bassini versus Shouldice inguinal hernia repair. *Br J Surg* 1994; **81**:1531–4.

22 Kux M, Fuchsjager N. Shouldice is superior to Bassini inguinal herniorrhaphy. *Am J Surg* 1994; **168**:15–18.

23 Hay JM, Boudet MJ, Fingerhut A, *et al.* and the French Association for Surgical Research. Shouldice inguinal hernia repair in the male adult: the gold standard? A multicenter trial in 1578 patients. *Ann Surg* 1995; **222**:719–27.

24 Barwell NJ. Results of conventional inguinal hernia surgery in England. In Buchler MW, Farthmann EH, eds. *Progress in Surgery,* vol. 21. Basel and London: Karger 1996; 100–104.

25 Simons MP, Kleijnen J, van Geldere D, Hoitsma HF, Obertop H. Role of the Shouldice technique in inguinal hernia repair: a systematic review of controlled trials and a meta-analysis. *Br J Surg* 1996; **83**:734–8.

26 Neubauer E, Troidl H, Kum CK, Eypasch E, Miserez M. The E.A.E.S. Consensus development Conferences on laparoscopic cholecystectomy, appendectomy, and hernia repair. *Surg Endosc* 1995; **9**:550–63.

27 Stoker DL, Spiegelhalter DJ, Singh R, Wellwood JM. Laparoscopic versus open inguinal hernia repair: randomized prospective trial. *Lancet* 1994; **343**:1243–5.

28 Lawrence K, McWhinnie D, Goodwin A, *et al.* Randomized controlled trial of laparoscopic versus open repair of inguinal hernia: early results. *BMJ* 1995; **311**:981–5.

29 Barkun JS, Wexler MJ, Hinchey EJ, Thibeault D, Meakins JL. Laparoscopic versus open inguinal herniorrhaphy: preliminary results of a randomized controlled trial. *Surgery* 1995; **118**:703–10.

30 Lichtenstein IL, Shulman AG, Amid PK, Montilier M. The tension-free hernioplasty. *Am J Surg* 1989; **157**:188–93.

31 Rutten P, Ledecq M, Hoebeke Y *et al.* Hernia inguinal primaire; hernioplastic ambulatoire selon Lichtenstein: premiers resultats cliniques et implications economiques etude des 130 premiers cas operes. *Acta Chir Belg* 1992; **92**:168–71.

32 Kux M, Fuchsjager N. Lichtenstein-patch versus Shouldice-Technik bei primassen Leistenhernien mit hoher rezidivgefahrdung. *Chirurgie* 1994; **65**:59–62.

33 Davies N, Thomas MG, McIlroy B, Kingsnorth AN. Early results with the Lichtenstein tension-free repair. *Br J Surg* 1994; **81**:1478–9.

34 Kark AE, Kurzer M, Waters KJ. Tension-free mesh repair: review of 1098 cases using local anaesthesia in a day unit. *Ann R Coll Surg Engl* 1995; **77**:299–304.

35 Fitzgibbons RJ, Camps J, Cornet DA *et al.* Laparoscopic inguinal herniorrhaphy; results of a multicenter trial. *Ann Surg* 1995; **221**:3–13.

36 Williams MH, Blazeby JM, Eachus JI. Current challenges for outcome measurement in surgical practice. *Ann R Coll Surg Engl* 1995; **77**:401–3.